NUMBER
21

Recent Advances in

Anaesthesia and Analgesia

Edited by

A. P. Adams MB BS PhD FRCA FANZCA DA

Professor of Anaesthetics, University of London; Honorary Consultant Anaesthetist, Guy's, King's and St Thomas' Hospitals, London, UK

J. N. Cashman BSc MB BS BA MD FRCA

Consultant Anaesthetist, St George's Hospital, London; Honorary Senior Lecturer, University of London, UK

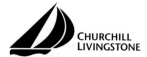
CHURCHILL
LIVINGSTONE

EDINBURGH LONDON NEW YORK PHILADELPHIA ST LOUIS SYDNEY TORONTO 2000

CHURCHILL LIVINGSTONE
An imprint of Harcourt Publishers Limited

First published 2000

ISBN 0-443-064253

ISSN 0309-2305

British Library Cataloguing in Publication Data
A catalogue record for this book is available from the British Library

Library of Congress Cataloging in Publication Data
A catalog record for this book is available from the Library of Congress

Medical knowledge is constantly changing. As new information becomes available, changes
in treatment, procedures, equipment and the use of drugs become necessary. The editors
and the publishers have, as far as possible, taken care to ensure that the information given
in this text is accurate and up to date. However, readers are strongly advised to confirm that
the information, especially with regard to drug usage, complies with current legislation and
standards of practice.

Commissioning Editor – Mike Parkinson
Project Editor – Michele Staunton
Project Controller – Frances Affleck
Designer – Sarah Cape
Printed in China

Recent

Anaesthesia
and Analgesia

Recent Advances in Anaesthesia and Analgesia 20
Edited by A.P. Adams and J.N. Cashman

ISBN 0-443-05988-8
ISSN 0309-2305

Contents

Preface

It is not completely by chance that this 21st edition of *Recent Advances in Anaesthesia and Analgesia* should be published at the very beginning of the 21st century. The speciality of anaesthesia as we know it was started 150 years ago and for the past 70 years *Recent Advances in Anaesthesia and Analgesia* has been presenting reviews of recent developments in our speciality. As we enter the new millennium the pace of advance in anaesthesia shows no sign of abating and the editors have collected together a number of contributions from respected authorities in order to bring the reader up to date with developments in their respective fields.

The recognition that α_2-adrenergic agonists possess potent analgesic and sedative effects has resulted in the increasing use of these agents. The basic and clinical science evidence for the anaesthetic-sparing action of the first generation α_2-agonist clonidine and the subsequently introduced second generation. α_2-agonist dexmedetomidine is presented by Drs Kamibayashi, Harasawa and Professor Maze. In *Recent Advances in Anaesthesia and Analgesia* volume 19, Professor Jean-Louis Vincent discussed the role of cytokines in the development of septic shock. We make no apology for returning to the topic of cytokines so soon. As Dr Eileen Ingham states the 150 known cytokine molecules with their diverse functions present a daunting topic for anybody other than a molecular biologist. In an attempt to bring order to this topic, Dr Ingham presents a brief historical overview followed by a description of the relevant biological activities of the cytokines. The pro-inflammatory cytokines most relevant to anaesthesia and analgesia are discussed in detail. The inflammatory process and the changes in sensitivity of nociceptive pathways elicited by inflammatory mediators are the subject of Drs Farquhar-Smith and Rice's chapter. These authors consider mechanisms for attenuation of pro-inflammatory mediators and also enhancement of physiological analgesic control systems. In particular, the neuromodulatory role of the endogenous cannabinoid system is presented in detail.

The application of basic science to clinical practice in acute pain management is eloquently presented by Professor Stephan Schug and Dr Kieran Davis. In particular, the role of Acute Pain Services and the techniques employed are discussed.

Current concepts in cerebral resuscitation are also considered in this edition. Professor Werner and Dr Engelhard outline the physical and pharmacological strategies to protect the brain from ischaemic and/or hypoxic damage. Future concepts such as the use of nitric oxide, polymorphonuclear leukocytes and programmed cell death are also presented.

In the treatment of hypovolaemic shock, it would seem to be completely against all of our best instincts to allow patients to continue to bleed. However, Dr Bernard Riley presents the evidence for and against a beneficial effect of permissive hypotension on survival. Anaesthetists will be only too aware of the concerns regarding the safety of human donor blood and there remains the continual problem of shortage of blood supplies. Artificial blood would seem to be the logical solution to the problem. Initial enthusiasm for artificial blood was tempered by disappointment. However, as Drs Frietsch, Lenz and Waschke point out, the latest artificial blood products are entering phase III trials and likely to be available soon. Albumin is one blood product that has been widely used in clinical practice, but which since the systematic reviews by the Cochrane Collaboration has been deemed to have a detrimental effect on outcome. Dr Neil Soni reviews the evidence and presents a perceptive overview.

Every anaesthetist will be familiar with the American Society of Anesthesiologists' (ASA) classification of physical status, but as Dr van Besouw points out risk assessment will surely play a greater part in all of our professional lives. Most risk assessment schemes focus on cardiovascular and to a lesser extent on respiratory risk. However, the choice of anaesthetic will also influence outcome and this is the subject of another chapter by Professor Hugo Van Aken.

Society is enlarging. Since Professor Anthony Adams first reviewed the problems facing the anaesthetist confronted by a morbidly obese patient requiring surgery, the prevalence of obesity in industrialised countries has continued to increase. Professor Adams has been joined by Dr Jeremy Cashman and together they revisit this topic.

Central neuraxial block is now a thoroughly accepted part of modern anaesthesia, but these blocks pose a unique risk for inducing neurological injury. In the final chapter of this volume, Dr János Károvits and Dr Helena Scott focus on minor neurological complications and backache (rather than hypotension and post-dural puncture headache).

The editors hope that the reader, like themselves, will find the foregoing chapters interesting and educational. Moreover, continuing professional development is demanded by our patients and our professional bodies and the volumes of the *Recent Advances in Anaesthesia and Analgesia* series has long supported this pursuit. It is increasingly difficult to keep up-to-date with developments in our speciality and, if this book continues to help the reader to achieve that end, then both editors and authors will be genuinely pleased.

London
2000

A.P.A
J.N.C

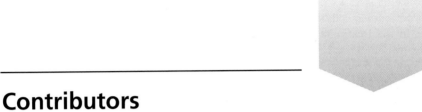

Contributors

Anthony P. Adams MBBS PhD FRCA FANZCA FFARACS DA
Professor of Anaesthetics in the University of London at the Guy's, King's and
St Thomas' Hospitals' School of Medicine, Honorary Consultant Anaesthetist,
Guy's and St Thomas' Trust, and Honorary Consultant Anaesthetist, King's
College Hospital NHS Trust, London, UK

Jeremy N. Cashman BSc MBBS BA MD FRCA
Consultant Anaesthetist, Department of Anaesthetics, St George's Hospital,
London; Honorary Senior Lecturer, University of London, UK

Kieran Davis MBChB FRCA
Pain Fellow, The Auckland Regional Pain Service, Auckland Hospital,
Auckland, New Zealand

Kristin Engelhard MD
Resident in Anaesthesiology, Klinikum rechts der Isar, Klinik für
Anaesthesiologie, Technische Universität München, München, Germany

Paul Farquhar-Smith MA MBBChir FRCA
Royal College of Anaesthetists' Jubilee Research Fellow, Imperial College
School of Medicine, Pain Research Group, Department of Anaesthetics, St
Mary's Hospital, London, UK

Thomas Frietsch MD
Research Assistant and Staff Anaesthetist, Institut für Anästhesiologie und
Operative Intensivmedizin, Fakultät für Klinische Medizin Mannheim der
Ruprecht-Karls-Universität Heidelberg, Universitäts-Klinikum Mannheim,
Mannheim, Germany

Katsumi Harasawa MD
Department of Anesthesiology and Acute Critical Medicine, Osaka
University Graduate School of Medicine, Osaka, Japan

Eileen Ingham BSc PhD
Reader in Medical Immunology, Department of Microbiology, University of
Leeds, Leeds, UK

Takahiko Kamibayashi MD PhD
Assistant Professor, Department of Anesthesiology and Acute Critical Medicine, Osaka University Graduate School of Medicine, Osaka, Japan

János Károvits MD PhD
Consultant Anaesthetist and Honorary Senior Lecturer, Department of Anaesthetics, Guy's Hospital, London, UK

Christian Lenz MD
Staff Anaesthetist, Institut für Anästhesiologie und Operative Intensivmedizin, Fakultät für Klinische Medizin Mannheim der Ruprecht-Karls-Universität Heidelberg, Universitäts-Klinikum Mannheim, Mannheim, Germany

Michael Margarson FRCA
Specialist Registrar in Anaesthesia and Intensive Care Medicine, Chelsea and Westminster Hospital, London, UK

Mervyn Maze MB ChB FRCP FRCA
Professor of Anaesthetics, Imperial College School of Medicine, Magill Department of Anaesthetics, Chelsea & Westminster Hospital, London, UK

Andrew S.C. Rice MB BS MD FRCA
Senior Lecturer in Pain Research, Imperial College School of Medicine, Pain Research Group, Department of Anaesthetics, St Mary's Hospital, London, UK

Bernard Riley MBE BSc MBBS FRCA
Consultant in Adult Intensive Care, University Hospital, Nottingham, UK

Norbert Rolf MD PhD
Assistant Medical Director, Klinik und Poliklinik für Anästhesiologie und operative Intensivmedizin, Westfälische Wilhelms Universität, Münster, Germany

Stephan A. Schug MD FANZCA FFPMANZCA
Head, Discipline of Anaesthesiology, Faculty of Medicine and Health Sciences, University of Auckland, Auckland, New Zealand

Helena Scott MB BChir FRCA
Consultant Anaesthetist, Department of Anaesthetics, Guy's Hospital, London, UK

Neil Soni MD FFICANZCA FRCA
Consultant in Anaesthesia and Intensive Care Medicine, Chelsea and Westminster Hospital, London, UK

Hugo Van Aken MD PhD FRCA FANZCA
Director, Klinik und Poliklinik für Anästhesiologie und operative Intensivmedizin, Westfälische Wilhelms Universität, Münster, Germany

Jean-Pierre van Besouw BSc MBBS FRCA
Consultant Anaesthetist, Department of Anaesthetics, St George's Hospital, London, UK

Klaus F. Waschke MD
Assistant Professor, Institut für Anästhesiologie und Operative
Intensivmedizin, Fakultät für Klinische Medizin Mannheim der Ruprecht-
Karls-Universität Heidelberg, Universitäts-Klinikum Mannheim, Mannheim,
Germany

Christian Werner MD PhD
Professor of Anaesthesiology, Klinikum rechts der Isar, Klinik für
Anaesthesiologie, Technische Universität München, München, Germany

Takahiko Kamibayashi Katsumi Harasawa Mervyn Maze

Alpha-2 adrenergic agonists

The peri-operative use of α_2-adrenergic agonists is finally coming of age. Since the first reports in the literature on the utility of α_2-adrenergic agonists a decade ago, two drugs in this class have now been registered for clinical use, namely epidural clonidine (Duraclon) and dexmedetomidine (Precedex).[1] Initially, reports concentrated on the anaesthetic-sparing actions of α_2-adrenergic agonists; now, their efficacy in pain management (Duraclon), regional anaesthesia (Duraclon), and sedation in the Intensive Therapy Unit (Precedex) have dominated this field. Furthermore, there is a plethora of studies addressing the manner by which α_2-agonists can enhance the safety of other anaesthetic agents, as well as suggestions on how to improve the therapeutic window of its own administration which bodes well for its future use. In this review, we will draw attention to novel information which has accrued in both the basic and clinical sciences and reflect on the optimum use of this exciting class of compounds.

BASIC PHARMACOLOGY

Adrenergic receptors have been differentiated into α and β based on the rank order of potency of various natural and synthetic catecholamines in different physiological preparations.[2] Subsequently, the α adrenoceptor was separated into two subtypes, α_2 and α_1, depending on their sensitivity to the α_2-selective antagonist yohimbine or the α_1-selective antagonist prazosin.[3] New techniques have elucidated both the subtype specificity and efficacy of α_2 ligands. Scheinin's group[4] measured agonist-stimulated binding of the stable GTP-analogue, guanosine-5-O-3-[^{35}S]-thiotriphosphate ([^{35}S]-GTPγS), as a functional assay to

Prof. Takahiko Kamibayashi, Department of Anesthesiology and Acute Critical Medicine, Osaka University Graduate School of Medicine D7, 2-2 Yamada-oka, Suita, Osaka 565-0871, Japan

Dr Katsumi Harasawa, Department of Anesthesiology and Acute Critical Medicine, Osaka University Graduate School of Medicine D7, 2-2 Yamada-oka, Suita, Osaka 565-0871, Japan

Prof Mervyn Maze, Imperial College School of Medicine, Magill Department of Anaesthetics, Chelsea & Westminster Hospital, 369 Fulham Road, London SW10 9NH, UK (for correspondence)

monitor G-protein activation by recombinant human α_2-adrenoceptor subtypes (α_{2A}, α_{2B} and α_{2C}) expressed on Chinese hamster ovary cell membrane. Using noradrenaline as the reference full agonist in all receptor subtypes, dexmedetomidine was shown to be a full agonist at α_{2C}-adrenoceptors and a partial agonist at α_{2A} and α_{2C} subtypes. Brimonidine (UK14,304) was a full agonist at α_{2A} and a partial agonist at α_{2B} and was inactive at α_{2C}. Clonidine was a weak partial agonist at the α_{2B}, but appeared inactive at α_{2A} and α_{2C}. Using similar techniques, Jasper et al[5] also reported efficacy profiles for α_2 agonists on $\alpha_2$adrenoceptor-dependent [^{35}S]-GTPγS binding using membranes from transfected HEK293 cells. In their study, clonidine and oxymetazoline were clearly discernible from inactive compounds at α_{2A} and α_{2C}. The authors attributed this discrepancy with Scheinin's report to differences in the cell line employed for the assay (CHO versus HEK293 cells) and different assay conditions (especially the difference in the duration of incubation of the assay mixture: 10 min in this study versus 60 min in Jasper's study). [^{35}S]-GTPγS binding appears to be a convenient functional test to screen potential subtype-selective agonists and to discriminate between full and partial agonists.

Since several α_2 ligands have also been shown to have activity at the 5-HT$_{1A}$ serotonergic receptor, Millan's group[6] have examined the binding and activation of recombinant α_{2A}-adrenoceptor and 5-HT$_{1A}$ receptor by chemically diverse α_2-adrenoceptor ligands. The agonists included dexmedetomidine, clonidine, brimonidine (UK14,304), the benzopyrrolidine fluparoxan and the guanidines guanfacine and guanabenz, while the antagonists were 1-(2-pyrimidinyl)-piperazine (1-PP), (±)-idazoxan, benalfocin (SKF86,466), yohimbine and RX821,002. The agonist dexmedetomidine and the antagonist atipamezole are the ligands of choice to distinguish α_2-mediated from 5-HT$_{1A}$-mediated actions, whilst the other compounds including clonidine show only low or modest selectivity for α_2 over 5-HT$_{1A}$ receptors. Therefore, caution should be exercised in experimental and clinical interpretation of the actions of traditionally employed α_2 ligands, such as clonidine, yohimbine and (±)-idazoxan, which exhibit marked agonist activity at 5-HT$_{1A}$ receptors.

From these results, it is apparent that there are few available agonists or antagonists that exhibit significant subtype selectivity and none that has full agonist activity at the α_{2A}-adrenoceptor, the site of anaesthetic and analgesic action. Agonist-mediated [^{35}S]-GTPγS binding is a sensitive and relatively simple method to study α_2-adrenoceptor activation of G-proteins allowing one to distinguish compounds of differing intrinsic activity and potency.

An important question to be resolved relates to the signalling pathway used by the different receptor subtypes. To address this, Akerman and colleagues[7] transfected a PC12 cell line with cDNAs for either the rat α_{2A}- or α_{2B}-adrenoceptor subtypes and investigated Ca^{2+} currents recorded by the whole-cell patch-clamp technique. One interpretation of their data is that the α_{2B}-adrenoceptor activation leads to stimulation of dihydropyridine-sensitive (L-type) Ca^{2+} channels via pertussis toxin-insensitive mechanisms while α_{2A}-adrenoceptor activation leads to inhibition of dihydropyridine-insensitive (mainly N-type) Ca^{2+} channels via pertussis toxin-sensitive G-proteins (Gi/Go-type G-proteins). This difference could provide an opportunity to functionally achieve subtype-selective responses with non-selective agonists by manipulating the post-receptor effector pathway.

PHARMACEUTICS

CLONIDINE

Clonidine, an imidazole compound, is a selective partial agonist for α_2 adrenoceptors with a ratio of approximately 200:1 (α_2:α_1). Clonidine is rapidly and almost completely absorbed after oral administration and reaches a peak plasma level within 60–90 min by this route. Clonidine can also be delivered via a time-release transdermal patch although it takes a minimum of 2 days for therapeutic levels to be achieved by this route.[8] The elimination half-life of clonidine is between 8–12 h with ~50% of the drug being metabolized in the liver to inactive metabolites while the rest is excreted unchanged in the kidney. A single dose of clonidine 0.3 mg has the same pharmacokinetic and pharmacodynamic profile whether administered orally or sublingually.[9] Therefore, the sublingual route can be predictably used in fasting patients, those having difficulty swallowing, or those who are unable to absorb drugs through the gastrointestinal tract. Clonidine is now being used by the rectal route of administration in children with a 95% bioavailability and unchanged pharmacokinetic parameters.[10] With the availability of epidural clonidine, numerous studies have investigated its pharmacokinetics by this route of administration which has been the subject of an excellent review.[11]

MEDETOMIDINE

Medetomidine, 4(5)-1-2,3-dimethylphenyl[ethyl]imidazole, is the prototype of the novel superselective α_2 agonists. It is an order of magnitude more selective than clonidine and is a full agonist at this class of receptor.[12] Medetomidine is extremely potent, active at low nanomolar concentrations, and has been widely used in veterinary practice in Europe. Since the D-enantiomer of this racemate is the active ingredient, dexmedetomidine has been developed for clinical use. The pharmacokinetic profile is more favourable for peri-operative use than is clonidine because of its much shorter half-life of approximately 2 h.[13] Phase III studies with this compound are currently being conducted in North America, Europe and Japan to investigate its peri-operative utility.

OTHER COMPOUNDS

Some of the ligands have an imidazole ring which facilitates binding to non-adrenergic imidazole-preferring receptors[14,15] as well as to the α_2 adrenoceptor. The cardiovascular properties of α_2 ligands may vary considerably depending on whether the imidazole-preferring receptor is also activated.[16] Other imidazoline compounds which have been investigated for their α_2 agonist properties include tizanidine[17] and mivazerol.[18]

APPLIED PHARMACOLOGY

CARDIOVASCULAR SYSTEM

The quintessential action of α_2 agonists is sympatholysis, i.e. the ability to block the sympathetic arm of the autonomic nervous system. There are several well-documented sites for this activity including, inhibition of firing of the locus coeruleus (the important noradrenergic relay nucleus in the brainstem) and postganglionic, presynaptic inhibition of noradrenaline release. Using an isolated dog stellate ganglion preparation, Bosjnak's group have now demonstrated that very high concentrations of dexmedetomidine (in the micromolar range) attenuate ganglionic transmission at a postsynaptic site of action. Presynaptic inhibition of neurotransmitter release by dexmedetomidine was also observed, but this effect was not robust and disappeared at high frequency (5 Hz) stimulation. The results from this study indicate that the central and peripheral sympatholytic effects of α_2 adrenoceptor stimulation may be further augmented by inhibition of ganglionic transmission.[19]

Using L659,066, a peripherally restricted α_2 antagonist, the early pressor response to dexmedetomidine, a subtype-non-selective α_2 agonist can be blocked in awake instrumented dogs.[20] These data are consistent with the finding that α_{2B}-adrenoceptors, located on smooth muscle cells in the resistance vessels, mediate this potentially dangerous side-effect. Pretreatment with L659,066 before intravenous administration of dexmedetomidine may be a useful pharmacological strategy to allow advantageous sedative-hypnotic and central sympatholytic action while avoiding the haemodynamic effects.

CENTRAL NERVOUS SYSTEM

Accumulating evidence indicates that noradrenaline (NA) has an important influence on the spatial working-memory and attentional functions of the prefrontal cortex (PFC).[21] α_2-Adrenergic agonists improve performance of several cognitive tasks which rely on the PFC. Furthermore, this response appears to be mediated by the α_{2A}-adrenoceptor subtype since low doses of agonists such as guanfacine and UK14,304, which have higher affinity for this subtype, are more efficacious than weak partial agonists of this receptor subtype. This represents the first sedative/hypnotic class of agent which enhances, rather than decreases memory performance. Therefore, α_{2A} agonists are now being tested as potential cognitive enhancers in disorders with prominent PFC dysfunction, such as attention deficit hyperactivity disorder.

With the advent of genetically modified rats which either lack or over-express a specific receptor subtype, investigators are now able to ascribe complex behavioural actions of α_2 agonists to activation of individual subtypes. Mice with targeted inactivation of the gene encoding α_{2C}-adrenoceptors had enhanced startle responses, and shortened attack latency in the isolation-aggression test, whereas tissue-specific over-expression of α_{2C}-adrenoceptors was associated with opposite effects.[22] Thus, drugs acting via α_{2C}-adrenoceptors may have therapeutic value in disorders associated with enhanced startle responses and sensorimotor gating deficits such as schizophrenia, attention deficit hyperactivity disorder, post-traumatic stress disorder, and drug withdrawal.

Following emergence from general anaesthesia with a potent volatile anaesthetic agent, patients may exhibit a hyperdynamic state (termed 'emergence syndrome') which can be attenuated with α_2 agonists. Recently, Quintin's group demonstrated that the turnover of catecholamines, as reflected by in vivo voltammetry, is enhanced in the vasomotor centre during the period of withdrawal from halothane anaesthesia in rats and that this can be blocked by either clonidine or mivazerol.[23]

In a series of rat studies, mivazerol was shown to attenuate the increase in blood pressure and heart rate through α_2-adrenoceptors in the spinal cord.[24] Further studies suggested that the emergence response is mediated via glutamate release.[25]

In a rat model of focal cerebral ischaemia, tizanidine significantly reduced infarction volumes even when the drug is administered after the initiation of the ischaemic insult.[26]

PERIPHERAL NERVOUS SYSTEM

In a Bennet neuropathic pain model, the combination of sub-effective doses of MK801 (the NMDA antagonist) and clonidine resulted in a significant antihyperalgesic action.[27] The analgesia enhancing effect of clonidine was also effective at attenuating the neurotoxic effects of MK801.

In a Chung model of neuropathic pain, the antihyperalgesic action of dexmedetomidine could be blocked by L659,066 the peripherally-restricted α_2 antagonist. This antagonist is ineffective in blocking the analgesic action of dexmedetomidine in normal rats.[28] The analgesic potency of dexmedetomidine was enhanced after nerve injury with a site of action outside the central nervous system. The finding of increased analgesic efficacy for α_2 agonist after nerve injury is in contrast to numerous reports of diminished analgesic efficacy for opioids in neuropathic models. Peripherally restricted α_2 agonists may be useful in the management of neuropathic pain without sedative side effect. This was recently established in a study using clonidine by intravenous regional anaesthesia in patients with sympathetically-mediated pain *vide infra*.[29]

CLINICAL APPLICATIONS OF ALPHA-2 ADRENERGIC AGONISTS

PREMEDICATION

Since sedation, anxiolysis and antisialogogue action are attractive attributes in a premedication agent, administration of α_2 agonists suits this purpose well. Another benefit of α_2 agonists as a premedication is their ability to potentiate the anaesthetic action of other agents and to reduce anaesthetic requirements during surgery. Conversely, requirements for neuromuscular blocking agents remain unaffected by pretreatment with α_2 agonists.[30]

The elderly patient population appears to be one that is most likely to benefit from the sympatholytic effects of the drug because of the prevalence of coronary artery disease and hypertension.[31,32] However, it is well to be prudent since these patients may exhibit the most extreme cardiovascular changes with this drug especially in diabetic patients.

In patients between 4–12 years of age, the combination of 4 µg/kg clonidine and 30 µg/kg atropine orally, 105 min before coming to the operating theatre, was more effective than diazepam at promoting anxiolysis and sedation.[33] The pre-operative administration of clonidine, 4 µg/kg, decreased postoperative pain and analgesic requirements in a paediatric population.[34]

Clonidine significantly attenuated the rapid increases in blood pressure and heart rate during the transition between low and high doses of desflurane.[35,36] Similarly, the sympatho-excitatory response to ketamine 1.0 mg/kg i.v., was attenuated by clonidine, 5 µg/kg p.o., as evidenced by the smaller increment in blood pressure.[37] Clonidine premedication also blunted hypertension, tachycardia as well as increments in plasma catecholamine concentrations during stepwise increase in isoflurane concentration by mask anaesthesia.[38]

Clonidine (5 µg/kg) significantly decreased intra-operative sufentanil use and lowered catecholamine response while maintaining stable haemodynamics in coronary artery bypass graft surgery.[39] To determine whether the addition of clonidine to a standardized general anaesthetic could safely provide post-operative sympatholysis for patients with known or suspected coronary artery disease, Ellis and colleagues[40] randomly allocated patients undergoing elective major non-cardiac surgery to receive either placebo or clonidine by a combination of oral and transdermal routes. Clonidine reduced enflurane requirements, intra-operative tachycardia, and myocardial ischaemia. Lastly, a relative 'renal-sparing' effect was noted in CABG surgery patients who received clonidine, 4 µg/kg, before induction.[41] In a placebo-controlled dose-ranging study of 300 patients undergoing peri-operative sympatholysis with mivazerol, intra-operative myo-cardial ischaemia and postoperative tachycardia were significantly reduced.[42]

From these studies, it is apparent that α_2 agonists are being used for more specific indications and by a variety of routes for their sympatholytic effect. The need to pre-empt sympatho-excitatory responses in surgical patients with cardiovascular disease will likely become an important indication for the clinical uses of this class of drugs.

REGIONAL ANAESTHESIA

Clonidine, administered via a variety of routes has been shown to be useful in improving the analgesic properties of adjunctive agents. Thirty-six geriatric patients, undergoing knee replacement using continuous spinal anaesthesia, were randomly assigned to receive bupivacaine alone or combined with either clonidine or morphine and the duration of surgical anaesthesia was assessed.[43] Only 1/9 patients in the clonidine group received re-injection of bupivacaine for surgical pain compared with 8/11 patients in the morphine and 8/10 patients in the bupivacaine alone groups.

Patients undergoing Caesarean section were randomized to receive spinal anaesthesia with bupivacaine alone or supplemented with either clonidine or clonidine plus fentanyl intrathecally.[44] The addition of clonidine improved the spread of the sensory block and prolonged postoperative analgesia, but moderately increased sedation.

Murat's group reported that the addition of clonidine to a local anaesthetic mixture (bupivacaine and lidocaine) administered into the caudal epidural space provided equivalent analgesia to that seen when fentanyl was added to the same local anaesthetic regimen. However, significantly fewer episodes of arterial oxygen desaturation and vomiting were seen in the clonidine group compared to the fentanyl group.

Oral clonidine dose-dependently prolongs spinal anaesthesia with hyperbaric tetracaine in patients undergoing gynaecological and urological surgery.[45] When compared to intrathecal fentanyl, oral clonidine (200 µg), shortened the onset time of tetracaine's sensory block and prolonged the duration of sensory and motor block.[46] Although severe hypotension and/or bradycardia are slightly more likely to occur, the postoperative opiate narcotic analgesic requirements are diminished.[47] The onset time required to surgical anaesthesia is unaffected by clonidine, and the duration of spinal and epidural anaesthesia was increased more than 2-fold.[48]

From the data included in these studies, it is now possible to both qualitatively and quantitatively enhance conduction blockade with α_2 agonists by various routes of administration. Yet, our understanding of the mechanism by which these local anaesthetic enhancing qualities occur are still not known.

GENERAL ANAESTHESIA

Although α_2 agonists have been recognized to possess potent analgesic and sedative effects, these agents have not been used as sole anaesthetic agents and may reflect their limited efficacy when used alone. The combination of oral and transdermal clonidine (which maintained the plasma concentration of clonidine at therapeutic levels) provided lower anaesthetic requirements, greater haemodynamic stability, more rapid recovery from anaesthesia and less postoperative requirement for supplemental morphine for pain control in patients undergoing lower abdominal surgeries.[49] An issue which has been repeatedly raised is that the α_2 agonists may be decreasing the anaesthetic requirements not by a direct anaesthetic action but through their ability to alter the haemodynamic responses which are used to titrate anaesthetic doses. Gabriel and colleagues[50] showed that, in the presence of clonidine, the EEG spectral indices reflected a deeper anaesthetic state despite the fact the end-expiratory isoflurane concentration was reduced by 50%. MAC studies in both volunteers and surgical patients support the contention that these agents have a primary anaesthetic action.

Data from these studies continue to stress the anaesthetic-sparing qualities of the α_2 agonists in patients undergoing general anaesthesia. Whether the use of lower concentrations of the other anaesthetics will be associated with a better outcome is not addressed. However, it is anticipated that with lower doses of 'fixed agents', a faster emergence from general anaesthesia may be anticipated with a commensurate decrease in time in the post-anaesthesia care unit.

In a landmark manuscript, Scheinin and colleagues have reported on the ability of atipamezole, a selective α_2 adrenoceptor antagonist to reverse the sedative properties of dexmedetomidine in volunteers.[51] Both the sedative and sympatholytic effects of intramuscular dexmedetomidine were dose-dependently antagonized by intravenous atipamezole, although the sensitivity for reversal of these two responses may be different. Since the agonist and the antagonist have similar elimination half-lives, the likelihood of recurrence of dexmedetomidine's clinical effects after atipamezole reversal is small.

POSTOPERATIVE PAIN

In a study involving post-Caesarean section patients, Capogna and colleagues[52] showed a dose-dependent increase in the duration of epidural morphine/local anaesthetic analgesia when clonidine (75 or 150 μg) was included in the mixture. Also, the need for re-dosing was diminished in the patients who received clonidine. In a further study involving Caesarean section patients, the addition of either clonidine or epinephrine (which also activates α_2 adrenergic receptors) to epidural sufentanil decreased the number of administrations of sufentanil by PCA.[53]

Patients undergoing gastrectomy with a combined general/epidural technique received epidural morphine with or without clonidine (3 μg/kg) for postoperative analgesia.[54] The cumulative number of supplemental systemic morphine injections via PCA was less in those patients who received clonidine at each hour for 24 h postoperative period ($P < 0.05$) while the VAS for pain was lower. In the clonidine-treated patients, sedation score was higher, and mean blood pressures were lower.

Bernard's group[55] compared the analgesic efficacy, arterial blood gases, and pharmacokinetics of an intravenous infusion of fentanyl (75 μg/h) and a mixture of fentanyl (25 μg/h) plus clonidine 0.3 μg/h) after surgery. Pain relief, sedation, and supplemental ketoprofen requirements were similar in both groups. The number of episodes of arterial desaturation (less than 90% for more than 20 s) totalled 106 in four of the patients in the fentanyl group (versus none in the clonidine/fentanyl group). Mean arterial blood pressure, plasma clearance, and the elimination rate constant of fentanyl were lower in the clonidine/fentanyl group than in the fentanyl group.

In an interesting study, Rockemann and colleagues[56] compared the analgesic effects of epidural clonidine (8 μg/kg) alone, with a lower dose (4 μg/kg) in combination with morphine (2 mg), or morphine (50 μg/kg) alone in patients undergoing pancreatectomy. Patients who received epidural solutions containing clonidine had earlier onset and a longer duration of analgesia than when morphine alone was used. Haemodynamically, the clonidine-treated patients had a rate-dependent decrease in cardiac output.

The efficacy of α_2 agonists, alone, for postsurgical analgesia has yet to be shown in surgical patients other than in patients receiving quite high doses or in parturients. In other settings, the combination of α_2 agonists with opiate narcotics appears to provide very durable analgesia with fewer side-effects than if either were used alone.

In post-thoracotomy patients, the addition of clonidine (2 μg/kg) significantly enhanced both the postoperative analgesia obtained with an intercostal block of bupivacaine as well as arterial oxygenation.[57] Whether this means that a lower dose of bupicaine (with a lower potential for toxicity) can be used was not addressed.

The addition of clonidine (1 μg/kg) to a caudal epidural solution of bupivacaine, improved the duration of postoperative analgesia[58] without compromising ventilation.[59]

In a study of the sparing effect of clonidine on the PCA fentanyl demand in burns patients,[60] demand for fentanyl over a 24 h period was reduced by more than 50% when clonidine was infused. Furthermore, the hyperdynamic haemodynamic state was also attenuated.

MISCELLANEOUS ACTIONS

ANABOLISM

Peri-operative infusion of clonidine will increase the anabolic growth hormone levels.[61] This may be expected to have a positive effect on nitrogen wasting. Mertes and colleagues[62] demonstrated that nitrogen balance was well maintained in alcoholics undergoing radical cancer surgery when they were given clonidine peri-operatively; an age-matched (non-alcoholic) group of cancer surgery patients served as historical controls.

SHIVERING

Treatment of uncontrolled shivering in patients in labour receiving epidural analgesia often consists of administration of meperidine. Mercadante and colleagues[63] demonstrated that clonidine (0.15 mg, i.v.) was as effective as this standard therapy for shivering during labour. In a large double-blind study, the prophylactic use of clonidine (4 µg/kg, i.v.) immediately after induction of general anaesthesia, reduced the incidence, severity and duration of postoperative shivering without changing the incidence of sedation.[64]

In patients undergoing surgical procedures under general anaesthesia (induction with propofol and fentanyl and maintenance with isoflurane in nitrous oxide) the incidence of postoperative shivering can be reduced from 40% to 0% by administering clonidine (1.5 µg/kg) before emergence.[65] Similarly, intravenous clonidine (1 µ/kg) reduced the incidence of shivering from 38% to 6% in patients undergoing knee arthroscopy under epidural anaesthesia.[66]

SEDATION IN THE INTENSIVE THERAPY UNIT

In some European countries, clonidine has gained acceptance in the intensive care setting as a sedative agent. Dexmedetomidine appears to have additional advantages over clonidine as a sedative agent in the intensive care unit (ITU) because of its higher receptor selectivity. This selectivity would be expected to produce more predictable effects with dexmedetomidine, and the reduction in the incidence of undesirable adverse effects related to stimulation of the α_1 receptors. In a recent multicentre double-blind placebo-controlled study, ITU patients on dexmedetomidine were clinically sedated, but could be roused when stimulated, and returned to their sleep-like state when left alone.[67] The ability for patients to be rousable presents a new patient profile, because it facilitates patient involvement with their own care while at the same time making patient management easier on the intensive care staff. Therapeutic ranges for benzodiazepines and anaesthetics frequently allow clinicians to provide adequate sedation only at the expense of inducing patients into a deep sleep. Patients are routinely non-responsive or semi-anaesthetized. In contrast, dexmedetomidine-treated patients can be adequately sedated, yet rousable and responsive.

In a large percentage of dexmedetomidine-treated patients, it was sufficient to give dexmedetomidine alone allowing the patient to be sedated yet rousable and co-operative, and free of significant pain. If additional sedation and/or

Alpha-2 adrenergic agonists

analgesia were required (after dexmedetomidine was titrated to its highest indicated dose), it was not a problem to concomitantly add another sedative and/or analgesic to the therapeutic regimen to meet the patient's particular treatment requirement.

Tachycardia and arterial hypertension can cause severe problems in many postsurgical patients requiring intensive care, especially during the period of weaning from the respirator and when transitioning to the awake state; dexmedetomidine reduces these adverse effects. In addition to the haemodynamic stability and predictability of dexmedetomidine, the respiratory effects provided by dexmedetomidine are also stable. Dexmedetomidine does not cause clinically relevant respiratory depression like propofol, benzo-diazepines and opioids. Unlike these agents, dexmedetomidine does not need to be weaned prior to extubation. The dexmedetomidine infusion can continue through mechanical ventilation, during extubation and the postextubation period without having to be turned off to allow patients to return to normal respiration rates. This allows greater flexibility for removing patients from artificial ventilation, and it also allows patients to be calm, comfortable and pain-free during the extubation process.

Adverse effects associated with dexmedetomidine, especially cardiovascular system-related events, are predictable based on the pharmacological effects of the drug. The most prominent adverse effects on the cardiovascular system (bradycardia and reduction of sympatho-adrenergic hypertension) are desired effects in most postsurgical intensive care patients.

The use of α_2 agonists in the immediate emergence and early postoperative period appears to hold out great promise. This class of compound may represent the first of its kind to provide such a positive effect on nitrogen balance. If this feature is corroborated in other studies, the utility of α_2 agonists in the severely ill ICU patient may become *de rigeur*.

CHRONIC PAIN

In an 'enrichment' study design, transdermal clonidine could be shown to decrease pain in subjects with diabetic neuropathy.[68] Since phentolamine was ineffective, even in the most responsive patients, the mechanism for the clonidine response appears to be separate from its sympatholytic action. Anecdotally, it has been noted, in a patient suffering from pharyngeal cancer pain, that the addition of clonidine to intracerebroventricular doses of morphine enhanced the efficacy of the opiates.[69] Similarly, in a patient suffering from intractable pain following spinal cord injury, the addition of clonidine resulted in a rapid improvement.[70]

Reuben and colleagues[71] have reported on the resolution of sympathetically maintained pain with intravenous clonidine (1 μg/kg) by a Bier's block. Plasma concentrations of clonidine 30 min after deflation of the tourniquet were 0.12 ng/ml, which are significantly lower than those required for a central sympatholytic effect (1.5–2.0 ng/ml). The authors concluded that clonidine also possesses peripheral analgesic properties in patients with sympathetically maintained pain.

Eisenach's group investigated the thermal and mechanical anti-hyperalgesic efficacy of intrathecal versus intravenous administration of clonidine (150 μg) in capsaicin-induced pain in volunteers.[72] Only intrathecally-administered clonidine was efficacious and was without the sedative effects which were evident after intravenous clonidine. Therefore, this study suggests that the inflammatory component of the chronic pain state can only be interrupted at a central site with α_2 agonists as opposed to the neurogenic component which may also have a peripheral site of action (see Reuben et al[29,71] and Poree et al[28]).

COMPLICATIONS

An extension of the pharmacological properties of α_2 agonists is the development of bradycardia and hypotension.[10,73,74] Bradycardia can be pre-empted by the prophylactic use of an anticholinergic agents (atropine or glycopyrrolate) although the increment in heart rate which can obtain is significantly less in both an adult as well as a paediatric population.[75] Conversely, hypotension will respond in an exaggerated fashion to treatment with ephedrine.[76] The pressor response to adrenaline is enhanced following oral clonidine and thus restoration of blood pressure can be achieved effectively by either ephedrine or adrenaline.[77]

CONCLUSIONS

The use of α_2 agonists, either alone or in combination, is becoming widespread in anaesthesia. The original enthusiasm for this class of compound for its plethora of beneficial effects appears to have been justified based on the more recent clinical studies reported here. In the last year, the field has rapidly evolved with the clinical introduction of the second generation of α_2 agonists, notably dexmedetomidine, a more selective, specific and efficacious compound than the prototype, clonidine. Furthermore, formulations allowing several different routes of administration, ranging from transdermal to neuraxial, have further extended its clinical utility.

Key points for clinical practice

- The clinical responses to α_2 agonists are predictably based on the physiology of the α_2-adrenergic receptors. Adverse events are due to an extension of the pharmacological properties into the toxic range.

- The different receptor subtypes are potential targets for novel drug development since more selective actions can be produced.

- With the development of proteomics and genomics, alterations in responsiveness may be anticipated.

- Dexmedetomidine provides a clinically desirable sedation state in the mechanically-ventilated postoperative patient that cannot be matched by current alternative therapeutics options.

ACKNOWLEDGEMENTS

The authors gratefully acknowledge the support of the Uehara Foundation (TK), and the Medical Research Council, UK.

REFERENCES

1. Bachand RT, List W, Etropolski M, Martin E. A phase III study evaluating dexmedetomidine for sedation in postoperative patients. Anesthesiology 1999; 91: A296.
2. Ahlquist PR. A study of the adrenotropic receptors. Am J Physiol 1948; 153: 586–600.
3. Bylund DB, U'Pritchard DC. Characterization of alpha-1 and alpha-2 adrenergic receptors. Int Rev Neurobiol 1983; 24: 343–431.
4. Peltonen JM, Pihlavisto M, Scheinin M. Subtype-specific stimulation of [^{35}S]-GTPgammaS binding by recombinant alpha2-adrenoceptors. Eur J Pharmacol 1998; 355: 275–279.
5. Jasper JR, Lesnick JD, Chang LK et al. Ligand efficacy and potency at recombinant alpha2 adrenergic receptors: agonist mediated [^{35}S]-GTPgammaS binding. Biochem Pharmacol 1998; 55: 1035–1043.
6. Newman-Tancredi A, Nicolas JP, Audinot V et al. Actions of alpha2 adrenoceptor ligands at alpha2A and 5-HT1A receptors: the antagonist, atipamezole, and the agonist, dexmedetomidine, are highly selective for alpha2A adrenoceptors. Naunyn Schmiedebergs Arch Pharmacol 1998; 358: 197–206.
7. Soini SL, Duzic E, Lanier SM, Akerman KE. Dual modulation of calcium channel current via recombinant alpha2-adrenoceptors in pheochromocytoma (PC-12) cells. Pflügers Arch 1998; 435: 280–285.
8. Toon S, Hopkins KJ, Aarons L et al. Rate and extent of absorption of clonidine from a transdermal therapeutic system. J Pharm Pharmacol 1989; 41: 17–21.
9. Cunningham FE, Baughman VL, Peters J, Laurito CE. Comparative pharmacokinetics of oral versus sublingual clonidine. J Clin Anesth 1994; 6: 430–433.
10. Lonnqvist PA, Bergendahl HTG, Eksborg S. Pharmacokinetics of clonidine after rectal administration in children. Anesthesiology 1994; 81: 1097–1101.
11. Eisenach JC, de Kock M, Klimscha W. Alpha-2 adrenergic agonists for regional anesthesia. A clinical review of clonidine (1984–1995). Anesthesiology 1996; 85: 655–674.
12. Scheinin H, Virtanen R, MacDonald E et al. Medetomidine – a novel of alpha2-adrenoceptor agonist: a review of its pharmacodynamic effects. Prog Neuropsychopharmacol Biol Psychiatry 1989; 13: 635–651.
13. Dyck JB, Maze M, Haack C et al. The pharmacokinetics and hemodynamic effects of intravenous and intramuscular dexmedetomidine hydrochloride in adult human volunteers. Anesthesiology 1993; 78: 813–820.
14. Ernsberger P, Meeley MP, Mann JJ, Reis DJ. Clonidine binds to imidazole binding sites as well as alpha2-adrenoceptors in the ventrolateral medulla. Eur J Pharmacol 1987; 134: 1–13.
15. Zonnenchein R, Diamant S, Atlas D. Imidazoline receptors in rat liver cells: a novel receptor or a subtype of alpha2-adrenoceptors? Eur J Pharmacol 1990; 190: 203–215.
16 Tibirica E, Feldman J, Mernet D et al. An imidazoline-specific mechanism for the hypotensive effect of clonidine. A study with yohimbine and idazoxan. J Pharmacol Exp Ther 1991; 256: 606–613.
17. Miettunen TJ, Kanto JH, Salonen MA, Scheinin M. The sedative and sympatholytic effects of oral tizanidine in healthy volunteers. Anesth Analg 1996; 82: 817–820.
18. Noyer M, de Laveleye F, Vauquelin G, Gobert J, Wulfert E. Mivazerol, a novel compound with high specificity for alpha 2 adrenergic receptors: binding studies on different human and rat membrane preparations. Neurochem Int 1994; 24: 221–229.
19 McCallum JB, Boban N, Hogan Q, Schmeling WT, Kampine JP, Bosnjak ZJ. The mechanism of alpha2-adrenergic inhibition of sympathetic ganglionic transmission. Anesth Analg 1998; 87: 503–510.
20 Pagel PS, Proctor LT, Devcic A et al. A novel alpha 2-adrenoceptor antagonist attenuates the early, but preserves the late cardiovascular effects of intravenous dexmedetomidine in conscious dogs. J Cardiothorac Vasc Anesth 1998; 12: 429–434.

21. Arnsten AF, Steere JC, Jentsch DJ, Li BM. Noradrenergic influences on prefrontal cortical cognitive function: opposing actions at postjunctional alpha 1 versus alpha 2-adrenergic receptors. Adv Pharmacol 1998; 42: 764–767.

22. Sallinen J, Haapalinna A, Viitamaa T, Kobilka BK, Scheinin M. Adrenergic alpha2C-receptors modulate the acoustic startle reflex, prepulse inhibition, and aggression in mice. J Neurosci 1998; 18: 3035–3042.

23. Bruandet N, Rentero N, Debeer L, Quintin L. Catecholamine activation in the vasomotor center on emergence from anesthesia: the effects of alpha2 agonists. Anesth Analg 1998; 86: 240–245.

24. Guyaux M, Gobert J, Noyer M, Vandevelde M, Wulfert E. Mivazerol prevents the tachycardia caused by emergence from halothane anesthesia partly through activation of spinal alpha 2-adrenoceptors. Acta Anaesthesiol Scand 1998; 42: 238–245.

25. Zhang X, Kindel G, Wulfert E, Hanin I. Mivazerol inhibits intrathecal release of glutamate evoked by halothane withdrawal in rats. Acta Anaesthesiol Scand 1998; 42: 1004–1009.

26. Berkman MZ, Zirh TA, Berkman K, Pamir MN. Tizanidine is an effective agent in the prevention of focal cerebral ischemia in rats: an experimental study. Surg Neurol 1998; 50: 264–270; discussion 270–271.

27. Jevtovic-Todorovic V, Wozniak DF, Powell S, Nardi A, Olney JW. Clonidine potentiates the neuropathic pain-relieving action of MK-801 while preventing its neurotoxic and hyperactivity side effects. Brain Res 1998; 781: 202–211.

28. Poree LR, Guo TZ, Kingery WS, Maze M. The analgesic potency of dexmedetomidine is enhanced after nerve injury: a possible role for peripheral alpha2-adrenoceptors. Anesth Analg 1998; 87: 941–948.

29. Reuben SS, Steinberg RB, Madabhushi L, Rosenthal E. Intravenous regional clonidine in the management of sympathetically maintained pain. Anesthesiology 1998; 89: 527–530.

30. Takahashi H, Nishikawa T. Oral clonidine does not alter vecuronium neuromuscular blockade in anaesthetized patients. Can J Anaesth 1995; 42: 511–515.

31. Ghingnone M, Calvillo O, Quintin L. Anesthesia for ophthalmic surgery in the elderly: the effects of clonidine on intraocular pressure, perioperative hemodynamics, and anesthesia requirement. Anesthesiology 1988; 68: 707–716.

32. Kumar A, Bose S, Phattacharya A, Tandon OP, Kundra P. Oral clonidine premedication for elderly patients undergoing intraocular surgery. Acta Anaesthesiol Scand 1992; 36: 159–164.

33. Mikawa K, Maekawa N, Nishina K, Takao Y, Yaku H, Obara H. Efficacy of oral clonidine premedication in children. Anesthesiology 1993; 79: 926–931.

34. Mikawa K, Nishina K, Maekawa N, Obara H. Oral clonidine premedication reduces postoperative pain in children. Anesth Analg 1996; 82: 225–230.

35. Devcic A, Muzi M, Ebert TJ. The effects of clonidine on desflurane-mediated sympathoexcitation in humans. Anesth Analg 1995; 80: 773–779.

36. Weiskopf RB, Eger 2nd EI, Noorani M, Daniel M. Fentanyl, esmolol, and clonidine blunt the transient cardiovascular stimulation induced by desflurane in humans. Anesthesiology 1994; 81: 1350–1355.

37. Tanaka M, Nishikawa T. Oral clonidine premedication attenuates the hypertensive response to ketamine. Br J Anaesth 1994; 73: 758–762.

38. Tanaka S, Tsuchida H, Namba H, Namiki A. Clonidine and lidocaine inhibition of isoflurane-induced tachycardia in humans. Anesthesiology 1994; 81: 1341–1349.

39. Howie MB, Hiestand DC, Jopling MW, Romanelli VA, Kelly WB, McSweeney TD. Effect of oral clonidine premedication on anesthetic requirement, hormonal response, hemodynamics, and recovery in coronary artery bypass graft (CABG) surgery patients. J Clin Anesth 1996; 8: 263–272.

40. Ellis JE, Drijvers G, Pedlow S et al. Premedication with oral and transdermal clonidine provides safe and efficacious postoperative sympatholysis. Anesth Analg 1994; 79: 1133–1140.

41. Kulka PJ, Tryba M, Zenz M. Preoperative alpha2-adrenergic receptor agonists prevent the deterioration of renal function after cardiac surgery: results of a randomized, controlled trial. Crit Care Med 1996; 24: 947–952.

42. McSPI-EUROPE Research Group. Beneficial effects of the alpha$_2$ adrenoceptor agonist mivazerol on hemodynamic stability and myocardial ischaemia. Anesthesiology 1997; 86: 346–363.

43. Brunschwiler M, Van Gessel E, Forster A, Bruce A, Gamulin Z. Comparison of clonidine, morphine or placebo mixed with bupivacaine during continuous spinal anaesthesia. Can J Anaesth 1998; 45: 735–740.

44. Benhamou D, Thorin D, Brichant JF, Dailland P, Milon D, Schneider M. Intrathecal clonidine and fentanyl with hyperbaric bupivacaine improves analgesia during cesarean section. Anesth Analg 1998; 87: 609–613.

45. Ota K, Namiki A, Iwasaki H, Takahashi I. Dose-related prolongation of tetracaine spinal anesthesia by oral clonidine in humans. Anesth Analg 1994; 79: 1121–1125.

46. Singh H, Liu J, Gaines GY, White PF. Effect of oral clonidine and intrathecal fentanyl on tetracaine spinal block. Anesth Analg 1994; 79: 1113–1116.

47. Niemi L. Effects of intrathecal clonidine on duration of bupivacaine spinal anaesthesia, haemodynamics, and postoperative analgesia in patients undergoing knee arthroscopy. Acta Anaesthesiol Scand 1994; 38: 724–728.

48. Klimscha W, Chiari A, Krafft P et al. Hemodynamic and analgesic effects of clonidine added repetitively to continuous epidural and spinal blocks. Anesth Analg 1995; 80: 322–327.

49. Segal IS, Javis DJ, Duncan SR, White PF, Maze M. Clinical efficacy of oral-transdermal clonidine combinations during the perioperative period. Anesthesiology 1991; 74: 220–225.

50. Gabriel AH, Faryniak B, Sojka G, Czech T, Freye E, Spiss CK. Clonidine: an adjunct in isoflurane N_2O/O_2 relaxant anaesthesia. Effects on EEG power spectra, somatosensory and auditory evoked potentials. Anaesthesia 1995; 50: 290–296.

51. Scheinin H, Aantaa R, Anttila M, Hakola P, Helminen A, Karhuvaara S. Reversal of the sedative and sympatholytic effects of dexmedetomidine with a specific alpha2-adrenoceptor antagonist atipamezole: a pharmacodynamic and kinetic study in healthy volunteers. Anesthesiology 1998; 89: 574–584.

52. Capogna G, Celleno D, Zangrillo A, Costantino P, Foresta S. Addition of clonidine to epidural morphine enhances postoperative analgesia after cesarean delivery. Reg Anesth 1995; 20: 57–61.

53. Vercauteren MP, Vandeput DM, Meert TF, Adriaensen HA. Patient-controlled epidural analgesia with sufentanil following caesarean section: the effect of adrenaline and clonidine admixture. Anaesthesia 1994; 49: 767–771.

54. Anzai Y, Nishikawa T. Thoracic epidural clonidine and morphine for postoperative pain relief. Can J Anaesth 1995; 42: 292–297.

55. Bernard JM, Lagarde D, Souron R. Balanced postoperative analgesia: effect of intravenous clonidine on blood gases and pharmacokinetics of intravenous fentanyl. Anesth Analg 1994; 79: 1126–1132.

56. Rockemann MG, Seeling W, Brinkmann A et al. Analgesic and hemodynamic effects of epidural clonidine, clonidine/morphine, and morphine after pancreatic surgery – a double-blind study. Anesth Analg 1995; 80: 869–874.

57. Tschernko EM, Klepetko H, Gruber E et al. Clonidine added to the anesthetic solution enhances analgesia and improves oxygenation after intercostal nerve block for thoracotomy. Anesth Analg 1998; 87: 107–111.

58. Klimscha W, Chiari A, Michalek-Sauberer A et al. The efficacy and safety of a clonidine/bupivacaine combination in caudal blockade for pediatric hernia repair. Anesth Analg 1998; 86: 54–61.

59. Dupeyrat A, Goujard E, Muret J, Ecoffey C. Transcutaneous CO_2 tension effects of clonidine in paediatric caudal analgesia in patients. Paediatr Anaesth 1998; 8: 145–148.

60. Viggiano M, Badetti C, Roux F, Mendizabal H, Bernini V, Manelli JC. Controlled analgesia in a burn patient: fentanyl sparing effect of clonidine. Ann Fr Anesth Reanim 1998; 17: 19–26.

61. De Kock M, Merello L, Pendeville P, Maiter D, Scholtes JL. Effects of intravenous clonidine on the secretion of growth hormone in the perioperative period. Acta Anaesthesiol Belg 1994; 45: 167–174.

62. Mertes N, Goeters C, Kuhmann M, Zander JF. Postoperative α_2 adrenergic stimulation attenuates protein catabolism. Anesth Analg 1996; 82: 258–263.

63. Mercadante S, De Michele P, Letterio G, Pignataro A, Sapio M, Villari P. Effect of clonidine on postpartum shivering after epidural analgesia: a randomized, controlled, double-blind study. J Pain Symptom Management 1994; 9: 294–297.

64. Vanderstappen I, Vandermeersch E, Vanacker B, Mattheussen M, Herijgers P, Van Aken H. The effect of prophylactic clonidine on postoperative shivering. A large prospective double-blind study. Anaesthesia 1996; 51: 351–355.

65. Horn EP, Standl T, Sessler DI, von Knobelsdorff G, Buchs C, Schulte am Esch J. Physostigmine prevents postanesthetic shivering as does meperidine or clonidine. Anesthesiology 1998; 88: 108–13.

66. Sia S. I.v. clonidine prevents post-extradural shivering. Br J Anaesth 1998; 81: 145–146.

67. Bachand RT, List W, Etropolski M, Martin E. A phase III study evaluating dexmedetomidine for sedation in postoperative patients. Anesthesiology 1999; 91: A296.

68. Byas-Smith MG, Max MB, Muir J, Kingman A. Transdermal clonidine compared to placebo in painful diabetic neuropathy using a two-stage 'enriched enrolment' design. Pain 1995; 60: 267–274.

69. Loriferne JF, Souchal Delacour I, Rostaing S, N'Guyen JP, Bonnet F. Combined intraventricular morphine and clonidine administration for cephalic cancer pain relief. Ann Fr Anesth Reanim 1995; 14: 233–236.

70. Siddall PJ, Gray M, Rutkowski S, Cousins MJ. Intrathecal morphine and clonidine in the management of spinal cord injury pain: a case report. Pain 1994, 59: 147–148.

71. Reuben SS, Steinberg RB, Madabhushi L, Rosenthal E. Intravenous regional clonidine in the management of sympathetically maintained pain. Anesthesiology 1998; 89: 527–530.

72. Eisenach JC, Hood DD, Curry R. Intrathecal, but not intravenous, clonidine reduces experimental thermal or capsaicin-induced pain and hyperalgesia in normal volunteers. Anesth Analg 1998; 87: 591–596.

73. Carabine UA, Wright PMC, Moore J. Preanaesthetic medication with clonidine: a dose-response study. Br J Anaesth 1991; 67: 79–83.

74. Aantaa R, Kanto J, Scheinin M. Intramuscular dexmedetomidine, a novel alpha2 adrenoceptor agonist, as premedication for minor gynaecological surgery. Acta Anaesthesiol Scand 1991; 35: 283–288.

75. Nishikawa T, Dohi S. Oral clonidine blunts the heart rate response to intravenous atropine in humans. Anesthesiology 1991; 75: 217–222.

76. Nishikawa T, Kimura T, Taguchi N, Dohi S. Oral clonidine preanesthetic medication augments the pressor responses to intravenous ephedrine in awake or anesthetized patients. Anesthesiology 1991; 74: 705–710.

77. Inomata S, Nishikawa T, Kihara S, Akiyoshi Y. Enhancement of pressor response to intravenous phenylephrine following oral clonidine medication in awake and anaesthetized patients. Can J Anaesth 1995; 42: 119–125.

Eileen Ingham

Cytokines

To the reader who is new to cytokines, this particular group of molecules can appear extremely daunting. This is not surprising given the chaos that surrounds the nomenclature of the more than 150 molecules that have now been cloned and characterised and the diverse, often ambiguous functions that these molecules have been shown to carry out. Cytokines have a role to play in essentially all physiological processes in the human body and, as such, some understanding of their characteristics and functions are necessary for all human biologists and clinicians. The purpose of this chapter is to attempt to produce some basic order from the apparent chaos. The emphasis is on the biological activities of the cytokines, with particular reference to the pro-inflammatory cytokines that are of most relevance to anaesthesia and analgesia.

A BRIEF HISTORICAL OVERVIEW

In order to appreciate the confusion that exists in the nomenclature of cytokines, it is appropriate to take a brief look at the history and discovery of the molecules. When the first cytokines were described, researchers did not have the benefits of modern molecular techniques and the early descriptions were based on the measurement of a particular biological activity. These biological activities were identified in four different areas – cellular immunology, virology, cell biology and haematology – that did not really come together until the 1980s. The fact that the cytokines are produced in picogram to nanogram quantities and many have numerous diverse biological activities in vitro meant that the same molecule was often studied by different groups and given a different name because a different biological effect was used to assay the molecule.

Dr Eileen Ingham BSc PhD, Reader in Medical Immunology, Department of Microbiology, University of Leeds, Leeds LS2 9JT, UK

The first cytokines were actually discovered by two virologists, Issacs and Lindemann in 1957.[1] They reported on a soluble substance present in the culture fluid when chick chorio-allantoid membrane was incubated with killed influenza virus. This substance, which they named interferon (IFN), was shown to protect cells from subsequent infections by the live virus. It is now known that this IFN was IFN-β, now designated as a type 1 IFN along with 13 structurally distinct forms of IFN-α and one form of IFN-ω. Several years later, a related factor produced by mitogen stimulated lymphocytes was described[2] which is now recognised as IFN-γ. IFN-γ is classed as a type II IFN because it has no structural homology with the type 1 IFNs, but shares some biological activities.

During the 1960s, cellular immunologists were attempting to determine the in vitro correlates of cellular immunity. It had been recognised that the culture supernatant from antigen or mitogen stimulated lymphocytes could transfer immunity, so-called 'transfer factor'. In 1966, an activity present in the culture supernatant of antigen-stimulated lymphocytes that was able to inhibit the migration of macrophages was described. This factor was termed 'migration inhibition factor' (MIF)[3,4] That this was in fact IFN-γ was not recognised at that time. This was followed by the demonstration of another activity in the culture supernatants of antigen stimulated lymphocytes that was cytotoxic for some target cell lines[5,6] and this was named 'lymphotoxin'. In 1969, Dumonde[7] introduced the term 'lymphokines' which were defined as 'cell free soluble factors generated by the interaction of sensitised lymphocytes with specific antigen and expressed without reference to the immunological specificity'. At this time, it was generally thought that such activities would be unique to lymphocytes.

This was soon to change when the first 'monokine' was described by Gery in 1971[8] as a lymphocyte activating factor (LAF) produced by adherent cells from human peripheral blood. In 1975, another lymphokine, perhaps the most important factor in the development of cellular immunology was described and named T-cell growth factor (TCGF).[9] Various other biological activities were then described in macrophage supernatants which were given a variety of different names, based on the activity measured, for example leukocyte pyrogen, B-cell activating factor and endogenous pyrogen. It is now known that these were not separate molecules but all identical to LAF. Tumour necrosis factor-α (TNF-α) was one of the earlier monokines to be demonstrated[10] in the serum of animals treated with lipopolysaccharide. In 1979, The Second International Lymphokine Workshop was held at Interlaken in Switzerland where it was proposed that the term 'interleukin' (IL) be adopted to describe the activities of leukocytes that had a biological effect on other leukocytes.[11] The first two ILs were designated, IL-1, to replace LAF (and its other diverse names) and IL-2 to replace TCGF.

During the late 1970s, over 100 different biological activities were described. The first colony stimulating factor, granulocyte monocyte stimulating factor, was described [12] and the growth factors were first identified.[13] It became apparent that many lymphokines and monokines could be produced by cells other then lymphocytes and macrophages, such as epidermal keratinocytes. In 1974, Cohen and colleagues[14] had suggested the use of the term cytokine to replace lymphokine; however, the term was not readily accepted until the 1980s.

With the 1980s came the molecular biology revolution and the development of monoclonal antibody technology. The field of cytokine research exploded, driven by the availability of recombinant cytokines and the antibody tools to measure them. Research in this field during the 1980s was driven by the hope that cytokines and/or cytokine antagonists may have a role to play in the treatment of disease. Although, to date, the clinical applications of cytokines have been disappointing, there have been some success stories. The 1990s have seen developments in the understanding of cytokine receptors, and the potential therapeutic role of soluble forms of these molecules. The mechanisms by which cytokine signals are transduced by cells is now largely understood and structural studies are beginning to bring some order to the chaos by an understanding of the evolution of cytokines and cytokine receptors.

CYTOKINE NOMENCLATURE

There is still no unifying system for the nomenclature of cytokines. For a cytokine to be designated as an IL, there are established criteria.[15] The cytokine must be molecularly cloned and expressed, possess a unique nucleotide sequence and a neutralising monoclonal antibody must be available. In addition, the cytokine must be a natural product of cells of the immune system. The new IL must also mediate a potentially important function in the immune response and have other functions such that a simple functional name is inadequate to fully describe the activity. These characteristics must also be described in a peer-reviewed publication. To date, there are 20 cytokines that are designated as ILs and these are simply designated IL-1 to IL-20. The difficulty is that this, of course, tells the reader nothing of the characteristics and functions of the cytokine.

The majority of the remaining 130 or more cytokines still retain their older descriptive names. This makes it easier to remember them but does not necessarily convey their range of activities or structural/evolutionary relatedness to other cytokines. The various names currently designated to the cytokines are given in Table 1.

CHARACTERISTIC FEATURES OF CYTOKINES

The cytokines share a variety of features:

1. They are all simple proteins or glycoproteins with a molecular weight of less than 40 kDa. Although IL-12 is a heterodimer of two polypeptides.
2. Most are not produced constitutively by cells, but are induced by a stimulus. Induction is at the level of transcription or translation.
3. When cytokines are induced they are produced transiently in picogram to nanogram quantities. Most cytokines have a short half-life.
4. In order for a cytokine to exert its effect on a target cell, the cell must be expressing the specific cytokine receptor.
5. Interaction of the cytokine (ligand) with its specific receptor leads to transduction of the signal to the nucleus and this induces an altered pattern of gene expression. This may result in a variety of alterations in the behaviour of the target cell including increased mitosis, inhibition of mitosis, apoptosis,

Recent Advances in Anaesthesia and Analgesia 21

Table 1 A functional grouping of the major cytokines

Broup	Cytokine (CK)	Abbreviation
Anti-viral CK	Interferon-α (13 subtypes)	IFN-α
	Interferon-β	IFN-β
	Interferon-ω	IFN-ω
	Interferon-γ	IFN-γ
Pro-inflammatory CK	Interleukin-1α	IL-1α
	Interleukin-1β	IL-1β
	Interleukin-6	IL-6
	Tumour necrosis factor-α	TNF-α
Anti-inflammatory CK	Interleukin-1 receptor antagonist	IL-1ra
	Interleukin-10	IL-10
	Transforming growth factor-β	TGF-β
	Interleukin-13	IL-13
Immunological CK	Interleukin-2	IL-2
	Interleukin-4	IL-4
	Interleukin-5	IL-5
	Interleukin-6	IL-6
	Interleukin-9	IL-9
	Interleukin-12	IL-12
	Interleukin-13	IL-13
	Interleukin-15	IL-15
	Interleukin-16	IL-16
	Interleukin-17	IL-17
	Interleukin-18	IL-18
	Interferon-γ	IFN-γ
Cytotoxic CK	Tumour necrosis factor-α	TNF-α
	Tumour necrosis factor-β	TNF-β
	Lymphotoxin-β	LT
	Fas ligand	Fas ligand
	CD40 ligand	CD40 ligand
	TNF-related apoptosis inducing ligand	TRAIL
Haematopoietic CK	Colony stimulating factor	CSF-1
	Granulocyte colony stimulating factor	G-CSF
	Granulocyte-monocyte stimulating factor	GM-CSF
	Stem cell factor	SF
	Erythropoietin	EPO
	Flt3-ligand	Flt3-ligand
	Leukemia inhibitory factor	LIF
	Interleukin-1	IL-1
	Interleukin-3	IL-3
	Interleukin-6	IL-6
	Interleukin-7	IL-7
	Interleukin-11	IL-11
Growth factors	Epidermal growth factor	EGF
	Fibroblast growth factor (9 subtypes)	FGF-a,b,3–9
	Transforming growth factor-β (3)	TGF-β_{1-3}
	Bone morphogenetic proteins (9)	
	Insulin-like growth factor-I & II	IGF-I&II
	Nerve growth factor	NGF
	Oncostatin-M	OSM
	Platelet-derived growth factor-A, B	PDGF-A,B
	Transforming growth factor-α	TGF-α
	Vascular-endothelial cell growth factor	VEGF
	Hepatocyte growth factor	HGF
Chemo-attractant CK	C–X–C chemokines (11)	e.g. IL-8, NAP-2, GRO-α,β,γ
	C––C chemokines (25)	e.g. RANTES, eotaxin
	C chemokines (1)	Lymphotactin
	C-X$_3$-C chemokines(1)	Fractalkine
	Interleukin-16	IL-16
Function not yet possible to assign	Interleukin-14	IL-14
	Interleukin-19	IL-19
	Interleukin-20	IL-20

Some cytokines (CK) are listed in more than one group because of their multiple activities.

differentiation, attraction (chemotaxis) or the synthesis of inducible protein(s) depending upon the target cell and the particular cytokine.

6. Most cytokines act in a paracrine manner, exerting their effects on target cells within the same micro-environment as the producer cell. A few cytokines, notably IL-2, act in an autocrine manner, in which the producer cell and target cell are the same. Some, for example the pro-inflammatory cytokines, act in an endocrine manner, interacting with target cells in distant tissues after circulating systemically.

ACTION OF CYTOKINES IN VIVO

In vivo, a cell will rarely, if ever, encounter one cytokine in isolation at a time. The resultant biological action of a cytokine on a cell will reflect various synergistic and antagonistic interactions of other factors. The major factors that may influence cytokine action are: (i) the differentiation state and receptor expression by the target cell; (ii) other cytokines acting synergistically or antagonistically; (iii) nutrients available to fuel mitosis or differentiation; (iv) hormones acting on the cell at the same time; (v) neurotransmitters acting on the cell at the same time; (vi) the presence of pathogens or toxins; and (vii) the presence of inhibitors.

MODE OF ACTION OF CYTOKINES

In order to appreciate the manner by which cytokines exert their effects on cells, it is important to understand that they may show the following features.

Pleiotropy
This refers to the fact that many cytokines, in particular the pro-inflammatory cytokines, exert a number of different effects on a variety of different cell types as illustrated in Table 2. It is, therefore, impossible to assign a single biological effect to the protein.

Ambiguity
This refers to the fact that the same cytokine may have totally opposite effects on different cells, acting via the same receptor. For example, TGF-β stimulates the proliferation of osteoblasts and fibroblasts, but inhibits the division of T-cells and osteoclasts.

Redundancy
The apparent redundancy in the cytokine system is exemplified by the chemokines. Over 60 of these cytokines have been recognised and many share the same apparent biological activity. Redundancy may result in a more robust system and yet rarely in biology do we see this taken to such an extreme.

Synergy
Cytokines may act synergistically, a process by which the biological effect of two cytokines upon a target cell is greater than the sum of the effect generated by each cytokine acting independently. An example here is the combined effect of TNF-α and IFN-γ on the differentiation of mononuclear phagocytes.

Table 2 The major biological activities of IL-1, IL-6 and TNF-α. (ICAM-1, intracellular adhesion molecule 1; VCAM-1, vascular adhesion molecule 1)

	IL-1	IL-6	TNF-α
LEUKOCYTES			
Monocytes/macrophages	Induction of IL-1, IL-6, IL-8, TNF-α, PGE$_2$	Synergy with CSF-1 in differentiation	Activation, TNF-α, IL-1, IL-6, IL-8, GM-CSF, TGF-β, CSF-1, PGE$_2$ production Transmigration and chemotaxis
Lymphocytes	Induction of IL-2 and IL-2R in T-cells Clonal expansion of B-cells	Co-mitogenic for T-cells Regulation of IgG and IgA production Clonal expansion of B-cells	Induction apoptosis in mature T-cells T-cell activation
Neutrophils	Increased adherence	Synergy with G-CSF in differentiation	Increased adherence Release of granules Increased phagocytic activity Increased production superoxide
VASCULAR ENDOTHELIAL CELLS	Induction of IL-1, IL-8, G-CSF, CSF-1, ICAM-1, VCAM-1, P-and E-selectin Increased permeability		Induction of IL-1, G-CSF, GM-CSF, ICAM-1, VCAM-1, P-and E-selectin Increased permeability, rearrangement of cytoskeleton Increased expression of MHCI Modulation of angiogenesis
FIBROBLASTS	Proliferation		Induction of proliferation, IL-1, IL-6, IFN-β, LIF, metalloproteinases Inhibition of collagen synthesis, metalloproteinase inhibitor
OTHERS	Proliferation of epithelial cells Osteoclast activation Hepatocyte production of acute phase proteins	Proliferation of keratinocytes Osteoclast activation Hepatocyte production of acute phase proteins Growth factor for plasmacytoma and myeloma cells	Release of free fatty acids from adipocytes Stimulation of adrenocorticotrophin and prolactin Inhibition of thyroid stimulating hormone Osteoclast activation
IN VIVO			
Central nervous system	Fever, anorexia, somnolence, headache, nausea	Fever	Fever, anorexia
Cardiovascular system	Hypotension		Shock, acute respiratory distress syndrome Capillary leakage syndrome
Skin/gastrointestinal system	Inflammation	Local inflammation	Inflammation Ischaemia, colitis, hepatic necrosis
Metabolic	Increased circulating IL-6 Rise in C-reactive protein Increase in adreno corticotrophin- Decreased blood glucose	Increase in acute phase proteins Increase in adrenocorticotrophin, prolactin, growth hormone, luteinising hormone	Net protein and lipid catabolism Stress hormone release and insulin resistance

Antagonism

There are some cytokines that directly antagonise the effects of others. For example, IFN-γ inhibits the actions of IL-4 in the stimulation of IgE production by B-cells.

Transmodulation of cytokine receptors

The action of a cytokine on a target cell may be to induce the expression of receptors for another cytokine. Indeed, IL-1 was discovered because it activated T-cells. It is now known that IL-1 induces the expression of IL-2 receptors on T-cells which enables them to proliferate in response to IL-2.

CYTOKINE RECEPTORS

Biochemical studies of cytokine receptors, together with cloning of the genes which encode them, has led to the discovery that many cytokine receptors can be grouped into families with shared structural features. The largest group has been called the class 1 cytokine receptor family or haematopoietin family of receptors. Cytokines which act via class 1 receptors include: IL-2, IL-4, IL-5, IL-6, IL-7, IL-9, IL-12, IL-13, IL-15, G-CSF, GM-CSF, LIF, OSM and EPO (Table 1). Class II cytokine receptors are also known as the IFN family receptors and include receptors for IFN-α, IFN-β, IFN-γ and IL-10. The other families are the TNF-receptor family, the IL-1 receptor family, TGF-β receptors and chemokine receptors. The mechanism by which the cytokine signal is delivered from the receptor to the nucleus (signal transduction), is determined largely by the structural features of the cytokine receptors. However, a discussion of these pathways is beyond the scope of this overview.

CYTOKINE INHIBITORS

There are proteins that act as specific inhibitors of cytokines. The IL-1 receptor antagonist (IL-1ra) is classified as a cytokine in its own right as one of the IL-1 family. As indicated by the name, this cytokine competes with IL-1 for receptor binding and is discussed more fully below. Many serum proteins bind to cytokines in the blood and inhibit their activity, e.g. α_2-macroglobulin. Individuals may also produce anti-cytokine antibodies that neutralise cytokine actions. The group of inhibitors that has recently received a great deal of attention, however, are the soluble cytokine receptors. The generation of soluble cytokine receptors appears to be a mechanism for regulating cytokine activity in vitro, since their levels are often raised in certain disease states. They have been described for most of the major cytokines including TNF-α (sTNFR1 & II), IL-1 (sIL-1R1 & II), IL-2 (sIL-2R), IL-4 (sIL-4R), IL-6 (sIL-6R) and IFN-γ (sIFN-γR). The soluble cytokine receptors will bind to their specific cytokines in solution and prevent them from interacting with the cellular receptors and exerting their biological activities.

A FUNCTIONAL GROUPING

Knowledge of the structure of cytokines and their receptors has allowed the division of cytokines into families based on the homology of their protein sequence, or the structure of the cytokine receptor.[16]

These developments have been extremely useful for the cytokine biologist who is familiar with the activities and idiosyncratic nature of these molecules. However, the structure of cytokines and their receptors does not necessarily enable the reader to understand the cytokines in terms of their major functions.

As illustrated in Table 1, cytokines given the same family name often have functions that put them into a separate group. For example, IFN-γ is an immunological cytokine and shares no structural homology with the other interferons. IL-8 is a classical C–X–C chemokine and yet was originally designated an IL. In order to help the reader understand the major functions of the cytokines, what follows is a description of the major cytokines with an emphasis on their biological activities. It should be noted that most of our knowledge of cytokine activities is based on in vitro studies.

ANTI-VIRAL CYTOKINES

The anti-viral cytokines are the type 1 IFNs and include the many subtypes of IFN-α, IFN-β and IFN-ω. In the human there are 13 structural genes encoding for IFN-α, one for IFN-β and one for IFN-ω. The type 1 IFNs are all derived from the same ancestral gene and have structural homology with between 165–172 amino acids, enabling them to utilise the same receptor, although with varying affinities.[17] The type 1 IFNs can be produced by any cell type in the body. They are not normally produced without stimulation. Agents that stimulate IFN-α/β production by cells include double stranded RNA, viruses, facultative intracellular bacteria, lipopolysaccharide and other cytokines including IL-1, TNF-α and IL-2.[18]

The induced IFN-α/β binds to receptors on target cells and stimulates the production of a range of proteins that have a variety of anti-viral effects acting at different stages of the virus infectious cycle.[17] This essentially prevents the replication of the majority of viruses in the target cell. Some viruses have, however, evolved mechanisms for evading this anti-viral activity. In addition to their anti-viral activities, the type 1 IFNs exhibit other functions important in the defence of the host. These include: (i) inhibition of the replication of cells, including tumour cells; (ii) modulation of the expression of MHC class 1 molecules allowing enhanced presentation of endogenous antigens to cytotoxic T-cells; and (iii) up-regulation of macrophage, cytotoxic T-cell and natural killer cell activity.

PRO-INFLAMMATORY CYTOKINES

The pro-inflammatory cytokines, sometimes referred to as primary cytokines include two members of the IL-1 family (IL-1α and IL-1β), TNF-α and IL-6. These cytokines are multifunctional in that they have effects on numerous cell types in the body, playing an important role in the primary defence of the body against trauma and infection. The cytokines have many overlapping biological activities and are produced by numerous cell types. The most important source is the macrophage, the cell that is central to the initial non-specific response to infection or wounding. The major biological activities of the pro-inflammatory cytokines are compared in Table 2 from which it can be seen that many of the activities of these cytokines appear to overlap. The functions are mainly related

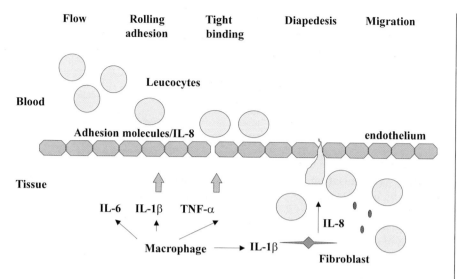

Figure 1 The role of pro-inflammatory cytokines in the attraction of leukocytes to sites of trauma/infection. The pro-inflammatory cytokines produced by macrophages in response to microbial products activate the endothelial cells in the local capillary vessels. The endothelial cells increase their expression of adhesion molecules (e.g. ICAM-1 and E-selectin) and synthesise chemokines such as IL-8. Leukocytes in the blood are activated by the chemokines, express the appropriate ligands for the adhesion molecules, begin to adhere to the endothelium and eventually migrate into the tissue where they are attracted by further chemokines produced by macrophages and fibroblasts (following activation by IL-1/IL-6) to the site where the microbial stimulus is located. The process acts to bring the cells to deal with the potential threat.

to the importance of these cytokines in the first-line defence of the body against threat, for example by invasion by a micro-organism. As shown in Figure 1, when a macrophage encounters a micro-organism it will produce all three pro-inflammatory cytokines. The effect that this has on the local tissue is to induce inflammation. The endothelial cells of the local microvasculature will increase their expression of the cellular adhesion molecules, ICAM-1, E-selectin and P-selectin allowing the adhesion and diapedesis of leukocytes from the blood into the tissue to deal with the threat. This is aided by the increased production of IL-8 and other chemokines. In addition, the pro-inflammatory cytokines have systemic effects that work to prepare the body for the worst case scenario, the spread of the microbe into the bloodstream (Fig. 2).

Essentially all of the effects mediated by these cytokines have some anti-microbial benefit. Microbes do not survive easily at elevated temperatures, the acute phase proteins such as C-reactive protein and the complement proteins are all anti-microbial. The metabolic activities of the cytokines provide fuel in the form of amino acids, fatty acids and glucose. This enables the specific immune system to mount an effective immune response against the stimulating microbe. The whole system provides the optimal chance of the organism being dealt with as efficiently as possible. Although the response appears to have evolved to deal with micro-organisms, it is a non-specific response and will be generated to some extent by any injurious agent. When

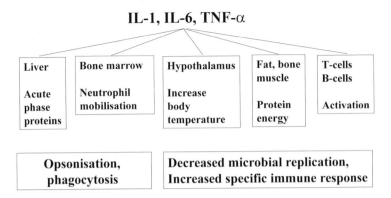

Figure 2 Pro-inflammatory cytokines in host defence. Although the pleiotropic activities of pro-inflammatory cytokines may directly result in disease symptoms such as elevated temperature, muscle loss, and weight loss, all these activities are in fact important in the host defence against infection.

the response is inappropriate or exaggerated, it may lead to pathology or even the mortality of the individual and, for this reason, the system is tightly regulated by antagonists and regulatory cytokines as explained below.

Interleukin-1

IL-1α and IL-1β have the same range of biological activity and have been shown to have effects on every cell type tested. There are in fact three members of the IL-1 family, the third being the IL-1 receptor antagonist. IL-1α and IL-1β are the agonists and IL-1ra the antagonist. This situation appears to be unique in cytokine biology and reflects the fact that IL-1 is a highly inflammatory cytokine and the activity of IL-1 has to be tightly controlled to prevent over-stimulation by IL-1 in disease. There is evidence that the three cytokines arose from the duplication of a common ancestral gene.[19]

Agents that stimulate the production of IL-1 in macrophages include most micro-organisms and their products; non-microbial substances can also induce synthesis of the IL-1 proteins.[19] IL-1 itself is also a potent inducer of IL-1. Prostaglandin E_2 is a major inhibitor of IL-1 synthesis. When IL-1α and IL-1β are synthesised by cells in response to appropriate stimulation, they are initially synthesised as 31 kDa precursor proteins without leader sequences. The cellular processing of IL-1α and IL-1β to mature biologically active secreted proteins of ~17 kDa requires specific cellular proteinases.[19] Pro-IL-1α is biologically active and when cells die they release pro-IL-1α which is then cleaved by extracellular proteinases to the 17 kDa form. Living cells can release IL-1α following membrane perturbation; the pro-IL-1α is then cleaved by membrane-bound proteinases into the 17 kDa form.[19] It is believed that IL-1α is mainly a cell-associated cytokine, since it is found in serum at very low levels during acute inflammatory disease. The tissue levels have been shown to correlate with inflammatory processes.[19] IL-1α is found at very high levels in the epidermis. It is synthesised constitutively by keratinocytes. Normally, the epidermal IL-1α is sequestered from the underlying dermis, but, if the epidermis is traumatised, high levels of IL-1α will be released into the dermis and activate the microvascular endothelial cells, initiating inflammation.[20] As such, epidermal IL-1α constitutes an important 'alarm' mechanism, informing components of the host defence mechanism that the skin barrier has been breached.

Pro-IL-1β, in contrast, is not biologically active. In order for IL-1β to be secreted in an active form, the pro-IL-1β must be cleaved by the IL-1β converting enzyme (ICE). ICE is a member of the caspase group of cysteine proteinases.[21]

There are two forms of the IL-1 receptor. These are termed IL-1RI and IL-1RII. The IL-1 receptor system also involves a further protein, the receptor accessory protein, IL-1R AcP.[22] These proteins share homology and are all members of the immunoglobulin supergene family of molecules. The binding of IL-1α/β to IL-RII does not produce a signal. A signal is transduced to the cell nucleus only when IL-α/β binds to IL-IRI in association with the IL-1R Acp. IL-1ra competes with IL-1α/β for binding to IL-1RII. The IL-1R1 is expressed by virtually every cell type in the body and is the primary signal transducing receptor. IL-1RII is also expressed by the same range of cell types and acts as a decoy receptor, binding IL-1α/β but failing to produce a signal. Both receptors are released as soluble cytokine receptors and can be found in normal human serum. Soluble IL-1R1 (sIL-1R1) is present normally at very low levels 10–20 pM) but levels can rise during inflammatory disease. sIL-1R1 binds IL-Ira with higher affinity than IL-1α and IL-1β. In contrast, sIL-1RII is normally present in serum at high concentrations (100–200 pM) and it has the highest affinity for IL-1β and lowest affinity for IL-1ra. Thus the soluble IL-1 receptors may also contribute to the overall availability of biologically active IL-1 in normal physiology and during inflammatory disease with IL-1R1 increasing and IL-1RII decreasing the availability of IL-1.[19]

Interleukin-6

IL-6 is produced by cells of the immune system and cells of non-lymphoid origin. IL-6 has a role to play in the regulation of immune responses, haematopoiesis and acute phase reactions. IL-6 is a glycoprotein of 21–28 kDa. The major cell types involved in IL-6 production are T-cells, macrophages and fibroblasts. T-cell production of IL-6 is regulated by antigenic stimulation in the context of other immunological cytokines. The production of IL-6 by macrophages and fibroblasts is stimulated by a variety of agents including lipopolysaccharide (LPS), numerous viruses and other cytokines such as IL-1, TNF-α IFN-β and PDGF.[23] The IL-6 receptor consists of two molecules, an IL-6 binding protein 80 kDa (α-chain) and a signal transducing molecule, gp130 (β-chain). IL-6Rα may also be released from cells in a soluble form and bind free IL-6. Although this may play a role in the regulation of IL-6 activity, it is thought that the IL-6/IL-6Rα may bind to gp130 on cells to mediate signal transduction.[24]

Tumour necrosis factor-α

TNF-α, often referred to as simply TNF and also known as cachectin, is a primary mediator of the inflammatory response and is also involved in the regulation of immunity. TNF-α can be synthesised by all types of white blood cell and a variety of mesenchymal and epithelial cells including fibroblasts, smooth muscle cells, osteoblasts, neuronal cells and keratinocytes. Many tumour cells also synthesise TNF-α. TNF-α synthesis can be induced by a whole range of stimuli including: (i) bacteria and their products; (ii) viruses (iii) parasites and their products; and (iv) chemical and physical stimuli. TNF-α synthesis is also regulated by other cytokines including IL-1, IL-2, IFN-γ, LIF, GM-CSF, CSF-I and TNF-α itself. Inhibitors of TNF-α production include prostaglandin E$_2$, TGF-β, INFα/β, IL-4, IL-6, IL-10 and G-CSF.[25]

There are two forms of TNF-α, a 26 kDa trans-membrane pro-form and a 17 kDa secreted form. The protein is initially displayed on the cell membrane surface and then cleaved to release the mature TNF-α protein. Both the mature extracellular form and the membrane bound form of TNF-α are biologically active. The transmembrane form can mediate cell cytotoxicity via cell-to-cell contact with cells expressing the TNF-α receptor. Bioactive secreted TNF-α exists as a trimer in serum. The multiple biological activities of TNF-α are mediated through two distinct but structurally related receptors. Called type 1 (p60–65) and type II (p75–80) TNF-α receptors. These receptors are present on all cell types except for mature red blood cells. TNFRI is the most abundantly expressed, but TNFRII is the most highly expressed on endothelial and haematopoietic cells. Soluble forms of both receptors are released from cells by proteolytic cleavage. They both bind and neutralise the effects of TNF-α. The soluble TNF-α receptors are present in normal human serum, but the levels increase dramatically in inflammatory disease processes.

Cleavage of macrophage TNF receptors is stimulated by IL-1 and LPS. This indicates that stimulation of TNF-α and the soluble receptor inhibitors will occur simultaneously to regulate the effects of this very potent pro-inflammatory cytokine.[26]

ANTI-INFLAMMATORY CYTOKINES

As indicated above, one of the major anti-inflammatory cytokines is a member of the IL-1 family, IL-1ra. IL-1ra is produced by cells in response to agents that stimulate IL-1 production and antagonises the effects of IL-1 by competing for the IL-1R signal transducing receptor.

A second important anti-inflammatory cytokine is IL-10. IL-10 was initially named, 'cytokine synthesis inhibitory factor',[27] and later 'macrophage deactivating factor' as its capacity to inhibit the activation of cells of the mononuclear phagocyte lineage was described.[27] Human IL-10 is an 18 kDa protein. IL-10 is produced by T-cells, B-cells, macrophages, epithelial cells and human placental cytotrophoblasts. Lymphocytes secrete IL-10 upon appropriate antigenic stimulation. Macrophages secrete IL-10 in response to LPS, α-melanocyte stimulating hormone, PGE$_2$, and macrophage production of IL-10 is inhibited by IL-4, IL-10 itself, IL-13, TGF-β and IFN-γ. Keratinocytes produce IL-10 in response to UV light, whereas other epithelial cells have been reported to produce IL-10 constitutively.[27] The IL-10 receptor is a member of the interferon receptor family of proteins and is found on cells of myeloid and lymphoid origin. The effects of IL-10 on macrophages are to modulate the expression of pro-inflammatory, haematopoietic, immunological cytokines and chemokines. IL-10 has also been shown to increase the expression of the IL-1ra by macrophages, demonstrating the potent anti-inflammatory activity of this cytokine. IL-10 also inhibits the activities of neutrophils and eosinophils. It is, therefore, believed to be an important cytokine in the regulation of inflammatory responses.[28]

IL-13 also has anti-inflammatory effects on macrophages, and inhibits IL-1 and TNF-α production whilst enhancing IL-1ra production by these cells, although the primary function of this cytokine is believed to be in the regulation of IgE production by B-cells. Another cytokine with anti-inflammatory activity is TGF-β. TGF-β is a fascinating cytokine since it can have completely opposite effects on cells depending on the cell lineage and differentiation-state of the target cells. TGF-β can decrease the expression of pro-inflammatory cytokines and enhance the expression of IL-1ra by macrophages, but this is highly dependent upon the differentiation state of the target macrophage and the presence/absence of other cytokines. TGF-β is produced by a variety of cell types in three forms known as TGF-β1, TGF-β2 and TGF-β3. When produced, it is not biologically active but secreted as a latent molecule in the form of a protein complex consisting of a TGF-β homodimer and two pro-segments. TGF-β is present in this latent form in the extracellular matrix. It can be released as the active form by proteases, and plasmin is currently believed to be the major enzyme involved in vivo. The full range of activities and the mechanisms of control and regulation of TGF-β are beyond the scope of this chapter and the reader is referred to an excellent overview of this cytokine.[29]

IMMUNOLOGICAL CYTOKINES

The cytokines that have a role to play in specific immunity include IL-2, IL-4, IL-5, IL-6, IL-10, IL-12, IL-13, IL-15, IL-18, and IFN-γ. It is not possible to discuss the molecular details of all of these cytokines, their receptors and regulation in this short chapter. Therefore, the role of these cytokines in the regulation and expression of the specific immune response will be covered in order that the reader gains an overview of our current knowledge of cytokine regulation of immunity.

The immune response

During the initiation of a specific immune response, the foreign material or antigen is taken up by a professional antigen presenting dendritic cells. These cells are specialised in their capacity to express high levels of MHC class I and class II molecules. They also express the necessary co-stimulatory molecules for the stimulation of naive T-cells. In order to initiate a specific immune response, antigen in the form of a processed peptide epitope must be presented in association with an MHC class II molecule to the corresponding specific CD4+ T-cell, or T-helper cell (Th-cell).

The Th-cell then becomes activated and expresses the IL-2 receptor and begins to synthesise and secrete IL-2. This process is enhanced by cytokines that activate Th-cells, such as IL-1, and IL-6 produced by the antigen presenting cell. What follows is unique in cell biology; the Th-cell derived IL-2 stimulates the Th-cell to clonally expand by interacting with the IL-2 receptor. The clonal expansion of the Th-cell will continue as long as there is sufficient antigenic stimulation to prevent the daughter cells differentiating into memory cells or terminally differentiated effector cells.

The activation of Th-cells is essential to provide help for the clonal expansion and differentiation of antigen specific B-cells and CD8+ cytotoxic T-cells. B-cells are concerned in the expression of humoral immunity in the form of specific antibodies, whereas CD8+ cytotoxic T-cells are concerned in killing cells expressing epitopes of antigens in association with MHC class I molecules in the cell-mediated immune response. Effector CD4+ Th-cells are also concerned in the expression of cell-mediated immunity by elaborating cytokines that regulate the response of other leukocytes such as macrophages.

Cytokines in the regulation of the quality of the immune response

It is now widely held that cytokines play an important role in regulating these responses.[30] Moreover, it is thought that cytokines made during the initial phase of the inflammatory response influence the functional differentiation of Th-cells into cells which will produce cytokines needed for the effective phagocytosis of antigen or become regulators of phagocyte independent immune reactions. Based largely on studies carried out in murine models, there is evidence for the existence of two subsets of Th-cell, namely the Th1-cell and the Th2-cell. Th1-cells secrete IL-2, LT-α (lymphotoxin) and IFN-γ. Th2-cells secrete IL-4, IL-5, IL-6 and IL-10. The two cell types secrete IL-3, IL-13 and GM-CSF.[30] T-cells with an intermediate cytokine profile have also been described (Th0-cells). Protective immunity is believed to result from the balanced activation of different types of Th-cell and over-stimulation of a given type of Th1- or Th2-cell may lead to immunopathology.

IL-12 and IL-18 are thought to play an important role in promoting the differentiation of naïve Th-cells into Th1-type cells. IL-12 is produced by dendritic cells and macrophages when the interact with Th-cells during antigen presentation. IL-12 was initially described by its potent capacity to synergise with IL-2 in the induction of IFN-γ producing Th-cells.[31] IL-18 is also a macrophage derived cytokine. IL-18 was initially named IFN-γ inducing factor because of its effects on inducing T-cells to secrete this cytokine. IL-12 and IL-18 act synergistically to promote the formation of IFN-γ secreting Th-cells.[32] It is, therefore, believed that if a naïve Th-cell (Th0) is presented with antigen appropriately, in the presence of IL-12 and IL-18, that the Th-cell will differentiate into a Th1-type T-cell concerned in cell mediated immune responses and the generation of opsonising antibodies.

On the other hand, IL-4 has been shown to be important in the generation of Th2-type T-cells. IL-4 is produced by a variety of cell types including basophils, mast cells and Th2-cells. Hence if a naïve T-cell is stimulated appropriately by antigen in the presence of IL-4, the differentiation of a Th2-type T-cell will ensue. The regulation of immunity is further complicated by cross-regulation of the cytokines generated by the Th1- and Th2-cells. IL-10 produced by Th2-cells inhibits IL-12 and IL-18 production by dendritic cells and macrophages. IL-10 and IL-4 inhibit the differentiation of Th1-cells and IFN-γ, a Th1-derived cytokine inhibits the generation of Th2-cells.[30] Thus the regulation of the expression of immunity is complex.

Cytokines and the expression of specific cell-mediated immunity

The major cytokines elaborated by effector Th1-cells are IL-2, IFN-γ and LT-α. The production of these cytokines is largely restricted to T-cells. IL-2 plays an important role in the expression of cell-mediated immunity by stimulating the proliferation of CD8+ cytotoxic T-cells and their subsequent expansion into cytotoxic effector cells capable of killing target cells expressing their specific epitope in association with MHC class I molecules. This is particularly important in the host defence against virus infected cells. IL-2 is also concerned in the proliferation and cytotoxicity of natural killer cells which are important in the non-specific recognition of virus infected and tumour cells. IL-2 also stimulates the production of a group of cells known as lymphokine activated killer (LAK) cells from a population of lymphoid cell precursors that have potent cytotoxic activity against fresh tumour cells.[33]

IFN-γ enhances the expression of MHC class II molecules on cells of the immune system including monocytes/macrophages, dendritic cell and B-cells. IFN-γ can also induce MHC class II expression on cells that do not normally express these proteins such as T-cells, epithelial cells, endothelial cells and many tumour cells. The advantages of this are the increased recognition of antigen expressing cells by CD4+ T-cells. However, the most important role of IFN-γ in the cell mediated response is its capacity to activate macrophages. Normal inflammatory macrophages do not have the capacity to kill some facultative intracellular bacteria and parasites. Activation by IFN-γ induces a microbicidal differentiation of macrophages, enhancing their ability to kill the intracellular organisms. This is the only mechanism of host defence against bacteria and parasites that adopt this virulence strategy. IFN-γ is also able to prime to prime macrophages for tumouricidal activity, although this activity is not unique to the cytokine. IFN-γ has also been shown to synergise with IL-2 in the activation of tumour cell killing by natural killer cells.[34]

LT-α (also known as TNF-β) and LT-β are members of the TNF family of cytokines and share many biological activities. LT-α binds to the TNFRI and TNFRII receptors on cells and stimulates apoptosis, proliferation or differentiation depending on the cell type and differentiation state. Like TNF-α, it is a tumouricidal cytokine. LT-β binds to a different receptor, named the LT-β receptor. Following binding to the receptor, apoptotic cell death is initiated in various cell types.[35]

IL-17 is a cytokine inducing agent and stimulates the production of IL-6, IL-8 and GM-CSF by fibroblasts. It may play a role in augmenting inflammation during the TH1-cell response. However, as one of the newly discovered cytokines, it may yet be found to have other activities.[36] Other cytokines that may be involved in specific cell mediated immune reactions include IL-15, a cytokine produced by macrophages, dendritic, epidermal and stromal cells. IL-15 has many features in common with IL-2 and binds to the IL-2 receptor on T-cells. It is a potent activator of the proliferation and cytokine production by T-cells. However, its physiological role is not yet fully understood.[37]

Cytokines and the expression of specific humoral immunity
The expression of humoral immunity (i.e. production of antibodies) is dependent upon the interaction between antigen specific sensitised CD4+ T-cells and a B-cell that recognise epitopes of the same antigen. The B-cell presents an epitopes of the antigen in association with MHC class II to the sensitised T-cells in a manner analogous to the interaction of CD4+ T-cells with macrophages. The T-cell then delivers the appropriate cytokines to enable the

B-cell to expand clonally and differentiate into memory cells and plasma cells. Plasma cells then synthesise and secrete the soluble antibody molecules specific to the antigen epitope recognised by the B-cell. The plasma cells will synthesise one of five major classes of antibody; IgD, IgM, IgG (IgG$_{1-4}$), IgA, IgE as soluble proteins to combat the antigen. IgM is always produced upon initial encounter with an antigen. There are many cytokines that have been implicated in the clonal expansion and differentiation of B-cells, including IL-2,[38] IL-4,[39] IL-5,[40] IL-6,[41] and IL-13.[42] It is believed that the class switching of B-cells as they develop into memory cells is dependent upon the cytokine signals received from the CD4+ T-cell.[38] IgG$_1$ and IgG$_3$ are concerned with the opsonisation of pathogens and activation of the complement system. IgG$_2$ and IgG$_4$ do not possess these properties. All the IgG subclasses are effective in neutralisation of toxins and viral infectivity. IgA is involved in mucosal immunity and IgE is responsible for activating mast cells and important in the immune defence against parasitic worms, but is also the cause of type 1 immediate-type hypersensitivity reactions. It is believed that a B-cell that receives Th1-cytokines, IL-2 and IFN-γ will switch the antibody class to IgG. IL-4 promotes class switching to IgE and IgG$_4$[39] as does IL-13.[42] IL-5 is an eosinophil growth and differentiation factor; therefore, it plays a role in the protective immune response against parasitic worms together with IL-4 and IL-13.[43] Both IL-6 and IL-5 have been reported to augment the production of IgA,[40,41] but these cytokines will not induce class switching to IgA. The factors that control B-cell class switching in vivo may include not only the correct 'soup' of cytokines but also the micro-environment of the particular lymphoid tissue, for example spleen or mucosal-associated tissues.

CYTOTOXIC CYTOKINES

The cytotoxic cytokines include the members of the TNF-α family as shown in Table 1. These cytokines are produced by CD4+ Th1-cells or cytotoxic CD8+ T-cells and interact with receptors on target cells that mediate death by apoptosis as discussed above for LT-α.

HAEMATOPOIETIC CYTOKINES

There are a limited number of cytokines designated as colony stimulating factors (CSF-1, GM-CSF and G-CSF) and these, together with other haematopoietic factors (SCF, EPO, LIF, IL-1, IL-3, IL-7 and IL-11) are concerned with the growth and differentiation of cells in the bone marrow. Stem-cell factor is a growth factor for primitive lymphoid and myeloid haematopoietic stem cells and is produced by bone marrow stromal cells and fibroblasts.[44] Erythropoietin (EPO) is the erythroid growth factor concerned in the differentiation of erythroid precursor cells into mature red blood cells. EPO is produced by cells in the kidney and liver in response to hypoxia or anaemia and works back to the bone marrow to stimulate the production of more oxygen carrying cells, the red blood cells.[45] IL-3 is a haematopoietic growth factor that promotes colony formation of erythroid, megakaryocyte, neutrophil, eosinophil, basophil, mast cell and monocyte lineages. Most of the activities of IL-3 are enhanced by other cytokines and indeed its production is largely dependent upon stimulation of mesenchymal and epithelial cells by IL-1α/β.[46]

LIF allows stem cells to remain in an undifferentiated state and can maintain their proliferation in culture. LIF can have profound effects on haematopoiesis, particularly in combination with other cytokines such as IL-3. It is produced by mononuclear phagocytes and fibroblasts.[47] IL-7 is a stromal cell derived growth factor for cells of the lymphoid lineage and promotes the proliferation of pre-T and pre-B-cells. In addition to acting in the bone marrow, IL-7 is important in the development of T-cells in the thymus.[48]

CSF-1 is also known as M-CSF or macrophage colony stimulating factor. This cytokine is produced by mononuclear phagocytes, neutrophils, endothelial cells and fibroblasts. The major actions of M-CSF are to stimulate the growth of monocyte precursors into monocytes and the differentiation of monocytes into macrophages.[49] In an analogous manner, G-CSF, or granulocyte colony stimulating factor, is produced by the same range of cell types, but promotes the maturation of granulocyte stem cells and activates mature polymorphonuclear leukocytes.[50] G-CSF synergises with IL-3 to stimulate the growth of haematopoietic progenitors. Granulocyte/macrophage colony stimulating factor is a survival and growth factor for haematopoietic progenitor cells. It also acts as an activating and differentiation factor for mature mononuclear phagocytes and granulocytes.[51]

CHEMO-ATTRACTANT CYTOKINES

The chemokines constitute a super-family of small cytokines that play a critical role in inflammatory and immune responses. The first chemokine to be identified was IL-8 and since then more than 60 different human chemokines have been described.[52] They are classified into subfamilies according to having only one cysteine residue C, or the position of the first two cysteine residues which are separated by one amino acid (C–X–C), three amino acids (C–X$_3$–C) or are adjacent (C–C).[53] Most of the chemokines cause attraction of leukocytes, but these cytokines also affect angiogenesis, collagen production and the proliferation of haematopoietic precursors.

The C–X–C chemokines include: IL-8, PF-4 (platelet factor 4), NAP-2 (neutrophil activating peptide-2), GRO-α/β/γ, ENA-78 (epithelial cell derived neutrophil attractant-78), GCP-2 (granulocyte chemotactic protein-2), IP-10, (IFN-γ inducible protein-10), Mig (monokine induced by IFN-γ) and SDF-1α/β (stromal cell-derived factor-1α/β).[54] With the exception of IP-10 and Mig, they are mainly active on neutrophils and many are active on lymphocytes. The C–C chemokines exert their action on several leukocytes, but they are generally inactive on neutrophils. The chemokines with the most restricted actions are the eotaxins that only attract eosinophils and basophils. Fractaline is the only chemokine described to have the C–X$_3$–C motif, and it is active on T-cells, NK-cells and monocytes. Similarly, there is only one chemokine with the C motif, lymphotactin, which attracts T-cells and NK-cells.[55]

IL-8 can be produced by virtually every cell type tested. It is produced in response to stimulation by IL-1, IL-2, IL-3, IL-7, IL-13, TNF-α, IFN-γ and GM-CSF. It is also produced in response to microbial products including LPS and FMLP (formyl-methionine-leucine-phenylalanine). The production of the other chemokines is more restricted, although IL-1, TNF-α and LPS are good inducers of numerous chemokines by many cell types.

Chemokines interact with G-protein coupled receptors. Fewer chemokine receptors than chemokines appear to exist. There are 8 C–C chemokine receptors (called CCR1–8), five C–X–C chemokine receptors (CXCR1–5) and one C–X–C receptor (CXCR1) that have been identified. The ability of a cell to express chemokine receptors is a crucial determinant of their spectrum of actions. The chemokines are able to interact with more than one of their respective subgroup of receptors and have thus been described as promiscuous.[55] In addition, the chemokine system appears to have a great deal of redundancy, with a single cell type, for example the macrophage, producing multiple chemokines with overlapping activities in response to stimulation. In addition, macrophages express several chemokine receptors that are recognised in a promiscuous way. It has been proposed that the reason there are so many chemokines with overlapping activities is to provide a robust system such that inactivation of any single component (chemokine or receptor) allows the minimal level of leukocyte trafficking to maintain fundamental functions.[55]

A chemo-attractant cytokine that does not share structural features with the other members of this family is IL-16 which has a specific role in attracting CD4+ T-cells.

GROWTH FACTORS

The growth factors now encompass a large number of cytokines including families such as the TGF-β family that has 30 members including the bone morphogenetic proteins. These cytokines have been classed as growth factors because their primary action appears to be to stimulate the proliferation of a cell or group of cell-types. However, it should be noted that the actions of some of the growth factors are ambiguous, for example TGF-β_{1-3} will inhibit the proliferation of lymphocytes. In addition, many of the other cytokines discussed above have growth promoting activity. IL-2 is a growth factor for lymphocytes and has been classed as an immunological cytokine. Perhaps a better working definition of a growth factor is a cytokine that promotes the proliferation of cells that are not of haematopoietic origin.

The major growth factors are listed in Table 1 and they are largely named according to their origin or activity. TGF-β and the bone morphogenetic proteins act as growth factors for mesenchymal cells, such as fibroblasts and osteoblasts.[29] The fibroblast growth factors (FGFs of which there are 9) are produced by fibroblasts and stimulate angiogenesis by their action on endothelial cells.[56] The three platelet derived growth factors (PDGF) are found in platelets and, when released, have many activities including acting as growth factors for connective tissue cells.[57] Transforming growth factor-α (TGF-α) is made as an integral membrane protein by mononuclear phagocytes, keratinocytes of the skin and many mesenchymal and tumour cells. The mature cytokine is released from these cells by proteolytic cleavage and acts as an auto-inductive growth factor. TGF-α is closely related to EGF (epidermal growth factor) and shares the same receptor.[58] Vascular cell growth factor is produced by mononuclear phagocytes, smooth muscle cells and keratinocytes. It acts as a growth factor for vascular endothelial cells, enhances vascular permeability and is a pro-coagulant.[59] The

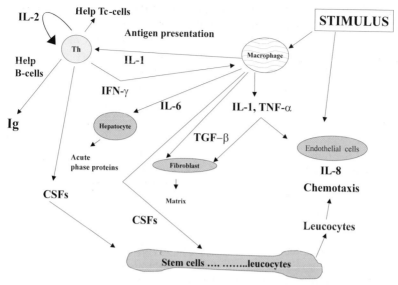

Figure 3 How the cytokine network operates in the immune defence of the body to an exogenous stimulus. Pro-inflammatory cytokines set the cascade into motion. Immunological cytokines regulate the specific response, ensuring (in most instances) that the appropriate response is mounted. Haematopoietic cytokines provide the leukocytes needed for defence against the exogenous agent. Chemokines attract the cells to the tissue site and, when the agent has been eliminated, growth factors stimulate tissue repair and regeneration.

insulin-like growth factors (IGFs) were originally isolated from serum and had insulin-like activities that could not be neutralised by anti-insulin antibodies. The IGFs are produced by a variety of mesenchymal cell types and are mitogenic for mesenchymal cells.[60] Nerve growth factor is produced in the brain and nervous system and enhances the survival, growth and neurotransmitter biosynthesis of sympathetic and sensory neurons.[61] The cytokine known as oncastatin-M or OSM was so named because of its biological activity in inhibiting the growth of melanoma cell lines. This cytokine is produced by activated T-cells and macrophages and is a growth factor for fibroblasts and smooth muscle cells. It has many activities in common with LIF and IL-6.[62]

CASCADES/NETWORKS

It is generally believed that, in vivo, cytokines act in cascades or, as more commonly described, networks. This means that the induction of a primary cytokine such as IL-1 by macrophages in response to an exogenous stimulus, will lead to the IL-1 inducing further cytokines to be produced by target cells, such as IL-6 and IL-8 by fibroblasts and so on. Cytokine networks are believed to act in vivo in the bone marrow (control of haematopoiesis) during embryogenesis (control of development) in the control of the wound healing response, inflammation and the regulation of specific immunity.

Perhaps the most pertinent example of this is to consider how cytokines from all of the functional groups may be involved in the host response to infection, as summarised in Figure 3. The initial pro-inflammatory cytokine response activates the endothelial cells to allow recruitment of leukocytes to the tissue site. Their migration is guided by chemokines. Colony stimulating factors released by macrophages during the inflammatory response act to increase the production of leukocytes from the bone marrow. The pro-inflammatory cytokines prepare the bloodstream for invasion by the organism by providing acute phase proteins and a supply of amino acid building blocks and fatty acids from protein and lipid stores to fuel the host response. The elevated temperature is anti-microbial. The macrophages also form a link between the non-specific and specific immune response. The appropriate Th-cell response is initiated and the immunological cytokines regulate the generation of the appropriate type of response. Cytokines produced by the Th-cell activate the appropriate cells, and the organism is eliminated. Growth factors and chemokines produced by the macrophages then regulate the wound healing response to restore homeostasis. Anti-inflammatory cytokines work to modulate the response to prevent excessive immunopathology.

Although this is a gross over-simplification, it serves to illustrate how the cytokine network system may function in vivo. This example also demonstrates the potential pitfalls of attempting to understand cytokines in isolation.

Key points for clinical practice

- Cytokines are simple proteins or glycoproteins that act as chemical messengers between cells.

- Cytokines are concerned in inflammation, immunity, development, wound healing and haematopoiesis.

- Cytokines work in networks.

- A cell will rarely receive a single cytokine message in isolation in vivo.

- In order for a cell to respond to a cytokine, it must be expressing the specific cytokine receptor.

- Most cytokines act in a paracrine manner, affecting only target cells within their micro-environment. They have very short half-lives.

- The major pro-inflammatory cytokines that have systemic actions are IL-1, TNF-α and IL-6.

- The major anti-inflammatory cytokines are IL1ra and IL-10.

- Soluble cytokine receptors are often increased in serum in disease processes and will bind and inhibit their specific cytokine ligand.

- Cytokines regulate the quality of specific immune responses to antigens.

REFERENCES

1. Issacs A, Lindemann J. Virus interference. 1. The Interferon. Proc R Soc Lond 1957; 147: 258–267.

2. Wheelock EF. Interferon-like virus-inhibitor induced in human leukocytes by phytohaemagglutinin. Science 1965; 149: 310–311.

3. Bloom BR, Bennett B. Mechanism of a reaction in vitro associated with delayed-type hypersensitivity Science 1966; 153: 80–82.

4. David JR. Delayed hypersensitivity in vitro: its mediation by cell-free substances formed by lymphoid cell-antigen interaction. Proc Natl Acad Sci USA 1966; 52: 72–77.

5. Ruddle NH, Waksman BH. Cytotoxicity mediated by soluble antigen and lymphocytes in delayed hypersensitivity. 3. Analysis of mechanism. J Exp Med 1968; 128: 1267–1279.

6. Williams TW, Granger GA. Lymphocyte in vitro cytotoxicity: lymphotoxins of several mammalian species. Nature 1968; 219: 1076–1077.

7. Dumonde DC, Wolstencroft RA, Panayi GS et al. Lymphokines: non-antibody mediators of cellular immunity generated by lymphocyte activation. Nature 1969; 224: 38–42.

8. Gery I, Gershon RK, Waksman BH. Potentiation of cultured mouse thymocyte responses by factors released by peripheral leucocytes. J Immunol 1971; 107: 1778–1780.

9. Morgan DA, Ruscetti FW, Gallo R. Selective in vitro growth of T lymphocytes from normal human bone marrows. Science 1976; 193: 1007–1008.

10. Carswell EA, Old LJ, Kassel RL et al. An endotoxin-induced serum factor that causes necrosis of tumors. Proc Natl Acad Sci USA 1975; 72: 3666–3670.

11. Aarden LA, Brunner TK, Cerottini JC et al. Revised nomenclature for antigen-non-specific T cell proliferation and helper factors. J Immunol 1979; 123: 2928–2929.

12. Burgess T, Hiddemann W, Wormann B et al. Purification and properties of colony stimulating factor from mouse lung conditioned medium. J Biol Chem 1977; 252: 1998–2003.

13. De Larco JE, Todara GJ. Growth factors from murine sarcoma virus-transformed cells. Proc Natl Acad Sci USA 1978; 75: 4001–4005.

14. Cohen S, Bigazzi PE, Yoshida T. Commentary. Similarities of T cell function in cell mediated immunity and antibody production. Cell Immunol 1974; 12: 150–159.

15. Paul WE, Kishimoto T, Melchers F et al. Sub-committee of the nomenclature committee of the International Union of Immunological Societies. Clin Exp Immunol 1992; 88: 367.

16. Vilcek J. The cytokines: an overview. In: Thompson A. (ed) The Cytokine Handbook, 3rd edn. London: Academic Press, 1998; 1–20.

17. De Maeyer E, De Maeyer-Guignard J. Interferons. In: Thompson A. (ed) The Cytokine Handbook, 3rd edn. London: Academic Press, 1998; 491–516.

18. Reis LFL, Lee TH, Vilcek J. Tumour necrosis factor acts synergistically with autocrine interferon-β and increases interferon-β mRNA levels in human fibroblasts. J Biol Chem 1989; 264: 16351–16354.

19. Dinarello CA. Interleukin-1. In: Thompson A. (ed) The Cytokine Handbook, 3rd edn. London: Academic Press, 1998; 35–72.

20. Barker JNWN, Mitra RS, Griffiths CEM et al. Keratinocytes as mediators of inflammation. Lancet 1991; 337: 211–217.

21. Wilson KP, Black JA, Thomson JA et al. Structure and mechanism of interleukin-1β converting enzyme. Nature 1994; 370: 270–275.

22. Greenfeder SA, Nunes P, Kwee L et al. Molecular cloning and characterisation of a second subunit of the interleukin-1 receptor complex. J Biol Chem 1995; 270: 13757–13765.

23. Hirano T. The biology of interleukin-6. Chem Immunol 1992; 51: 153–180.

24. Hibi M, Nakajima K, Hirano T. IL-6 cytokine family and signal transduction: a model of the cytokine system. J Mol Med 1996; 74: 1–12.

25. Zhang M, Tracey KJ. Tumor necrosis factor. In: Thompson A. (ed) The Cytokine Handbook, 3rd edn. London: Academic Press, 1998; 35–72.

26. Aderka D. The potential biological and clinical significance of the soluble tumour necrosis factor receptors. Cytokine Growth Factor Rev 1996; 7: 231–240.

27. Ho AS, Moore KW. Interleukin-10 and its receptor. Ther Immunol 1994; 1: 173–185.

28. De Waal Malefyt R, Moore KW. Interleukin-10. In: Thompson A. (ed) The Cytokine

Handbook, 3rd edn. London: Academic Press, 1998; 333–364.

29. Massague J, Attisano L, Wrana JL. The TGF-β family and its composite receptors. Trends Cell Biol 1994; 4: 172–178.

30. Romagnani S. The Th1/Th2 paradigm. Immunol Today 1997; 18: 263–266.

31. Gately MK, Wilson DE, Wong HL. Synergy between interleukin-2 (rIL-2) and IL-2 depleted lymphokine-containing supernatants in facilitating allogeneic human cytolytic T lymphocyte responses in vitro. J Immunol 1986; 136: 1274–1282.

32. Kohno K, Kataoka J, Ohtsuki T et al. IFN-inducing factor (IGIF) is a co-stimulatory factor on the activation of Th1 but not Th2-cells and exerts its effect independently of IL-12. J Immunol 1997; 158: 1541–1550.

33. Yannelli JR, Nakata M, Azuma A et al. Growth of tumor-infiltrating lymphocytes from human solid cancers: a summary of a 5-year experience. Int J Cancer 1996; 65: 413–421.

34. Thomas SM, Garrity LF, Brandt CR et al. IFN-γ-mediated antimicrobial response. J Immunol 1993; 150: 5529–5534.

35. Ware CF, Santee S, Glass A. Tumor necrosis factor-related ligands and receptors. In: Thompson A. (ed) The Cytokine Handbook, 3rd edn. London: Academic Press, 1998; 549–592.

36. Yao Z, Painter SL, Fanslow WC et al. Human IL-17: a novel cytokine derived from T cells. J Immunol 1995; 155: 5483–5486.

37. McInnes IB, Liew FY. Interleukin-15: a pro-inflammatory role in rheumatoid arthritis synovitis. Immunol Today 1998; 2: 75–79.

38. Nakanishi K, Hirose S, Yoshimoto T et al. Role and regulation of interleukin-2 receptor α and β chains in IL-2 driven growth. Proc Natl Acad Sci USA 1992; 89: 3551–3555.

39. O'Garra A, Spits H. The immunobiology of interleukin-4. Res Immunol 1993; 144: 567–643.

40. Purkerson JM, Isakson PC. Interleukin-5 (IL-5) provides a signal that is required in addition to IL-4 for isotype. J Exp Med 1992; 175: 973–982.

41. Muraguchi A, Hirano T, Tang B et al. The essential role of B cell stimulatory factor 2 (BSF-2/IL-6) for the terminal differentiation of B-cells. J Exp Med 1988; 67: 332–344.

42. Defrance T, Carayon P, Billian G et al. Interleukin 13 is a B cell stimulating factor. J Exp Med 1994; 179: 135–143.

43. Lopez AF, Sanderson CJ, Gamble JR et al. Recombinant human interleukin 5 is a selective activator of human eosinophil function. J Exp Med 1988; 167: 219–224.

44. Molneux G, McNiece IK. Stem cell factor. In: Thompson A. (ed) The Cytokine Handbook 3rd edn. London: Academic Press, 1998; 713–725.

45. Tabbara IA. Erythropoietin. Biology and clinical applications. Arch Intern Med 1993; 153: 298–304.

46. Frendl G, Interleukin 3: from colony–stimulating factor to pluripotent immunoregulatory cytokine. Int J Immunopharmacol 1992; 14: 421–430.

47. Gearing DP. Leukemia inhibitory factor: does the cap fit? Ann N Y Acad Sci 1991; 628: 9–18.

48. Callard R, Gearing A. IL-7. In: The Cytokine Facts Book. London: Academic Press, 1994; 70–74.

49. Hamilton JA. The biochemistry of colony stimulating factor-1 action. In: Thompson A. (ed) The Cytokine Handbook, 3rd edn. London: Academic Press, 1998; 689–712.

50. Demetri GD, Griffin JD. Granulocyte colony stimulating factor and its receptor. Blood 1991; 78: 2791–2808.

51. Aman MJ, Stockdreher K, Thews A et al. Regulation of immunomodulatory functions by granulocyte-macrophage colony stimulating factor and granulocyte stimulating factor in vivo. Ann Haematol 1996; 73: 231–238.

52. Baggiolini M, Dewald B. Moser B. Human chemokines: an update. Annu Rev Immunol 1997; 15: 675–705.

53. Bacon KB, Greaves DR, Dairaghi DJ, Schall TJ. C, CX_3C and CC chemokines. In: Thompson A. (ed) The Cytokine Handbook, 3rd edn. London: Academic Press, 1998; 753–775.

54. Wuyts A, Proost P, Van Damme J. Interleukin-8 and other CXC chemokines. In: Thompson A. (ed) The Cytokine Handbook, 3rd edn. London: Academic Press, 1998; 271–311.

55. Mantovani A. The chemokine system: redundancy for robust outputs. Immunol Today 1999; 20: 254–257.

56. Burgess WH, Maciag T. The heparin-binding (fibroblast) growth factor family of proteins. Annu Rev Biochem 1989; 58: 575–606.

57. Callard R, Gearing A. PDGF. In: The Cytokine Facts Book. London: Academic Press, 1994; 214–222.

58. Derynck R. The physiology of transforming growth factor-α. Adv Cancer Res 1992; 58: 27–52.

59. Connolly DT. Vascular permeability factor: a unique regulator of blood vessel function. J Cell Biochem 1991; 47: 219–223.

60. Cohick WS, Clemmons DR. The insulin-like growth factors. Annu Rev Physiol 1993; 55: 131–153.

61. Callard R, Gearing A. NGF. In: The Cytokine Facts Book. London: Academic Press, 1994; 191–198.

62. Callard R, Gearing A. OSM. In: The Cytokine Facts Book. London: Academic Press, 1994; 207–209.

W. Paul Farquhar-Smith Andrew S.C. Rice

CHAPTER 3

Peripheral mechanisms of inflammatory pain: towards the discovery of novel analgesics

THE PAIN PATHWAY

THE PLASTICITY OF PAIN PROCESSING

Physiological mechanisms which detect injurious threats and initiate a behavioural avoidance response are found throughout the animal kingdom. The classical description of this system includes structures which detect nociceptive energy, transduce them into electrophysiological signals which are transmitted to perceptive apparatus. These signals can be modulated. It is apparent that the pain pathway is not hard wired, but is plastic and undergoes profound functional changes under conditions of persistent stimulation, such as tissue damage inflammation (for example postoperative pain) or nerve injury. Inflammatory mediators elicit changes in sensitivity of nociceptive pathways which profoundly influence the processing of nociceptive traffic. Adjustments in nociceptive sensitivity are thought to be responsible for changes in the extent, intensity and quality of pain perception, and provide a mechanism for pain perception.

PRIMARY AND SECONDARY HYPERALGESIA: THE IMPORTANCE OF PERIPHERAL MECHANISMS

Inflammation is associated with a shift in the stimulus-response function of primary afferent neurons (Fig. 1), and expansion of nociceptor receptive fields (Fig. 2) within the zone of tissue inflammation.[1] Enhanced excitability of existing nociceptors is only one element of this primary hyperalgesia.

Dr W.P. Farquhar-Smith MA MBBChir FRCA, Royal College of Anaesthetists' Jubilee Research Fellow, Imperial College School of Medicine, Pain Research Group, Department of Anaesthetics, St Mary's Hospital, Praed Street, Paddington, London W2 1NY, UK
Dr A.S.C. Rice MB BS MD FRCA, Senior Lecturer in Pain Research, Imperial College School of Medicine, Pain Research Group, Department of Anaesthetics, St Mary's Hospital, Praed Street, Paddington, London W2 1NY, UK (for correspondence)

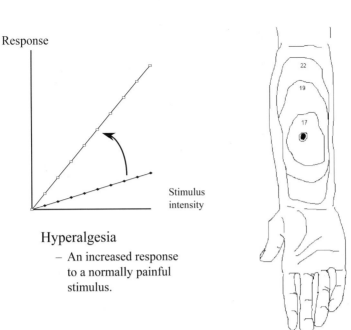

Response

Stimulus
intensity

Hyperalgesia
– An increased response
to a normally painful
stimulus.

Figure 1 Theoretical portrayal of changes in stimulus intensity–biological response relationship representative of hyperalgesia.

Figure 2 The development of a spreading secondary hyperalgesia in the minutes (labels) following a cutaneous injury with dry ice (hatched central area). Reproduced with permission from Fields H. Pain: Mechanisms and Management. New York. McGraw-Hill Publishers.

Recruitment of previously unresponsive primary sensory neurons (silent nociceptors) that become responsive to both noxious and non-noxious stimuli, is another.[2] The overall effect of these changes is to increase the total nociceptive afferent barrage to the spinal cord. This barrage provokes a state of enhanced excitability in spinal nociceptive neurons (secondary hyperalgesia). Furthermore, there is evidence to suggest that, under certain circumstances, this state of hyperexcitability may become self-sustaining, so that pain continues to be perceived in the absence of on-going tissue injury; a cardinal feature of many chronic pains.[3] In addition, spinal neuronal receptive fields expand and stimulation thresholds fall. The excitatory amino acid glutamate plays a central role both via the AMPA ion-channel linked receptor in acute pain transmission, and via the N-methyl-D-aspartate (NMDA) receptor to mediate the sensitising effects.[3,4] NMDA is activated by the removal of Mg^{2+} blocking the channel, and is facilitated by AMPA activation. Substance P acts synergistically with AMPA via neurokinin (NK_1) receptors, but clinical trials of NK_1 antagonists for analgesia have been largely disappointing.

Both peripheral and spinal mechanisms contribute to the plasticity of pain processing. Peripheral mechanisms occur 'upstream' in pain processing, and suggest not only an inherently more efficient and powerful site of analgesic action, but also offer the possibility of separating beneficial peripheral effects from central side effects. Therefore, although central nociceptive processing is of paramount importance, it has been discussed elsewhere,[3,4] and this review will be limited to new mechanisms of peripheral analgesia for both somatic and visceral inflammatory pain.

In the development of novel peripherally acting analgesics it is important to identify the key players. Some of the most important chemical mediators that participate directly or indirectly in inflammatory pain processes, include neurotrophins, kinins, cytokines and prostanoids.[5] Cyclo-oxygenase-1(COX-1) and COX-2 inhibition by non-steroidal anti-inflammatory drugs (NSAIDs) reduces algogenic prostanoids PGE_2 and PGI_2, and, although important for currently available analgesics, this will not be discussed further. In addition, endogenous modulatory systems exist to counteract these pro-inflammatory changes, and intensification of these processes presents a further avenue for therapeutic intervention.

NOCICEPTIVE SPECIALISATION

As well as exhibiting the concept of plasticity, it is becoming abundantly clear that anatomical and biochemical specialisation is manifest at all levels of nociceptive processing. The complexity of this system is reflected by the presence of a plethora of chemical mediators peripherally and spinally, comparable in number and intricacy to neurotransmitters in the brain. This is exemplified by the division of nociceptive cells into classes based on specific trophic factor dependence and biochemical properties. Particular nociceptors may express different receptors or chemical mediators and project to separate pain processing areas of the spinal cord dorsal horn. Specialisation for pain also means a potential for specialisation for analgesia.

PERIPHERAL NOCICEPTION: PATHWAYS AND IMMEDIATE PROCESSING

Somatic nociceptors

Specialised detectors, nociceptors, respond to noxious stimuli of many modalities, including thermal, chemical and mechanical. Somatic nociceptors have been classified according to anatomical features and physiological characteristics. Nociceptors comprise free nerve endings and fall into two groups: (i) unmyelinated C polymodal nociceptors (CPMN) are activated by many tissue-damaging modalities, are associated with prolonged 'burning' pain, and are slowly conducting (0.5–2 m/s); and (ii) thinly myelinated Aδ mechano-heat receptors, which are thought to mediate a briefer 'sharp' pain – these larger fibres are more rapidly conducting (5–20 m/s).

However, nociceptors can also be classified by the patterns of their central terminations, trophic factor sensitivity and biochemical properties which have more relevance to investigation of novel analgesics than the traditional classification above. During development, 70–80% of dorsal root ganglion (DRG) cells express the high affinity nerve growth factor (NGF) receptor, trkA (a tyrosine kinase), and are dependent upon the neurotrophin NGF for survival. These neurons include most unmyelinated, small diameter neurons that project to laminae I and II of the superficial dorsal horn of the spinal cord. In the post-natal period, half of these cells lose trkA, develop a distinct histochemistry and become sensitive to glial cell line-derived neurotrophic factor (GDNF).[6] Thus, in the adult, 40–45% of DRG neurons express trkA and

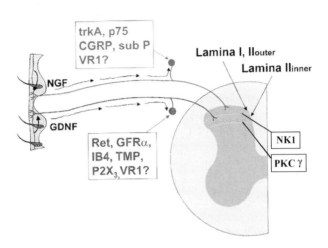

Figure 3 Peripheral and central target fields, trophic factor dependence, and biochemical properties of the two major classes of cutaneous receptors. Adapted from Snider and McMahon.[7]

also co-express the neuropeptides substance P and calcitonin gene-related peptide (CGRP).[6] These nociceptors project to lamina I and IIouter (IIo; Fig. 3). The GDNF-dependent neurons express another receptor, tyrosine kinase (Ret), bind the lectin IB4, and project centrally to lamina IIinner (IIi; Fig. 3). There is evidence to suggest the peptidergic, NGF-dependent projections are important in inflammatory pain, whilst the non-peptidergic, GDNF dependent projections of the latter may be important in neuropathic pain states.[7]

Some receptors, such as the vanilloid VR1 receptor which is the site of action of capsaicin, are expressed on both classes of nociceptor and occupy a position of great nociceptive potential. Thus, the signalling of specific noxious stimuli is carried out by specific sensory neurons which selectively express key nociceptive molecules.

Visceral nociceptors

Much less is known about visceral sensory innervation, but there is considerably less specialisation. The majority of visceral afferent neurons are of the intensity coding type, whereby innocuous and noxious traffic is encoded by the same neurons. Qualitative aspects of sensation are extrapolated by firing rate and the pattern of discharge. However, there is some evidence that there are specific visceral nociceptors which respond to the differing visceral stimuli of distension, inflammation and ischaemia that warn of internal disease.[8] The biochemical properties of these afferents have not yet been fully elucidated, but it is likely that they express specifically nociceptive molecules similar to other primary sensory afferents.

A deluge of neurochemical mediators act peripherally and centrally to alter the 'gain' or sensitivity of nociceptive systems, and it is important to identify the key molecular mediators of inflammatory hyperalgesia to offer targets for therapeutic exploitation.

MEDIATORS OF PRO-INFLAMMATORY MECHANISMS

NERVE GROWTH FACTOR: A PIVOTAL MOLECULE

Evidence for NGF as a mediator of inflammatory pain

NGF is a target-derived growth factor that in development is responsible for the survival of most nociceptive primary afferent neurons and phenotypic maturation of a population of NGF-dependent nociceptors. NGF is produced by many tissues, particularly connective tissue cells, but also in the peripheral nervous system. NGF mRNA is expressed by both the sciatic nerve and the DRG, and is probably manufactured by Schwann cells.[9] In peripheral non-neuronal tissue, the level of NGF expression correlates with the sympathetic innervation of that tissue.[10] In skin, the bulk of NGF production occurs in fibroblasts, keratinocytes and with tissue damage, inflammatory cells such as the mast cell.[11]

In the adult, NGF acts on trkA expressing neurons and serves a pivotal role peripherally (and centrally) in the regulation of nociceptive function.[12,13]

There are many data to support the importance of NGF in somatic and visceral pain models:

1. In animals and humans, NGF and its mRNA are found in inflamed tissue.[14–17] Up-regulation of NGF levels is a common component of the inflammatory response.

2. Administration of exogenous NGF not only reproduces hyperalgesic responses similar to those observed in inflammatory pain models,[18–20] but also evokes persistent pain and hyperalgesia in human volunteers.[21]

3. Reduction of available NGF by molecules that sequester NGF, is associated with a hypoalgesia in normal animals and attenuates hyperalgesia in inflammatory pain models.[19,22]

4. Electrophysiological investigation has demonstrated that NGF directly sensitises cutaneous and visceral primary afferent neurons.[23] NGF also facilitates the development of novel mechanosensitivity or spontaneous activity in previously unresponsive unmyelinated afferents. This is known as recruitment of 'silent nociceptors'.[8]

5. Although its precise physiological significance is unknown, expression of the immediate early onset gene *c-Fos* in the spinal cord is said to be a marker of sustained noxious sensory input[24] and is induced by administration of exogenous NGF.[25] NGF sequestration also reduces *c-Fos* expression in somatic[26] and visceral[25] inflammatory pain.

6. Mice in which encoding of the gene for NGF has been disrupted (NGF 'knockout' mice), not only fail to develop nociceptive neurons, but exhibit elevated thresholds to noxious stimuli.[27] Conversely, animals which are genetically modified to over-express NGF are hypersensitive to sensory stimuli.[28]

NGF and visceral hyperalgesia

Specifically, the key role of NGF in an established and clinically relevant model of visceral pain has been demonstrated.[19] In this model, chemical cystitis is induced by intravesical installation of turpentine[29] and exhibits many of the

Box 1. Direct and indirect mechanisms of NGF action

How are pro-hyperalgesic actions of NGF mediated at a local level (Figures 4 & 5)? Following tissue injury, NGF is released by connective tissue and mast cells in response to cytokines (e.g. interleukin-1β, IL-1β and tumour necrosis factor-α, TNF-α).[1,2] NGF may also induce cytokine production and increase mast cell proliferation.[3] Cytokines and growth factors increase levels of NGF mRNA by activating intracellular mechanisms, most important of which is the protein kinase C (PKC) pathway.[4] Manipulation of these NGF-dependent intracellular processes is possible[5] and may warrant further deliberation.

NGF facilitates peripheral neuroplastic changes in nociceptive processing. This occurs primarily via activation of trkA receptors causing direct sensitisation of primary afferent nociceptors to thermal and chemical stimuli.[6] Sympathetic efferents may also be involved since they not only express trkA receptors[7] but surgical or chemical sympathectomy can attenuate NGF-evoked hyperalgesia.[8] NGF action on the low affinity neurotrophin receptor, p75, is important for the regulation of at least some aspects of nociceptor excitability.[9,10]

Also significant are other cellular elements in peripheral tissues which express trkA and cause sensitisation indirectly. NGF liberated from mast cells can itself precipitate further mast cell degranulation via trkA receptors, thus amplifying NGF activity. TrkA mediated mast cell degranulation by NGF also liberates other pro-hyperalgesic molecules, such as histamine and serotonin (5HT). The importance of NGF-induced mast cell degranulation is highlighted by the finding that pre-treatment with mast cell degranulators reduces hyperalgesia and attenuates up-regulation of NGF expression in inflammation.[11]

NGF may also indirectly sensitise nociceptive afferents by interaction with the 5-lipoxygensase pathway (not shown) and promotion of leukotriene production. Inhibitors of this pathway attenuate thermal hyperalgesia from intraplantar NGF administration.[12]

Antagonism of any one of these indirect mechanisms of NGF action has a potentially analgesic capability. This circular process of escalating NGF-induced pro-inflammatory processes, unless checked, could be deleterious. It is conceivable and advantageous that natural antagonistic mechanisms exist and the position of both CB_1 and CB_2 receptors is indicative of such a role.

REFERENCES

1. Woolf CJ, Safieh-Garabedian B, Ma Q-P, Crilly P, Winters J. Nerve growth factor contributes to the generation of inflammatory sensory hypersensitivity. Neuroscience 1994; 62: 327–331.
2. Lewin GR, Mendell LM. Nerve growth factor and nociception. Trends Neurosci 1993; 16: 353–359.
3. Bullock ED, Johnson EM. Nerve growth factor induces the expression of certain cytokine genes and BLC-2 in mast cells – potential role in survival promotion. J Biol Chem 1996; 271: 27500–27508.
4. Bennett DLH, McMahon SB, Rattray M et al. Nerve growth factor and sensory nerve function. In: Brain SD, Moore PK. (eds) Pain and Neurogenic Inflammation. Basel: Birkhauser, 1999; 167–193.
5. Berg MM, Sternberg DW, Parada LF, Chao MV. K-252a inhibits nerve growth factor-induced trk proto-oncogene phosphorylation and kinase activity. J Biol Chem 1992; 267: 13–16.

6. McMahon SB, Armanini MP, Ling LH, Phillips HS. Expression and coexpression of trk receptors in subpopulations of adult primary sensory neurons projecting to identified peripheral targets. Neuron 1994; 12: 1161–1171.

7. Smeyne RJ, Klein R, Schnapp A et al. Severe sensory and sympathetic neuropathies in mice carrying a disrupted Trk/NGF receptor gene. Nature 1994; 368: 246–249.

8. Andreev NY, Dmitrieva N, Koltzenburg M, McMahon SB. Peripheral administration of nerve growth factor in the adult rat produces a thermal hyperalgesia that requires the presence of sympathetic post-ganglionic neurones. Pain 1995; 63: 109–115.

9. Petersen M, Segond von Banchet G, Heppelmann B, Koltzenburg M. Nerve growth factor regulates the expression of bradykinin binding sites on adult sensory neurons via the neurotrophin receptor p75. Neuroscience 1998; 83: 161–168.

10. Bennett DLH, Koltzenburg M, Priestley JV, Shelton DL, McMahon SB. Endogenous nerve growth factor regulates the sensitivity of nociceptors in the adult rat. Eur J Pharmacol 1998; 10: 1282–1291.

11. Woolf CJ, Ma Q-P, Allchorne A, Poole S. Peripheral cells types contributing to the hyperalgesic action of nerve growth factor in inflammation. J Neurosci 1996; 16: 2716–2723.

12. Amann R, Schuligoi R, Lanz I, Bernhard A, Peskar A. Effect of 5-lipoxygenase inhibitor on nerve growth factor-induced thermal hyperalgesia. Eur J Pharmacol 1996; 306: 89–91.

NGF-induced phenomena discussed above. Indeed, vesical inflammation can be reproduced by intravesical installation of NGF itself. Two NGF-induced manifestations are particular to visceral inflammation: (i) viscero-visceral hyper-reflexia (VVH; an increase in reflex bladder motility that mirrors clinical features of cystitis); and (ii) a referred hyperalgesia.[30]

Referred pain, common and difficult to treat in many visceral pain states, has also been shown to be NGF-induced.[30] Exploitation of this NGF-induced phenomenon could improve clinical management of chronic abdominal pain, syndromes characterised by visceral hyperalgesia.

Interaction with nociceptive peptides and neurotrophins

NGF up-regulates the expression of certain nociceptive peptides and neurotrophins. NGF promotes substance P and CGRP expression in DGR cells[31] and increases their subsequent release in the spinal cord.[32] NGF indirectly and directly influences other neurotrophins. NGF may indirectly influence trk-neurotrophin signalling via a second receptor, the low affinity neurotrophin receptor, p75 (see Box 1).[11] Directly, NGF up-regulates the expression of brain-derived neurotrophic factor (BDNF).[13] Although the participation of BDNF in pain has not been fully elucidated, it appears to be synthesised in trkA expressing cells and is anterogradely transported to axon terminals in the spinal cord[33] where it increases the excitability of second order neurons.[34] However, the actions of BDNF do not only promote central sensitisation, but may sensitise nociceptors peripherally and evoke a heat hyperalgesia.[35] Both of these phenomena were blocked in mast cell depleted preparations, suggesting a mechanism of action not dissimilar to NGF. The role of another neurotrophin, GDNF, also remains elusive although evidence is emerging to suggest it is neuroprotective to the IB4-binding class of nociceptors after nerve damage.[36,37] Bearing in mind the pivotal role of NGF in

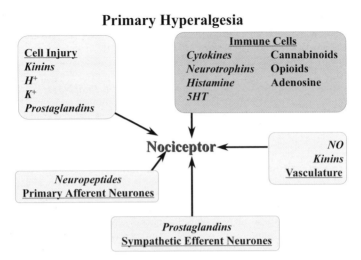

Figure 4 Contributory mechanisms of primary hyperalgesia (focus on highlighted panel).

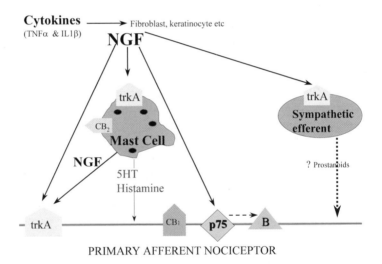

Figure 5 Neuroimmune interactions of NGF.

inflammatory pain, further investigation into peripheral actions of these other neurotrophins may provide potential analgesic mechanisms.

Possibilities for therapeutic antagonism of NGF actions

It is clear that NGF plays a pivotal role in the neuroplasticity of sensory systems in inflammation, and offers a potent analgesic target. However, because there has been little success in the development of competitive antagonists at the trkA receptor, alternative methods to reduce NGF available for binding to trkA have been developed. A novel molecule, manufactured by dimerisation of the extracellular domain of the trkA receptor and fused to an IgG, acts by sequestering NGF and has proven to be analgesic in animal models of inflammation.[19,22] Antibodies raised against NGF have also proved to be effective in reducing pain measures.[26] The leading role of NGF in inflammation-induced nociceptive plasticity points to pharmacological manipulation of NGF as a new and powerful analgesic strategy. However, an alternative tactic is to augment endogenous systems physiologically antagonistic to NGF. The endogenous cannabinoid system attenuates some NGF-mediated inflammatory processes and will be discussed later.

BRADYKININ: STIMULATION AND SENSITISATION

Kinins are released locally by damaged tissue, including bradykinin and its kinase I metabolite, des-Arg^9-bradykinin, and are manufactured from immune cells, in particular mast cells.[38] Complex synergy occurs between members of the 'inflammatory soup'. Bradykinin not only stimulates nociceptors directly, but it also indirectly promotes sensitisation of primary afferents.[39] Bradykinin activates nociceptors via the constitutive G protein-coupled bradykinin B$_2$ receptor. This may also stimulate prostanoid, cytokine and nitric oxide (NO) production which then mediate the sensitisation of nociceptors and induce expression of the bradykinin B$_1$ receptor. The induction and subsequent function of B$_1$ receptors become more important in inflammation of longer duration,[40,41] and this may be mediated by NGF via release of kallikreins from mast cells.[42] Indeed, in inflamed tissue, the B$_1$ selective des-Arg^9-bradykinin is found in greater concentration than bradykinin. Thus, B$_2$ receptor antagonists are analgesic by attenuating nociceptor stimulation, whilst B$_1$ receptor antagonist-mediated analgesia is facilitated by indirectly inhibiting afferent sensitisation.[43]

At least part of these actions are mediated by via G proteins to generate, amongst other substances, diacylglycerol (DAG). DAG then activates a protein kinase C (PKC) causing phosphorylation of various intracellular proteins that promote calcium mobilisation.[44] Manipulation of PKC, an intracellular effector of some bradykinin and NGF-induced actions, would be therefore expected to have a decisive analgesic action. This opportunity may be exploited.

Bradykinin is important in the previously discussed clinically relevant model of visceral pain. When the inflammatory hyperalgesia was well established, both B$_1$ and B$_2$ antagonists reduced signs of hyperalgesia. However, only administration of B$_2$, but not B$_1$, antagonists at the onset of inflammation attenuated development of hyperalgesia.[41] B$_1$ and B$_2$ receptors offer a novel 'up-stream' analgesic target, an action exemplified by the anti-nociceptive effects of the peptide analogue B$_2$ and B$_1$ antagonists.[45] However, peptide analogues suffer from potential problems of immunogenicity and short duration of action and non-peptide antagonists are being developed.[46]

CYTOKINES: INTERACTIVE PERIPHERAL INFLAMMATORY MEDIATORS

Inflammation-driven release of cytokines from immune cells provokes hyperalgesia through stimulation and production of other pro-inflammatory agents. Interleukin-1β (IL-1β) and tumour necrosis factor-α (TNF-α) are the main stimulus to NGF release from connective tissue cells, underlining the importance of NGF in inflammatory hyperalgesia. IL-1β prompts hyperalgesia, at least in part, by B_1 receptor induction.[47] TNF-α-induced hyperalgesia may itself be mediated by IL-1β release.[48] Obviously, development of antagonists to these molecules affords another putative analgesic target. Evidence exists to support a beneficial effect of anti-TNF-α antibody treatment on the synovitis of rheumatoid arthritis.

Another approach has been to reduce production of cytokines at a transcription level with cytokine-suppressive anti-inflammatory drugs (CSAIDs). CSAIDs decrease IL-1β and TNF-α production by interaction with a specific type of protein kinase, which could be a possible analgesic target itself.[49] However, TNF-α and other inflammatory cytokines perform specific functions combating infection and tumours, which could pose problems for long-term treatment. The employment of endogenous anti-inflammatory cytokines has also been investigated. The neuroimmune signalling molecule, leukaemia inhibitory factor (LIF) is up-regulated by experimental inflammation and may attenuate IL-1β expression.[50] This anti-inflammatory role of LIF suggests a more congruous cytokine target to exploit for analgesic gain, although some evidence suggests a LIF may have a potentially pro-nociceptive function.[51]

NOCICEPTIVE ION CHANNELS

Manipulation of inflammatory mediators affects nociceptive mechanisms at one level, yet nociceptive specificity also exists anatomically. One recent line of inquiry considers whether there are ion channels that are unique to nociceptors and thus open to a precision strike for analgesia.[52]

Sodium channels revisited

One family of channels has been the focus of a large body of research into the nature of modulation of nociceptor excitability: voltage gated Na^+ currents (VGSCs). Not only is there evidence to support the role of VGSCs in control of neuronal excitability, but therapeutic compounds that block these channels may also be effective in treating hyperalgesia.[53,54] The Na^+ current evoked from sensory neurons is made up of activation of a number of distinct ion channels, which are divided into two types: (i) tetrodotoxin (TTX)-sensitive current; and (ii) TTX-resistant current. VGSCs associated with TTX-sensitive currents are present on all sensory neurons, whilst the TTX-resistant current is largely restricted to neurons with nociceptive characteristics.[54] Hyperalgesic inflammatory mediators increase the magnitude of TTX-resistant currents,[54] which may involve phosphorylation via protein kinase C.[52] Furthermore, a sub-population of these channels has been coined sensory nerve specific (SNS) and undergoes increased expression in certain models of inflammation.[55] Experiments with mice in which the *sns* gene, responsible for encoding the SNS TTX-resistant channel has been disrupted, demonstrated that all slow TTX-resistant currents are encoded by this gene. These animals exhibited a pronounced analgesia to noxious mechanical stimuli and delayed development of inflammatory hyperalgesia.[56] The specificity of TTX-resistant currents, and their putative up-regulation in inflammatory and neuropathic pain states, is an obvious site for analgesic action.

Heat, capsaicin and the VR1 receptor

The discovery of a heat-sensitive ion channel on sensory neurons, which was not only activated by heat, but also by the algogen, bradykinin, provided a possible candidate for a nociceptive specific channel.[57] This channel is insensitive to conventional sodium and calcium channel blockers, although ruthenium red selectively blocks capsaicin-induced activation of the channel and prevents intracellular effects by preventing the increased calcium entry into the cell.[58] Further interest into examination of this channel was provoked by the cloning of the vanilloid capsaicin receptor, VR1. Cells transfected with the VR1 receptor exhibit a non-selective cation channel with high Ca^{2+} permeability that is activated by sudden increases in temperature.[59] It is unclear if the VR1 receptor is identical to the previously described ion channel. Nevertheless, it has been postulated that heat is the endogenous 'ligand' for this receptor, and protons or acid moieties (such as from the tissue acidity of inflammation) have a profound effect on the nociceptive activation of VR1.[59]

The VR1 receptor is expressed by both NGF- and GDNF-dependent classes of nociceptor[60] and, accordingly, both are sensitive to capsaicin. Capsaicin acts by evoking a functional desensitisation of these ion channels to other stimuli. as well as attenuating the subsequent effect of additional capsaicin.[58] Further investigation may lead to development of agents that alter these ion channels directly, but without problems of pain precipitation and possible neuronal damage caused by capsaicin. However, the situation is likely to be more complicated, as proven by the discovery of another heat sensitive ion channel receptor, VRL-1.[61] Still, these ion channels may provide sites for novel analgesic approaches.

ATP and adenosine

Investigation into the recently characterised adenosine triphosphate (ATP)-gated ion channels have re-fuelled interest into the role of ATP and pain.[52] Similar to the heat-sensitive ion channels, ion channels that opened in response to ATP had previously been described on sensory neurons.[62] Concentrations of ATP needed to open these channels are not only present in all tissues, but so are the necessary enzymes to remove ATP after release. ATP has also been shown to be nociceptive in animal[63] and human experiments.[64] The large family of ion channels that are opened by ATP are termed P2X purinoceptors, of which $P2X_3$ may be important in nociception, and may even be selectively expressed on nociceptors.[52] Furthermore, $P2X_3$ is expressed on the central terminals of those nociceptors in lamina IIi of the superficial dorsal horn, and exhibits co-localisation with IB4 lectin-staining nociceptors.[65] There is growing evidence that ATP and $P2X_3$ are crucial in the development of inflammatory pain, and offer a template for development of highly selective analgesics.

Adenosine is related to ATP, yet occupies an intriguing position of being associated with hyperalgesia as well as analgesia. Adenosine A_1 receptor activation can produce antinociception. The best characterised analgesic effects occur at the spinal cord level,[66] but there are also peripheral antinociceptive actions which may be mediated by endogenous adenosine.[67,68] Yet, adenosine induces pain in human after intravenous administration, and sensitises nociceptors.[69] These latter effects are possibly A_2 receptor mediated.[68] This paradox demonstrates that even pharmacological clarification of specialised endogenous systems does not necessarily reveal an in vivo function. Nevertheless, exogenous adenosine or the manipulation of endogenous levels of adenosine by adenosine kinase inhibitors, may provide analgesic opportunities.[67,70]

INHIBITORY MECHANISMS

Antagonism of pro-hyperalgesic molecules affords one mechanism of investigating novel analgesia. Enhancement of physiological analgesic control systems is another.

PERIPHERAL OPIOIDS

Classically, the analgesic effects of opioids have been ascribed to purely central actions in the spinal cord and the brain.[71] Certainly, opioid receptors and endogenous opioids are located centrally at key junctures in nociceptive pathways. Opioid receptors modulate nociceptive input into the dorsal horn of the spinal cord both presynaptically and postsynaptically,[4] as well as being instrumental in analgesic descending inhibitory systems. The discovery of a central endogenous opioid system proved conclusively that endogenous antinociceptive systems exist. More recently still, evidence has been mounting that reveals a peripheral opioid action on receptors without the CNS, raising the possibility of divorcing analgesic action from unwanted central side-effects.[72,73] Numerous clinical, experimental and anecdotal reports had insinuated peripheral opioid actions, but methodological problems hampered aspirations of claiming these effects as receptor specific. Separating central from genuinely peripheral actions has fuelled much debate on this subject, typified by the discussions on intra-articular morphine.

It appears that the presence of an on-going inflammatory response is crucial to the full activation of the peripheral system. The augmentation of the potency of peripheral opioid analgesia after inflammation, is secondary principally to opioid peptide release from inflammatory cells.[72] Functionally active μ, δ, and κ opioid receptors exist in peripheral tissue.[74] Indeed, opioid receptor mRNA is present in DRGs and the receptors themselves have been found on peripheral terminals of thinly myelinated and unmyelinated primary afferent sensory neurons.[75] Anterograde (i.e. from DRG to the periphery) axonal transport of opioid receptors does increase in later stages of inflammation. This receptor up-regulation enhances the analgesic potential of opioids in the periphery, particularly in chronic inflammatory pain states. Peripheral opioids not only reduce propagation of nociceptive action potentials, but diminish the release of other excitatory neuropeptides, contributing to an additional anti-inflammatory effect.[76] Furthermore, increased levels of endogenous opioids available for antinociception have been found in inflamed tissue (such as synovitis). They are produced by immune cells[75] and their release is elicited by many factors including IL-1β.

Data from human studies, although generally supportive of the animal findings, have not been of sufficient methodological quantity or quality to demonstrate unequivocally the effectiveness of a peripheral opioid system. Further investigation into analgesia from systemically inactive doses of opioid agonists is required. Nonetheless, the discovery of a peripheral opioid analgesic system should facilitate development of novel opioids that do not cross the blood brain barrier and, therefore, do not cause unwanted central side-effects which mitigate current opioid usage. Some such compounds are in development and are showing early promise.[77] Although opioids are amongst the longest established analgesics, not only are they still the most effective, but also appear to have hidden endogenous, peripheral talents.

A system of endogenous agonists acting upon specific receptors to modulate nociceptive processes is not unique. Nor are peripheral endogenous opioids the only anti-inflammatory mediator to be released by inflammation or tissue damage. The pharmacology of derivatives of the plant *Cannabis sativa* has only recently been elucidated, and it appears that an extensive neuromodulatory endogenous cannabinoid system exists. NGF is a pivotal molecule in inflammatory hyperalgesia and cannabinoids may act by enhancing the physiological control of NGF-induced hyperalgesia.

CANNABINOIDS

Cannabinoids have been used empirically for thousands of years, both for therapeutic and recreational ends, yet there is, at present, little sound evidence to support their clinical use.[78] Political and legal concerns, as well as a problematic lipophilic pharmacology, have until relatively recently curtailed detailed clinical and scientific investigation. Since herbal cannabis is a complex and variable product containing over 60 different active compounds, investigation of selective and specific agonists appears to be the most prudent approach.[78] As with morphine, the discovery and subsequent cloning of a receptor (CB_1) for cannabinoids raised the possibility of endogenous ligands.[79,80] This possibility was realised by the discovery of a putative endogenous agonist, aptly named anandamide (ANA) after the Sanskrit word for 'bliss'.[81] The characterisation and cloning of a second and quite different receptor (CB_2) soon followed.[82]

An analgesic role for the CB_1 receptor

The CB_1 receptor is constitutively expressed on neurons, predominantly within the brain and spinal cord,[83–85] yet there is evidence that the receptor is expressed in the peripheral nervous system.[85,86] The CB_1 receptor is not only expressed on the cell bodies of the NGF-dependent class of primary afferent neurons,[87] but is also axonally transported to the periphery, analogous to the movement of peripheral opioid receptors after long-term inflammation.[88] Other data implicate the presence of pre-junctional CB_1 receptors in urinary bladder.[89] The development of a selective CB_1 receptor antagonist[90] has shown that many of the analgesic effects of cannabinoids are mediated via the CB_1 receptor. Bearing in mind the distribution of the CB_1 receptor, it is not surprising that much of the data supports an analgesic role for cannabinoids at a spinal[91–93] and supraspinal level.[94,95] Nevertheless, CB_1 receptor agonists are also analgesic peripherally.[96–98] The cellular effects of CB_1 receptor activation offer a peripheral analgesic mechanism for cannabinoids on NGF-dependent nociceptors: agonists at the CB_1 receptor promote the inhibition of certain calcium currents[99] and enhance an inwardly rectifying potassium current,[100] both of which reduce cellular excitability. Cannabinoids could provide physiological opposition to attenuate NGF-induced nociceptor sensitisation. ANA also reduces peripheral capsaicin-evoked release of CGRP,[98] again suggestive of a peripheral effect to counteract inflammatory changes on NGF-dependent nociceptors. Because of the lipophilic nature of cannabinoids, development of a centrally inactive CB_1 agonist is unlikely; yet improvement of peripheral administration techniques could be utilised.

The peripheral CB_2 receptor

The CB_2 receptor also has a role in the physiological attenuation of peripheral NGF-induced inflammatory changes. The CB_2 receptor is expressed peripherally on components of the immune system, including the mast cell.[101–104] As previously discussed, the action of NGF on trkA receptors to provoke mast cell degrannulation further amplifying available NGF, typifies NGF as a pivotal molecule in the neuro-immune interactions of inflammation. Unregulated, this process of amplification of inflammation could be potentially damaging, indicating the likely existence of an endogenous means of defence. Autacoid local inflammation antagonism (ALIA) has been postulated, whereby autacoids, released by inflammation, lessen pro-inflammatory processes. Palmitoyl-ethanolamide (PEA), an endogenous CB_2 agonist, by acting at the mast cell CB_2 receptor, reduces NGF-mediated mast cell degranulation and thus inflammatory hyperalgesia. Indeed, PEA and other N-acylethanolamides accumulate in tissues following injury[105] and down-modulate mast cells in vitro.[106] The case for PEA and its congeners is strong enough for them to be coined 'ALIAmides'.[104] Other inflammatory cells may also be involved in ALIA; for example leukocytes both biosynthesise and degrade ANA and PEA.[107] Thus CB receptors are suitably positioned on trkA receptor expressing neuro-immune elements to be endogenous physiological antagonists to NGF.

Potential analgesic mechanisms for cannabinoids

The manipulation of endogenous cannabinoids (endocannabinoids) for analgesic gain, is also feasible. Endocannabinoids are broken down by fatty acid amide hydrogenase (FAAH), so the concentration of endocannabinoids could be raised by FAAH inhibition.[108] Certain non-steroidal anti-inflammatory (NSAID) drugs act similarly to increase local levels of anandamide.[109] This may explain the observed central analgesic effects of these drugs in the absence of inflammation, suggesting a novel mechanism outside the traditional explanation. The biological effects of endocannabinoids are also limited by a re-uptake mechanism, inhibition of which could increase local concentration and augment cannabinoid effects[110] including analgesia.[111] Other arachidonic acid metabolites have also been postulated to be putative endogenous agonists.[112] They may act directly or increase levels of other endocannabinoids by competing for sites on inactivating enzymes.[108]

The exploitation of endogenous systems offers a framework for analgesic action for exogenous cannabinoids. Exogenous administration of PEA has been demonstrated to be analgesic in models of clinical somatic and visceral inflammatory pain.[96,97] as well as exhibiting anti-inflammatory actions.[113] PEA also appears to be particularly effective in NGF-induced inflammatory pain models.[114] However, not only does ANA bind to CB_2 receptors,[115] but this interaction is also analgesic.[114] The recent development of a CB_2 antagonist[116] and the development of CB_1 and CB_2 knockout mice (in which the gene encoding the CB receptor has been disrupted) should clarify to what extent the actions of PEA are CB_2 mediated.[117,118]

The CB_2 receptor is another site of powerful analgesic action which allows for separation of therapeutic from pyschotropic central effects of cannabinoids.

By manipulating the physiological effects of the cannabinoid system, endogenous cannabinoids offer new methods for analgesia acting via both peripheral CB_1 and CB_2 receptors as pharmacological antagonists to NGF-induced inflammatory and hyperalgesic effects. Cannabinoids propose novel analgesic strategies, either by increasing levels of endocannabinoids or by administration of exogenous cannabinoids that act selectively on peripheral receptors and avoid central side effects.

Key points for clinical practice

- The pain pathway is not hard-wired but, under conditions of persistent stimulation, undergoes changes in sensitivity which influences nociceptive processing.

- This is manifest by primary (peripheral) and secondary (central) hyperalgesia. Attenuation of 'up-stream' peripheral mechanisms offers a powerful position for analgesia.

- The nociceptive pathway is highly specialised both biochemically and anatomically, which augurs well for specific analgesic mechanisms.

- NGF is a key molecule in inflammatory hyperalgesia, and as such is a key target for analgesia.

- Attenuation of other pro-inflammatory mediators (bradykinins and cytokines) or inhibiting intracellular effector mechanisms may also provide novel approaches to pain relief.

- The endogenous peripheral opioid and cannabinoid systems can be exploited by either manipulation of levels of endogenous agonists, or by exogenous influence. Mechanisms exist whereby therapeutic analgesic effects can be separated from unwanted psychoactive central side effects.

- Specific nociceptive ion channels exist, highlighting the possibility of attenuating transmission of nociceptive traffic without affecting other sensory processes.

ACKNOWLEDGEMENT

WPF-S is supported by the Jubilee Fellowship of the Royal College of Anaesthetists, UK.

REFERENCES

1. Rice ASC. Recent developments in the pathophysiology of acute pain. Acute Pain 1998; 1: 27–36.
2. McMahon SB, Koltzenburg M. Silent afferents and visceral pain. In: Fields HL, Liebeskind JC. (eds) Pharmacological Approaches to the Treatment of Chronic Pain: New Concepts and Critical Issues. Seattle: IASP, 1994; 11–30.
3. Coderre TJ, Katz J, Vaccarino AL, Melzack R. Contribution of central neuroplasticity to pathological pain: review of clinical and experimental evidence. Pain 1993; 52: 259–285.
4. Dickenson AH. Spinal cord pharmacology of pain. Br J Anaesth 1995; 75: 193–200.
5. Dray A. Inflammatory mediators of pain. Br J Anaesth 1995; 75: 125–131.
6. Molliver DC, Wright DE, Leitner ML et al. IB-4 binding DRG neurons switch from NGF to GDNF dependence in early postnatal life. Neuron 1997; 19: 849–861.
7. Snider WD, McMahon SB. Tackling pain at the source: new ideas about nociceptors. Neuron 1998; 20: 629–632.
8. McMahon SB, Dmitrieva N, Koltzenburg M. Visceral pain. Br J Anaesth 1995; 75: 132–144.
9. Goedert M, Fine A, Hunt SP, Ullrich A. Nerve growth factor mRNA in peripheral and central rat tissues and in the human central nervous tissue: lesion effects in the rat and levels in Alzheimer's disease. Brain Res 1986; 387: 85–92.
10. Shelton DL, Reichart LF. Expression of the beta-nerve growth factor gene correlates with the density of sympathetic innervation in effector organs. Proc Natl Acad Sci USA 1984; 81: 7951–7955.
11. Bennett DLH, McMahon SB, Rattray M et al. Nerve growth factor and sensory nerve function. In: Brain SD, Moore PK. (eds) Pain and Neurogenic Inflammation. Basel: Birkhauser, 1999; 167–193.
12. Lewin GR, Mendell LM. Nerve growth factor and nociception. Trends Neurosci 1993; 16: 353–359.
13. McMahon SB, Bennett DLH. Growth factors and Pain. In: Dickenson AH, Besson. JM (eds) The Pharmacology of Pain. Berlin: Springer, 1997; 135–157.
14. Lowe EM, Anand P, Terenghi G, Williams-Chestnut RE, Sinicropi DV, Osborne JL. Increased nerve growth factor levels in the urinary bladder of women with idiopathic sensory urgency and interstitial cystitis. Br J Urol 1997; 79: 572–577.
15. Oddiah D, Anand P, McMahon SB, Rattray M. Rapid increase of NGF, BDNF and NT-3 mRNAs in inflamed bladder. Neuroreport 1998; 9: 1455–1458.
16. Anand P. Nerve growth factor regulates nociception in human health and disease. Br J Anaesth 1995; 75: 201–208.
17. Aloe L, Tuveri MA, Carcassi U, Levi-Montalcini R. Nerve growth factor in the synovial fluid of patients with chronic arthritis. Arthritis Rheum 1992; 35: 351–355.
18. Lewin GR, Rueff A, Mendell LM. Peripheral and central mechanisms of NGF-induced hyperalgesia. Eur J Neurosci 1994; 6: 1903–1912.
19. Dmitrieva N, Shelton D, Rice ASC, McMahon SB. The role of nerve growth factor in a model of visceral inflammation. Neuroscience 1997; 78: 449–459.
20. Amann R, Schuligoi R, Herzeg G, Donnerer J. Intraplantar injection of nerve growth factor into the rat hind paw: local edema and effects on thermal nociceptive threshold. Pain 1995; 64: 323–329.
21. Petty BG, Cornblath DR, Adornato BT et al. The effect of systemically administered recombinant human nerve growth factor in healthy human subjects. Ann Neurol 1994; 36: 244–246.
22. McMahon SB, Bennett DLH, Priestley JV, Shelton DL. The biological effects of endogenous nerve growth factor on adult sensory neurons revealed by a trkA–IgG fusion molecule. Nat Med 1998; 1: 774–780.
23. Rueff A, Mendell LM. Nerve growth factor and NT-5 induce increase thermal sensitivity of cutaneous receptors in vivo. J Neurophysiol 1996; 76: 3593–3596.
24. Hunt SP, Pini A, Evan G. Induction of c-fos-like protein in spinal cord neurons following sensory stimulation. Nature 1987; 328: 632–634.
25. Dmitrieva N, Iqbal R, Shelton D et al. c-Fos induction in a rat model of cystitis: role of NGF. Soc Neurosci Abstr 1996; 22: 301.6.
26. Woolf CJ, Safieh-Garabedian B, Ma Q-P, Crilly P, Winters J. Nerve growth factor

contributes to the generation of inflammatory sensory hypersensitivity. Neuroscience 1994; 62: 327–331.

27. Crowley C, Spencer SD, Nishimura MC et al. Mice lacking nerve growth factor display perinatal loss of sensory and sympathetic neurones yet develop basal forebrain cholinergic neurons. Cell 1994; 76: 1001–1011.

28. Davis BM, Lewin GR, Mendell LM, Jones ME, Albers KM. Altered expression of nerve growth factor in the skin of transgenic mice leads to changes in response to mechanical stimuli. Neuroscience 1993; 56: 789–792.

29. McMahon SB, Abel C. A model for the study of visceral pain states: chronic inflammation of the chronic decerebrate rat urinary bladder by irritant chemicals. Pain 1987; 28: 109–127.

30. Jaggar SI, Scott HCF, Rice ASC. Inflammation of the rat urinary bladder is associated with a referred thermal nerve growth factor hyperalgesia which is NGF dependent. Br J Anaesth 1999; 83: 442–448.

31. Donnerer J, Schuligoi R, Stein C. Increased content and transport of substance P and calcitonin gene-related peptide in sensory nerves innervating inflamed tissue: evidence for a regulatory function of nerve growth factor in vivo. Neuroscience 1992; 49: 693–698.

32. Malcangio M, Garrett NE, Tomlinson DR. Nerve growth factor treatment increases stimulus evoked release of sensory neuropeptides in the rat spinal cord. Eur J Neurosci 1997; 9: 1101–1104.

33. Michael GJ, Averill S, Nitkunan A et al. Nerve growth factor treatment increases brain-derived neurotrophic factor selectively in trkA-expressing dorsal root ganglion cells and in their central terminations within the spinal cord. J Neurosci 1997; 17: 8476–8490.

34. Thompson SWN, Bennett DLH, Kerr BJ, Bradbury EJ, McMahon SB. Brain-derived neurotrophic factor is an endogenous modulator of nociceptive responses in the spinal cord. Proc Natl Acad Sci USA 1999; 96: 7714–7718

35. Shu X-Q, Llinas A, Mendell LM. Effects of trkB and trkC neurotrophin receptor agonists on thermal nociception: a behavioral and electrophysiological study. Pain 1999; 80: 463–470.

36. Bradbury EJ, Burnstock G, McMahon SB. The expression of $P2X_3$ purinoreceptors in sensory neurons: effects of axotomy and glial derived neurotrophic factor. Mol Cell Neurosci 1998; 12: 256–268.

37. Bennett DLH, Michael GJ, Ramachandran N et al. A distinct subgroup of small DRG cells express GDNF receptor components and GDNF is protective for these neurons after nerve injury. J Neurosci 1998; 18: 3059–3072.

38. Dray A. Tasting the inflammatory soup: the role of peripheral neurons. Pain Rev 1994; 1: 153–171.

39. Dray A, Perkins MN. Bradykinin and inflammatory pain. Trends Neurosci 1993; 16: 99–104.

40. Davis AJ, Perkins MN. Induction of B_1 receptors in vivo in a model of persistent inflammatory mechanical hyperalgesia in the rat. Neuropharmacology 1994; 33: 127–133.

41. Jaggar SI, Habib S, Rice ASC. The modulatory effects of bradykinin B_1 and B_2 receptor antagonists upon viscero-visceral hyper-reflexia in a rat model of visceral hyperalgesia. Pain 1998; 75: 169–176.

42. Rueff A, Dawson AJLR, Mendell LM. Characteristics of nerve growth factor induced hyperalgesia in adult rats: dependence on enhanced bradykinin-1 receptor activity but not neurokinin-1 receptor activity. Pain 1996; 66: 359–372.

43. Perkins MN, Campbell E, Dray A. Antinociceptive activity of the bradykinin B1 and B2 receptor antagonists, des-Arg^9, [Leu^8]-BK and HOE 140, in two models of persistent hyperalgesia in the rat. Pain 1993; 53: 191–197.

44. Rang HP, Bevan S, Dray A. Nociceptive peripheral neurons: cellular properties. In: Wall PD, Melzack R. (eds) Textbook of Pain. Edinburgh: Churchill Livingstone, 1994; 57–78.

45. Steranka LR, De Haas CJ, Vavrek RJ, Stewart JM, Enna SJ, Snyder SH. Antinociceptive effects of bradykinin antagonists. Eur J Pharmacol 1987; 136: 261–262.

46. Regoli D, Nsa-Allogho S, Rizzi A, Gobeil FJ. Bradykinin receptors and their antagonists. Eur J Pharmacol 1998; 348: 1–10.

47. Perkins MN, Kelly D. Interleukin 1 beta induced des-arg[9]-bradykinin-mediated thermal hyperalgesia in the rat. Neuropharmacology 1994; 33: 657–660.

48. Watkins LR, Goehler LE, Relton J, Brewer MT, Maier SF. Mechanisms of tumor necrosis factor alpha (TNFalpha) hyperalgesia. Brain Res 1995; 692: 244–250.

49. Lee JC, Laydon JT, McDonnel PC et al. A protein kinase involved in the regulation of inflammatory cytokine synthesis. Nature 1994; 372: 739–745.

50. Banner LR, Patterson PH, Allchorne A, Poole S, Woolf CJ. Leukemia inhibitory factor is an anti-inflammatory and analgesic cytokine. J Neurosci 1998; 18: 5456–5462.

51. Thompson SWN, Dray A, Urban L. Leukemia inhibitory factor induced mechanical allodynia but not thermal hyperalgesia in the juvenile rat. Neuroscience 1996; 71: 1091–1094.

52. McCleskey EW, Gold MS. Ion channels of nociception. Annu Rev Physiol 1999; 61: 835–856.

53. Devor M, Wall PD, Catalan N. Systemic lidocaine silences ectopic neuroma and DRG discharge without blocking nerve conduction. Pain 1992; 48: 261–268.

54. Gold MS, Reichling DB, Shuster MJ, Levine JD. Hyperalgesic agents increase a tetrodo-toxin-resistant Na^+ current in nociceptors. Proc Natl Acad Sci USA 1996; 93: 1108–1112.

55. Tanaka M, Cummins TR, Ishikawa K, Dib-Hajj SD, Black JA, Waxman SG. SNA Na^+ channel expression increases in dorsal root ganglion neurons in the carrageenan inflammatory pain model. Neuroreport 1998; 9: 967–972.

56. Akopian AN, Souslova V, England S et al. The tetrodotoxin-resistant sodium channel SNS has a specialized function in pain pathways. Nat Neurosci 1999; 2: 541–548.

57. Caesare P, McNaughton P. A novel heat-activated current in nociceptive neurons and its sensitization by bradykinin. Proc Natl Acad Sci USA 1996; 93: 15435–15439.

58. Winter J, Bevan S, Campbell EA. Capsaicin and pain mechanisms. Br J Anaesth 1995; 75: 157–168.

59. Tominaga M, Caterina MJ, Malmberg AB et al. The cloned capsaicin receptor integrates multiple pain-producing stimuli. Neuron 1998; 21: 531–543.

60. Guo A, Vulchanova L, Wang J, Li X, Elde R. Immunocytochemical localisation of the vanilloid receptor 1 (VR1): relationship to neuropeptides, the P2X$_3$ purinoceptor and IB4 binding sites. Eur J Neurosci 1999; 11: 946–958.

61. Caterina MJ, Rosen TA, Tominaga M, Brake AJ, Julius D. A capsaicin-receptor with a high threshold for noxious heat. Nature 1999; 398: 436–441.

62. Krishtal OA, Marchenko SM, Obukhov AG. Cationic channels activated by extracellular ATP in rat sensory neurons. Neuroscience 1998; 27: 995–1000.

63. Sawynok J, Reid A. Peripheral adenosine 5′-triphosphate enhances nociception in the formalin test via activation of a purinergic P2X receptor. Eur J Pharmacol 1997; 330: 115–121.

64. Bleehen T, Keele CA. Observations on the algogenic actions of adenosine compounds on the human blister base preparation. Pain 1977; 3: 367–377.

65. Vulchanova L, Riedl MS, Shuster SJ et al. P2X$_3$ is expressed by DRG neurons that terminate in inner lamina II. Eur J Neurosci 1998; 10: 3470–3478.

66. Sawynok J. Adenosine receptor activation and nociception. Eur J Pharmacol 1998; 347: 1–11.

67. Sawynok J, Reid A, Poon A. Peripheral antinociceptive effect of an adenosine kinase inhibitor, with augmentation by an adenosine deaminase inhibitor, in the rat formalin test. Pain 1998; 74: 75–81.

68. Karlsten R, Gordh T, Post C. Local antinociceptive and hyperalgesic effects in the formalin test after peripheral administration of adenosine analogues in mice. Pharmacol Toxicol 1992; 70: 434–438.

69. Sollevi A. Adenosine for pain control. Acta Anaethesiol Scand Suppl 1997; 110: 135–136.

70. Belfrage M, Sollevi A, Segerdahl M, Sjolund KF, Hansson P. Systemic adenosine infusion alleviates spontaneous and stimulus evoked pain in patients with peripheral neuropathic pain. Anesth Analg 1995; 81: 713–717.

71. Millan MJ. Multiple opioid systems and pain. Pain 1986; 27: 303–347.

72. Stein C. Peripheral mechanisms of opioid analgesia. Anesth Analg 1993; 76: 182–191.

73. Stein C, Schafer M, Cabot PJ et al. Peripheral opioid analgesia. Pain Rev 1997; 4: 173–187.

74. Stein C, Hassan AHS, Lehrberger K, Giefing J, Yassouridis A. Local analgesic effect of endogenous opioid peptides. Lancet 1993; 342: 321–324.

75. Stein C. The control of pain in peripheral tissues by opioids. N Engl J Med 1995; 332: 1685–1690.

76. Stein C, Yassouridis A. Peripheral morphine analgesia. Pain 1997; 71: 119–121.

77. Giardina G, Clark GD, Grugni M, Sbacci M, Vecchietti V. Central and peripheral analgesic agents: chemical strategies for limiting brain penetration in kappa-opioid agonists belonging to different chemical classes. Farmaco 1995; 50: 405–418.

78. British Medical Association. Therapeutic Uses of Cannabis. Amsterdam: Harwood; 1997.

79. Devane WA, Dysarz III FA, Johnson MR, Melvin LS, Howlett AC. Determination and characterization of a cannabinoid receptor in rat brain. Mol Pharmacol 1988; 34: 605–613.

80. Matsuda LA, Lolait SJ, Brownstein MJ, Young AC, Bonner TI. Structure of a cannabinoid receptor and functional expression of the cloned cDNA. Nature 1990; 346: 561–564.

81. Devane WA, Hanus L, Breuer A et al. Isolation and structure of a brain constituent that binds to the cannabinoid receptor. Science 1992; 258: 1946–1949.

82. Munro S, Thomas KL, Abu Shaar K. Molecular characterisation of a peripheral receptor for cannabinoids. Nature 1993; 365: 61–65.

83. Herkenham M, Lynn AB, Johnson MR, Melvin LS, de Costa BR, Rice KC. Characterization and localization of cannabinoid receptors in rat brain: a quantitative in vitro autoradiographic study. J Neurosci 1991; 11: 563–583.

84. Tsou K, Brown S, Sanudo-Pena MC, Mackie K, Walker JM. Immunohistochemical distribution of cannabinoid receptors in the rat central nervous system. Neuroscience 1998; 83: 393–411.

85. Hohmann AG, Herkenham M. Localisation of cannabinoid receptor (CB1) mRNA in neuronal subpopulations of rat spinal cord and dorsal root ganglia. Soc Neurosci Abstr 1997; 23: 760.3.

86. Hohmann AG, Herkenham M. Localisation of central cannabinoid CB1 receptor messenger RNA in neuronal subpopulations of rat dorsal root ganglia: a double-label in situ hybridisation study. Neuroscience 1999; 90: 923–931.

87. Friedel RH, Schnurch H, Stubbusch J, Barde Y. Identification of genes differentially expressed by nerve growth factor and neurotrophin-3 dependent sensory neurones. Proc Natl Acad Sci USA 1997; 94: 12670–12675.

88. Hohmann AG, Herkenham M. Cannabinoid receptors undergo axonal flow in sensory nerves. Neuroscience 1999; 92: 1171–1175.

89. Pertwee RG, Fernando SR. Evidence for the presence of cannabinoid CB1 receptors in mouse urinary bladder. Br J Pharmacol 1996; 118: 2053–2058.

90. Rinaldi-Carmona M, Barth F, Heaulme M et al. SR141716A, a potent and selective antagonist of the brain cannabinoid receptor. FEBS Lett 1994; 350: 240–244.

91. Lichtman AH, Martin BR. Spinal and supraspinal components of cannabinoid-induced antinociception. J Pharmacol Exp Ther 1991; 258: 517–523.

92. Hohmann AG, Tsou K, Walker JM. Cannabinoid modulation of wide dynamic range neurons in the lumbar dorsal horn of the rat by spinally administered WIN55,212-2. Neurosci Lett 1998; 257: 119–122.

93. Welch SP, Huffman JW, Lowe J. Differential blockade of the antinociceptive effects of centrally administered cannabinoids by SR141716A. J Pharmacol Exp Ther 1998; 286: 1301–1308.

94. Martin WJ, Hohmann AG, Walker JM. Suppression of noxious stimuli evoke activity in the ventral posterolateral nucleus of the thalamus by a cannabinoid agonist: correlation between electrophysiological and antinociceptive effects. J Neurosci 1996; 16: 6601–6611.

95. Meng ID, Manning BH, Martin WJ, Fields HL. An analgesia circuit activated by cannabinoids. Nature 1998; 395: 381–383.

96. Jaggar SI, Hasnie FS, Sellaturay S, Rice ASC. The anti-hyperalgesic actions of the cannabinoid anandamide and the putative CB_2 receptor agonist palmitoyl-ethanolamide in visceral and somatic inflammatory pain. Pain 1998; 76: 189–199.

97. Calignano A, La Rana G, Guiffrida A, Piomelli D. Control of pain initiation by endogenous cannabinoids. Nature 1998; 394: 277–281.

98. Richardson JD, Kilo S, Hargreaves KM. Cannabinoids reduce hyperalgesia and inflammation via interaction with peripheral CB_1 receptors. Pain 1998; 75: 111–119.

99. Twitchell W, Brown S, Mackie K. Cannabinoids inhibit N- and P/Q-type calcium channels in cultured rat hippocampal neurons. J Neurophysiol 1997; 78: 43–50.

100. Deadwyler SA, Hampson RE, Mu J, Whyte A, Childers S. Cannabinoids modulate voltage sensitive potassium A-current in hippocampal neurons via a cAMP-dependent process. J Pharmacol Exp Ther 1995; 273: 734–743.

101. Galiegue S, Mary S, Marchand J et al. Expression of central and peripheral cannabinoid receptors in human immune tissues and leukocyte subpopulations. Eur J Biochem 1995; 232: 54–61.

102. Lynn AB, Herkenham M. Localization of cannabinoid receptors and nonsaturable high-density cannabinoid binding sites in peripheral tissues of the rat: implications for receptor-mediated immune modulation by cannabinoids. J Pharmacol Exp Ther 1994; 268: 1612–1623.

103. Pertwee RG. Pharmacology of cannabinoid CB_1 and CB_2 receptors. Pharmacol Ther 1997; 74: 129–180.

104. Levi-Montalcini R, Skaper SD, Dal Toso R, Petrelli L, Leon A. Nerve growth factor: from neurotrophin to neurokine. Trends Neurosci 1996; 19: 514–520.

105. Schmid HH, Schmid PC, Natarajan V. N-acylated glycerophospholipids and their derivatives. Prog Lipid Res 1990; 29: 1–43.

106. Facci L, Dal Toso R, Romanello S, Buriani A, Skaper SD, Leon A. Mast cells express a peripheral cannabinoid receptor with differential sensitivity to anandamide and palmitoylethanolamide. Proc Natl Acad Sci USA 1995; 92: 3376–3380.

107. Bisogno T, Maurelli S, Melck D, De Petrocellis L, Di Marzo V. Biosynthesis, uptake, and degradation of anandamide and palmitoylethanolamide in leukocytes. J Biol Chem 1997; 272: 3315–3323.

108. Di Marzo V. 'Endocannabinoids' and other fatty acid derivatives with cannabimimetic properties: biochemistry and possible physiopathological relevance. Biochim Biophys Acta 1998; 1392: 153–175.

109. Fowler CJ, Janson U, Johnson RM et al. Inhibition of anadamide hydrolysis by the enantiomers of ibuprofen, ketorolac, and fluriprofen. Arch Biochem Biophys 1999; 362: 191–196.

110. Calignano A, La Rana G, Beltramo M, Makriyannis A, Piomelli D. Potentiation of anandamide hypotension by the transport inhibitor AM404. Eur J Pharmacol 199; 337: R1–R2.

111. Di Marzo V, Fontana A, Cadas H et al. Formation and inactivation of endogenous cannabinoid anandamide in central neurons. Nature 1994; 372: 686–691.

112. Stella N, Schweitzer P, Piomelli D. A second endogenous cannabinoid that modulates long-term potentiation. Nature 1997; 388: 773–778.

113. Mazzari S, Canella R, Petrelli L, Marcolongo G, Leon A. N-(2-hydroxyethyl) hexadecanamide is orally active in reducing edema formation and inflammatory hyperalgesia by down-modulating mast cell activation. Eur J Pharmacol 1996; 300: 227–236.

114. Farquhar-Smith WP, Jaggar SI, Rice ASC. Cannabinoids attenuate NGF-induced viscero-visceral hyper-reflexia (VVH) via CB_1 and CB_2 receptors. Soc Neurosci Abstr 1999; 25: 373.2.

115. Felder CC, Joyce KE, Briley EM et al. Comparison of the pharmacology and signal transduction of the human cannabinoid CB1 and CB2 receptors. Mol Pharmacol 1995; 48: 443–450.

116. Rinaldi-Carmona M, Barth F, Millan J et al. SR 144528, the first potent and selective antagonist of the CB_2 receptor. J Pharmacol Exp Ther 1998; 284: 644–650.

117. Ledent C, Valverde O, Cossu G et al. Unresponsiveness to cannabinoids and reduced addictive effects of opiates in CB_1 receptor knockout mice. Science 1999; 283: 401–404.

118. Buckley NE, Mezey E, Bonner TI et al. CB_2 knockout mouse. In: 1998 Symposium on the Cannabinoids. Burlington, Vermont. International Cannabinoid Research Society, 1998; 36.

Stephan A. Schug Kieran Davis

Acute pain management

Acute pain came of age as a speciality in 1988 in Seattle, when Brian Ready published his concept of an Acute Pain Service (APS).[1] This was followed in 1990 with the joint colleges' report,[2] that recommended the setting up of acute pain services at all hospitals. Acute pain teams are now widespread in North America, Australasia and, increasingly, Europe; there is now even a journal dedicated solely to the sub-speciality (*International Journal of Acute Pain Management*, Saldatore Ltd, Bishop's Stortford, UK).

ACUTE PAIN PHYSIOLOGY

The physiology of acute pain is an area of great scientific endeavour, which to describe in its entirety would be impossible in this context; for detailed reviews, we recommend the following references.[3-6] The following is a summary of areas where pharmacological advances are currently being made or may be made in the near future.

NERVE GROWTH FACTOR

In fetal and early neonatal life, nerve growth factor (NGF) plays a vital part in neuronal development. Its function then changes and it develops a pivotal role in hyperalgesia and nerve transmission. NGF is released from connective tissue and inflammatory cells, its action is then mediated via trkA (tyrosine kinase) receptors.[7]

NGF has a role both peripherally and centrally; at the former it causes mast cell degranulation, which via a positive feedback mechanism stimulates further

Prof. Stephan A. Schug, Head, Discipline of Anaesthesiology, Faculty of Medicine and Health Sciences, University of Auckland, Private Bag 92019, Auckland, New Zealand (for correspondence)
Mr Kieran Davis, Pain Fellow, The Auckland Regional Pain Service, Auckland Hospital, Auckland, New Zealand

NGF production. NGF acts directly on afferent neurones and causes sensitisation of silent nociceptors, thereby increasing the number of nerves involved in pain transmission. It is transported axonally and causes 'intermediate early gene' expression and an increase in levels of substance P and calcitonin gene related peptide (GGRP) in the spinal cord. It is thus thought to be involved in the propagation of secondary hyperalgesia.[8]

There are no antagonists as yet available; however, a molecule consisting of two trkA receptors has been used to sequester NGF with some success.[5]

BRADYKININ

Bradykinin is both released from mast cells and produced locally in response to tissue injury. It acts directly on nerve endings to cause a potent algesic effect and is also involved in sensitising silent nociceptors.[3]

There are two bradykinin receptors described, named B_1 and B_2. The B_2 receptor is directly involved in neuronal activation; inhibition of the B_2 receptor attenuates acute nociceptive events.[7] The B_1 receptor has a more complicated role in hyperalgesia, which has not yet been fully explained.

There are no bradykinin antagonists presently available for clinical use. Those that have been tried experimentally have been successful in reducing pain and hyperalgesia. However, they are all peptide based and consequently have a short duration of action.[9]

NOCICEPTIN (ORPHANIN FQ)

Nociceptin, also called orphanin FQ, is a novel opioid peptide that acts on the opioid-like receptor 1 (ORL1). Both the receptor and ligand are similar in structure to their opioid counterparts; however, the classical opioid agonists have little activity at the ORL1 receptor and vice versa with nociceptin and the opioid receptors. The location and role of ORL1 receptors within the central nervous system is significantly different to the opioid receptors.[10]

ORL1 receptors are found both centrally and in the superficial areas of the dorsal horn. Centrally, they are found in areas associated with neuroendocrine secretion, instinctive behaviours, emotions, auditory processing and nociception. When nociceptin is injected into the cerebral ventricles, it reverses the actions of other opioids, both indigenous and exogenous. Its other actions are to cause exploratory behaviour but, importantly, it is not associated with the mid-brain pathways that mediate reward.[10,11]

In the dorsal horn, ORL1 receptors are found in areas adjacent to the location of the conventional opioid receptors; however, they are located on intrinsic spinal neurones and not stimulated by descending afferents. Nociceptin inhibits C-fibre induced wind-up but not baseline responses at a spinal level; this means it is involved in pain modulation and not the suppression of the initial signal. Morphine, in contrast, is involved in both processes.[11]

The lack of cross-tolerance between nociceptin and morphine indicates that it may prove to be a useful adjunct or alternative to opioid analgesia.[10]

ORAL ANALGESICS

The degree of intervention needed to manage acute pain is graded to the severity of the patient's pain. The aim for the practitioner is to provide the best analgesia in the simplest and cheapest manner; oral analgesics are often all that are required.

ORAL NON-OPIOIDS

The vast majority of patients passing through a surgical department can be managed with simple analgesics administered orally.

Which analgesics these patients should receive has been extensively reviewed by Moore and McQuay, who have examined systematically all randomised controlled trials in this area. The concept they used is a 'number needed to treat' (NNT) approach.[12] The NNT is defined as the number of patients with moderate or severe pain needing to receive a particular drug for 50% relief to be obtained. This work resulted in tables of analgesic efficacy for various drugs, with low NNTs equating to good analgesic efficacy.[13] The tables show 1000 mg paracetamol (NNT = 4) and 400 mg ibuprofen (NNT = 2) to provide best analgesia of all non-opioids and weak opioids investigated.

These data suggest that paracetamol should be the first-choice analgesic for universal usage in view of its excellent side effect profile.

Non-steroidal anti-inflammatory drugs (NSAIDs) such as ibuprofen are clearly very useful analgesics; they have been shown to have opioid sparing effects of 15–60% when used concomitantly with opioids via patient controlled analgesia (PCA) devices,[14–16] but are also very effective on their own.[17] There is no evidence that giving NSAIDs either by injection or rectally has any advantage over the oral route.[18] However, NSAIDs also pose potential risks to patients, including the risk of gastrointestinal side-effects, renal complications and interference with haemostasis.[19] Even in patients who have been carefully screened for contra-indications to NSAIDs, there is a small risk of serious adverse effects with short-term peri-operative use.[20]

In conclusion, NSAIDs are widely used in the peri-operative setting both for day-case and in-patient surgery; but, despite their proven analgesic efficacy, anaesthetists must be aware of their potential to cause morbidity. Paracetamol is a slightly less effective, but safer, alternative.

ORAL MORPHINE

Morphine can be given orally as either an immediate release preparation or in a sustained release formulation. If a patient has no contra-indication to oral intake, then a combination of short- and long-acting morphine or short-acting morphine on demand alone can provide analgesia equivalent to intravenous PCA.[21] The longer duration of action provides the advantage to the patient that they do not have to wake up to use their PCA. In converting patients from intravenous to oral morphine, a conversion ratio in the range of 1:2 to 1:3 needs to be considered.

ORAL TRAMADOL

Tramadol, which was first introduced in Germany in 1977, offers a useful alternative to conventional opioids and has recently become available world-wide. It is an atypical, centrally acting analgesic; the analgesic effect is the result of a weak opioid agonistic effect by one of its major metabolites, but also inhibition of re-uptake of serotonin and noradrenaline. It has a high bioavailability exceeding 80%, which means that dose conversion for different routes of administration (oral, rectal, intravenous or intramuscular) is unnecessary.[22] It has a half-life of approximately 6 h, which means a 3–4 times-a-day dosing schedule is appropriate. Its advantage over conventional opioids is that it causes less respiratory depression, less sedation, less constipation and has limited abuse potential.[23–26]

The analgesic efficacy of tramadol has been compared favourably to aspirin 650 mg plus codeine 60 mg,[27] paracetamol 650 mg plus propoxyphene 100 mg,[28] and recently to ketorolac 10 mg.[29] Direct comparisons with oral morphine in the postoperative setting are not available, but our clinical experience would indicate that a ratio of 1:5, morphine:tramadol, with a ceiling effect for tramadol when more than approximately 150 mg of morphine equivalent is required.

INTRAVENOUS PATIENT CONTROLLED ANALGESIA (PCA)

Since its inception in the mid 1980s, there have been over 1100 papers, reviews and handbooks published on PCA.[30] The concept of patient determined dosing of opioids enables individual titration to subjective pain relief with the safety feature of no further drug administration in case of sedation.[31]

The best-documented protocol utilises a 1 mg bolus dose of morphine, a 5 min lock-out period and no background infusion.[31] However, morphine is not the only drug that can be used. Woodhouse and colleagues, in a well constructed study, showed that neither patients nor observers could distinguish between morphine, pethidine and fentanyl.[32] This suggests, that individualisation of drug choice with consideration of patient characteristics and comorbidities might improve efficacy and safety of PCA; in the following, we describe various drug options for use with intravenous PCA.

FENTANYL VIA INTRAVENOUS PCA

Although not a new idea, the use of fentanyl in PCA devices has always been limited by the concern that its brief duration of action would lead to poor analgesia. This concern is related to a misunderstanding of the pharmaco-kinetics of fentanyl; its high lipid solubility provides rapid onset followed by rapid redistribution. Once a steady state has been reached, it is the elimination half-life, which determines how often the patient has to push the PCA control button; fentanyl and morphine then have a similar elimination half-life. It is, therefore, not surprising that most patients generally require 1–3 bolus doses per hour, at a typical dose of 20 µg.[33]

Background infusions have often been added because of concern over the rapid redistribution of fentanyl. Although no study has directly compared fentanyl PCA alone with PCA plus background infusion, experience with other opioids would indicate that there is no analgesic benefit, but complication rates are increased.

Side-effects reported include nausea and vomiting in 30–40% and pruritus in 7–13% of patients. There are no reports of clinically significant respiratory depression; however, all the studies so far reported have used respiratory rate as the sole indicator.[33]

As fentanyl, in contrast to morphine, has no active metabolites, which are retained in renal insufficiency or failure, we use it in patients with these medical problems to avoid untoward sedation and possible respiratory depression, in particular with long-term use.

TRAMADOL VIA INTRAVENOUS PCA

The use of tramadol in PCA has been studied by both the intravenous and subcutaneous routes.[34,35] Two studies have shown it to have equi-analgesic properties to morphine after gynaecological and abdominal surgery[25,26] and to pethidine after orthopaedic surgery.[24] The study by Langford and colleagues particularly considered the risk of hypoxaemia associated with the two drugs and found that tramadol produced significantly less arterial hypoxaemia than morphine.[26] The dose ratio of morphine to tramadol has been estimated at between 1:10 and 1:12. However, Vickers hypothesized that a bolus dose of 50 mg with a lock-out period of 15 min would be appropriate if the relevant pharmacokinetics were rationalized.[21]

In a multicentre study by Stamer and colleagues, 66.7% of patients responded to initial loading doses of tramadol within the first 30 min, whereas 75% responded to morphine.[35] Nausea is more common with tramadol, 34% compared to 25% with morphine; however, vomiting has a similar incidence.[21]

In conclusion, tramadol via PCA can provide analgesia equivalent to morphine with less respiratory depression in most, but not all, circumstances. Prediction of tramadol failures is currently not possible, but it is not related to intensity of initial pain.[35] In our practice, tramadol is used if concern about sedation or respiratory depression is raised or previous morphine use has lead to such complications. The possibility of improved recovery of bowel function after surgery by use of tramadol instead of morphine is unanswered.

ADJUVANT ANALGESICS IN COMBINATION WITH INTRAVENOUS PCA

Morphine PCA is the gold standard of systemic opioid administration, against which all other regimens are compared. However, even morphine PCA as the sole analgesic regimen has been shown to provide inadequate pain relief in a considerable number of patients. In a study by Sidebotham and colleagues involving over 300 patients, 42% receiving morphine PCA had inadequate analgesia on the first postoperative day.[31] Similarly, 38% of surgical patients in another survey had inadequate analgesia during the first postoperative day.[36] In both studies, inadequate analgesia was further reflected in patients' inability to comply with physiotherapy (18% and 22% of patients on the first postoperative day, respectively). Much research has, therefore, been aimed at trying to improve the quality of the analgesia provided by PCA techniques.

Paracetamol

Paracetamol combined with morphine PCA has been shown to improve efficacy and patient satisfaction, while permitting early withdrawal of the PCA device.[37] In our practice, paracetamol is given routinely on a regular basis to all postoperative patients using morphine PCA.

NSAIDs

NSAIDs, as mentioned above, have an opioid sparing effect, if used concomitantly with opioid PCA. However, the evidence that this opioid sparing effect translates into improved analgesia, or a reduction in either, postoperative nausea and vomiting, or respiratory depression is equivocal. In view of their potential to cause side-effects, sometimes of a serious nature, they should only be used if specific indications and no contra-indications exist.

Clonidine

Clonidine, an α_2-adrenoreceptor agonist, may be useful in decreasing PCA morphine requirements peri-operatively. In a study by Park and colleagues, 44 elective orthopaedic patients were randomised to receive either placebo or clonidine 5 µg/kg, 90 min before surgery and 12 and 24 h after the first dose.[38] The clonidine group used 37% less morphine and also had less postoperative nausea and vomiting; however, these patients were also more sedated pre-operatively, and had lower mean arterial blood pressures throughout the study period.

Midazolam

In a study by Gilliland and colleagues, premedication with midazolam led to lower pain scores and morphine consumption postoperatively, without any increased postoperative sedation.[39] Although midazolam is analgesic at a spinal level, it is probably acting as an anxiolytic in these circumstances.

Ketamine

Several studies have looked at the analgesic effects of ketamine when given prior to surgical incision, as a postoperative infusion or combined with PCA.[40–42] Roytblat and colleagues gave 0.15 mg/kg of ketamine or placebo to 22 patients pre-incision for open cholecystectomy and showed a reduction in pain intensity for up to 4 h.[40] Ketamine, in doses of 0.3–0.5 mg/kg/h by infusion, gives significant analgesic effects.[41] The combination of ketamine 1 mg/ml with morphine 1 mg/ml via a PCA device in patients undergoing microdiscectomy resulted in significant reduction in morphine consumption.[42] When used in the doses already mentioned, the psychomimetic effects of ketamine occurred in 20–30% of patients and were more common when given as an infusion than when given as a single dose before operation.

ADJUVANT MEDICATION TO REDUCE PCA INDUCED NAUSEA AND VOMITING

The options for reducing the incidence and severity of nausea and vomiting associated with PCA are prophylactic or combined administration of anti-emetics, and the use of naloxone.

Droperidol

Droperidol has been shown to be most effective in reducing the incidence of PCA-induced nausea and vomiting; however, the debate over its co-administration with morphine continues. In a study by Klahsen and colleagues involving women undergoing abdominal hysterectomy, patients who received droperidol (1 mg) at induction of anaesthesia and 0.04 mg droperidol/mg morphine in their PCA pump had significantly less vomiting than the control group.[44] In a dose finding study, increasing doses of droperidol, added to the PCA, were associated with improvements in nausea and vomiting but more side-effects when the dose exceeded 0.05 mg droperidol/mg morphine.[45] The approach of combined administration of morphine and droperidol via the PCA device clearly values further investigation.

Naloxone

Naloxone for the treatment of nausea and vomiting appears a surprising, but promising, strategy. In a study by Gan and colleagues, infusions of 0.25 µg/kg/h of naloxone reduced nausea and vomiting and pruritis associated with PCA in 60 patients who underwent abdominal hysterectomy.[43] Morphine consumption was also reduced. This requires further consideration, but adds increasing doubts about the role of naloxone as a simple opioid antagonist.

EPIDURAL AND INTRATHECAL ANALGESIA

Continuous epidural analgesia is now common-place on the general wards of many hospitals, and provides more effective analgesia with less adverse events than PCA after major abdominal, thoracic and orthopaedic surgery.[36] Despite the wide use and the excellent results with regard to safety and efficacy, several areas of debate and concern remain.

MODE OF DELIVERY

Although the use of continuous epidural analgesia is still probably the most frequently used technique, there is an increasing trend towards patient-controlled epidural analgesia (PCEA). In two large studies in the US and Germany, involving 1030 and 1799 patients, respectively, PCEA was shown to be safe and effective in a general ward setting.[46,47] However, a number of issues regarding PCEA remain to be answered. Most importantly, it needs to be established whether PCEA provides increased analgesic efficacy or reduced requirements for corrective intervention in comparison to continuous infusion. Current results offer only a suggestion that PCEA may be dose sparing and reduce the need for further analgesic intervention, but there may also be more pain on movement, especially if no or low background rates are used. Last, but not least, more research on ideal infusion rate and bolus size is needed.

CHOICE OF AGENTS

Local anaesthetic

Local anaesthetic effects are necessary to achieve adequate pain control for early mobilisation and compliance with physiotherapy. They provide, also, the added benefits of decreased surgical stress response, improved myocardial protection, fast recovery of bowel function and the reduced risk of thrombo-embolic events. Bupivacaine is still the most widely used agent world-wide. However, there are a number of important advantages in favour of the new long-acting local anaesthetic, ropivacaine; it provides a favourable balance between sensory and motor block,[48,49] with reduced cardiotoxicity[50] (e.g. in case of dosing error or intravacular catheter migration) and established pharmacokinetics for prolonged infusions for up to 72 h.[51] Clearly the role of ropivacaine in epidural anaesthesia warrants further assessment, particularly with regard to the use of low concentration infusions to provide postoperative analgesia.

Opioids

Opioids, added to local anaesthetic, offer improved analgesia and may reduce the frequency of unilateral and patchy blocks.[52] There remains the unresolved issue of the relative merits of lipophilic versus hydrophobic opioids. A recent review of the data suggested that hydrophobic agents, such as morphine, are the best for single agent use and that lipophilic agents, such as fentanyl, offer enhanced analgesia when combined with local anaesthetics.[53] The dose-response curves for combinations of local anaesthetics and opioid in the epidural space have not been described; however, the most commonly used concentrations of fentanyl would appear to be 2–4 μg/ml of bupivacaine 0.125%.[52]

Clonidine

Clonidine is now registered for intrathecal use in the US after having undergone extensive testing without any signs of neurotoxicity. It has been shown to produce a segmental epidural block,[54] and to be effective as a single agent.[55] In combination with local anaesthetics and opioids, it has been shown to have a dose-dependent effect in reducing pain scores on coughing and reducing additional analgesic requirements.[56] However, the same study also showed that the higher doses of clonidine were associated with more haemodynamic changes and greater vasopressor requirements. Current data do not permit a definitive assessment on the value of using clonidine in a routine setting; nevertheless, in our practice it is clearly a useful adjunct in selected cases, e.g. patchy block, pain of neurogenic origin and complex regional pain syndrome (CRPS).

Ketamine

Ketamine represents another interesting agent with a potential use in epidural analgesia. Preservative-free ketamine has been shown to lack neurotoxic effects in contrast to the standard preparation containing preservatives.[57,58] It has been found to potentiate the effects of epidural opioids[59] and possibly the effects of epidurally administered local anaesthetics.[60] Data from a study by Choe and colleagues indicate that pre-operative administration of ketamine and morphine is more effective than when the combination is administered during surgery.[61] This finding is interesting with regard to the concept of 'pre-emptive analgesia'. Antagonism at the N-methyl-D-aspartate (NMDA) receptor, the mechanism of action of ketamine, is a likely way to inhibit 'wind-up' at a dorsal horn level.

INTRATHECAL AGENTS

The use of intrathecal opioids remains a controversial issue in view of the perceived risk of late respiratory depression. Data are still limited, with most of the evidence being in obstetric patients.[62] Even dose finding is not yet complete, as Milner and colleagues found that 0.1 mg of morphine produced similar postoperative analgesia to 0.2 mg of morphine in Caesarean section patients.[63] In a retrospective analysis by Gwirtz and colleagues in 5969 patients, there was an incidence of respiratory depression of 3% requiring naloxone infusions, there were no respiratory arrests and all cases of respiratory depression were detected by routine nursing observations.[64]

The use of intrathecal midazolam, although initially promising particularly for somatic pain,[65] has been curtailed due to fears of neurotoxicity.[66]

Although initially described as 'something to celebrate',[67] intrathecal neostigmine is associated with marked adverse effects including nausea and vomiting (16–67%), anxiety, somnolence and involuntary defaecation.[68,69] Further studies are required to discern whether the analgesic properties of neostigmine can be utilised, either in lower doses or in combination with other agents, without the adverse effects.

CONCOMITANT THROMBOPROPHYLAXIS

The use of concomitant anticoagulants and neuroaxial blocks has been an area of such concern that it was the subject of an entire journal supplement in the US recently.[70] The reason for this was a series of more than 40 epidural haematomas secondary to epidural anaesthesia with the use of higher doses of low molecular weight heparin (LMWH).[71] This has led to the establishment of guidelines for the use of LMWH in neuroaxial blocks,[70] similar to guidelines previously established in Germany, which are summarised below.[72]

1. NSAIDs or aspirin would appear safe on their own, but the risk is significantly increased when combined with heparins.

2. Warfarin should be considered an absolute contra-indication.

3. With low dose simple heparin (SH), there should be a minimal interval of 4 h between SH dose and neuroaxial block; there should then be a further 1 h before the next dose of SH.

4. Therapeutic anticoagulation with SH is an absolute contra-indication against use of neuraxial blocks. Catheter removal should be performed on patients receiving therapeutic doses of SH, when the SH was stopped for at least 4 h and appropriate laboratory tests had normalised.

5. Neuraxial blocks and catheter removal should not be performed within 12 h of LMWH administration and subsequent doses should not be given for at least a further 2 h after the procedure. There may also be an increased risk if dextrans are concomitantly used.

THE ACUTE PAIN SERVICE (APS)

In the 10 years since its inception, two different formats for acute pain teams have developed; these can be summarised in principle as anaesthetist-based and nurse-based. The former, which is based on the original service as described by Ready and colleagues, is now common in North America and Australasia.[1] The more common practice in Europe is a nurse-based, anaesthetist supervised service described by Rawal at the Orebro Medical Centre in Sweden.[73] The two forms of APS have developed simultaneously for various reasons including, responsibility, culture, cost, remuneration and accountability.

Although in both the UK[2] and also in Germany,[74] surgeons and anaesthetists orchestrated the original guidelines that proposed the setting up of an APS, most APS have been set up and run by anaesthetists. This can be clearly seen from a survey conducted in 1000 surgical units in Germany, where 99% of surgical departments had not established an APS, but 39% of their partners in anaesthesiology had done so.[75]

The role of the anaesthetist is pivotal. In the North American model, senior anaesthetists supervise more junior anaesthetists who manage the day-to-day functioning of the team, whereas in Europe they are more the adviser and teacher as well as the head of the team and exerting interdepartmental influence. The direct clinical role of the nurse specialist within the European model is often as a roving trouble-shooter, ensuring that PCAs and epidural blocks are being used effectively.

The objectives of the acute pain team are to: (i) prevent or minimise pain; (ii) facilitate the recovery process after surgery; (iii) avoid or effectively manage the side effects of therapy; and (iv) reduce or eliminate risk.[76] Achieving these objectives involves four steps.

PROMOTION OF PAIN ASSESSMENT

It has been demonstrated that nurses and doctors regularly under-estimate patients' pain.[77] There are several reasons for this. The most common reason is that patients are not asked directly about their pain. Any outside assessment will then only reflect the patient's level of distress, and people vary in the amount of distress they exhibit for a given amount of pain. Patients have a wide variability in their perceptions and expectations of analgesia and pain. It is, therefore, essential that pain assessment begins before surgery. Pre-operative assessments, by doctors and nurses, are a time to allay fear, anxiety and to explain and provide information about proposed analgesic regimens.[77]

The role of the nurse specialist is to ensure that ward staff make regular assessments of patients' pain scores, as well as nausea and sedation levels; these should then be recorded with the routine observations. It is worth remembering that, in the absence of formal documented pain assessment, many nurses will continue to believe that patients, who do not report pain, do not feel pain. However, these observations can be made using simple four point assessment scores. Although this process appears simple it has been shown to be one of the fundamentals to improving pain management.[78]

EDUCATION AND INFORMATION

The importance of education for staff and patients was illustrated in an audit at the Freeman Hospital in Newcastle, UK.[79] They showed that the appointment of a nurse specialist with a key role in pain assessment and education, resulted in a substantial improvement in the efficacy of analgesic regimens. The importance of on-going education cannot be overstated and, although it is time consuming, it is essential in maintaining standards. The nurse specialist has to provide regular tutorials for both ward and theatre nurses, as well as orientation programmes for new nurses, junior medical staff, physiotherapists and anaesthetists. They are often also involved in undergraduate education for various health care professionals. For the nursing staff, this should include basic pathophysiology and pharmacology, as well as discussion about protocols and analgesic equipment. The nurse specialist is also a provider of information; this can be direct verbal advise or by providing information on drugs and analgesic techniques. Written information should be available for ward staff and should also be handed out to patients.

STANDARDISATION OF METHODS AND PROVISION OF GUIDELINES

Standardisation of equipment, assessment charts and prescription guidelines minimises risk and enables training to be simple and reproducible. In a recent study by Harmer and colleagues, the processes of assessment, education and the provision of analgesic guidelines were shown to improve pain at rest and with movement.[78] They also showed an improvement in nausea and vomiting using the same process. The standard analgesic protocol used involved morphine or pethidine given intramuscularly every hour, regular assessment of pain, respiratory rate, blood pressure and sedation until pain was controlled. However, there is increasingly a move away from intramuscular injection to provide analgesia.[80] Analgesics should be given orally or, if this route is unavailable or the pain relief urgent, by intravenous titration. A standardised protocol has been used successfully in Auckland Hospital (New Zealand) for a number of years. It provides a standardised algorithm for nurses using similar doses and time constraints applicable to PCA, but with continuous assessment by the nurse until analgesia is provided.

Gould and colleagues showed that junior medical staff has a poor knowledge of analgesic regimens.[81] Here again, the provision of standardised guidelines by an APS increases safety and efficacy of analgesia.

AUDIT

Audit can be used in several ways:[79]

1. It can be used to ensure the effective use of analgesic tools, such as PCA, to enable limited resources to be targeted optimally.

2. Audit can also be used as part of the education process to demonstrate the effectiveness of regular pain assessment.

3. New protocols should always be audited before and after implementation.

4. Patients' understanding can be audited in order to direct written information to an appropriate level.

5. To justify the existence and the role of the pain team, and to highlight areas for future involvement.

CONCLUSIONS

Postoperative pain control progressed significantly since the first description of an acute pain service in 1988. Acute pain services are now a common feature of departments of anaesthesia all over the world. New techniques, such as PCA and continuous epidural analgesia, which were experimental then, are now well-established routine measures in many hospitals.

Despite these dramatic developments in little more than a decade, there is still much more to do. Future developments have to aim in two directions – spread of the currently available knowledge, techniques and organisational structures to all hospitals and improvement of these techniques and organisational structures. With regard to the first issue, it is of note, that despite all the data, guidelines and requirements stated by professional bodies, many hospitals have not yet developed policies on acute pain management, have not implemented policies they have, and have not established any organisational structures to provide postoperative pain relief on a hospital-wide basis. This deficit is not so much a result of lack of knowledge than of lack of commitment and needs to be overcome to improve the postoperative care of our patients.

With regard to future progress, the on-going research in physiology and pharmacology will yield new agents and new techniques to complement our

---

Key points for clinical practice

- Possible advances in the management of pain are to be expected with agents interfering with nerve growth factor, bradykinin and, possibly, nociceptin.

- Paracetamol is currently the non-opioid of first choice for acute pain management in view of its efficacy and minimal adverse effects.

- Tramadol offers a useful alternative to conventional opioids.

- There is no universally best opioid for use via patient controlled analgesia pumps; individualisation of drug choice might improve the side-effect profile of this technique.

- A combination of local anaesthetics and opioids provides the best compromise between high efficacy and low side-effect profile for epidural analgesia.

- Promotion of regular pain assessment is a fundamental step towards improvement of pain management on hospital wards.

- Provision of standardised guidelines by an Acute Pain Service increases safety and efficacy of pain management in the postoperative period.

- Future developments in acute pain management have to aim at spreading current knowledge and its application as well as at improving techniques, medications and organisational structures.

current armamentarium. The overall trend here goes towards a multimodal and multidisciplinary approach to postoperative care. Close co-operation of anaesthetists, surgeons, nurses, physiotherapists, pharmacists and others and integration of effective analgesia into a postoperative 'rehabilitation model' with early exercise and mobilisation and early enteral nutrition should lead to reduced hospital stay, improved outcome and reduced complications.[82]

REFERENCES

1. Ready LB, Oden R, Chadwick S et al. Development of an anesthesiology based acute pain service. Anesthesiology 1988: 68: 100–106.
2. The Royal College of Surgeons of England and The College of Anaesthetists. Report of the Working Party on Pain after Surgery. London: HMSO, 1990.
3. Dray A. Inflammatory mediators of pain. Br J Anaesth 1995; 75: 125–131.
4. Meyer RA, Campbell JN, Raja SN. In: Wall PD, Melzack R. (eds) Textbook of Pain, 3rd edn. Edinburgh: Churchill Livingstone, 1994; 13–44.
5. Rice ASC. Pathophysiology of acute pain. Acute Pain 1998; 1: 27–36.
6. Dickenson AH. Spinal cord pharmacology of pain. Br J Anaesth 1995; 75: 193–200.
7. McMahon SB, Dmitrieva N, Kolzenburg M. Visceral pain. Br J Anaesth 1995; 75: 132–144.
8. Annand P. Nerve growth factor regulates nociception in human health and disease. Br J Anaesth 1995; 75: 201–208.
9. Perkins MN, Campbell E, Dray A. Anti-nociceptive activity of B_1 and B_2 receptor antagonists des-Arg^{9}Leu^{8}Bk and HOE 140, in two models of persistent hyperalgesia in the rat. Pain 1993; 53: 191–197.
10. Darland T, Grandy DK. The orphanin FQ system: an emerging target for the management of pain? Br J Anaesth 1998; 81: 29–37.
11. Taylor F, Dickenson A. Nociceptin/orphanin FQ. A new opioid, a new analgesic? Neuroreport 1998; 12: R65–R70.
12. McQuay H, Moore A, Justins D. Treating acute pain in hospital. BMJ 1997; 314; 1531–1535.
13. McQuay H, Moore A. The concept of postoperative care. Curr Opin Anaesthesiol 1997; 10: 369–373.
14. Etches RC, Warriner CB, Basner N et al. Continuous intravenous administration of ketorolac reduces pain and morphine consumption after total hip or knee arthroplasty. Anesth Analg 1995; 81: 1175–1180.
15. Fredman B, Osfanger D, Jedeikin R. A comparative study of ketorolac and diclofenac on post laparoscopic cholecystectomy pain. Eur J Anaesthesiol 1995; 12: 501–504.
16. Dahl V, Raeder JC, Drosdal S, Wathne O, Brynildsrud J. Prophylactic oral ibuprofen-codeine versus placebo for postoperative pain after primary hip arthroplasty. Acta Anaesthesiol Scand 1995; 39: 323–326.
17. Moore A, McQuay H, Gavaghan D. Deriving dichotomous outcome measures from continuous data in randomised controlled trails of analgesics. Pain 1996; 66: 229–237.
18. Tramer M, Williams J, Carroll D, Wiffen PJ, Moore RA, McQuay HJ. Comparing the efficacy of non-steroidal anti-inflammatory drugs given by different routes in acute and chronic pain: a qualitative systematic review. Acta Anaesthesiol Scand 1998; 27: 466–475.
19. Strom BL, Taragin MI, Carson JL. Gastrointestinal bleeding from the non-steroidal anti-inflammatory drugs. Agents Actions 1990; 29 (Suppl): 27–38.
20. Merry AF, Holland RI, Middleton NG, Schug SA, Webster C. Peri-operative tenoxicam – safety and efficacy. A randomised controlled trial. Anaesth Intensive Care 1997; 25: 179.
21. Schug SA, Ritchie JE, Kanji K, Seay M. Evaluation of the use of sustained release morphine in subacute post-trauma pain. In: Abstracts 9th World Congress on Pain. Seattle: IASP Publications, 1999; 345.
22. Vickers MD. The efficacy of tramadol hydrochloride in the treatment of postoperative pain. Rev Contemp Pharmacother 1995; 6: 499–506.
23. Vickers MD, O'Flaherty D, Szekely SM, Read M, Yoshizumi J. Tramadol: pain relief by an opioid without depression of respiration. Anaesthesia 1992; 47: 291–296.

24. Tarradell R, Pol O, Farre M, Barrera E, Puig M. Respiratory and analgesic effects of meperidine and tramadol in patients undergoing orthopaedic surgery. Methods Find Exp Clin Pharmacol 1996; 18: 211–218.

25. Houmes R, Voets MA, Verkaaik A, Erdman W, Lachmann B. Efficacy and safety of tramadol versus morphine for moderate and severe postoperative pain with special regard to respiratory depression. Anesth Analg 1992; 74: 510–514.

26. Langford RM, Bakhshi KN, Moylan S, Forster JM. Hypoxaemia after lower abdominal surgery: comparison of tramadol and morphine. Acute Pain 1998; 1: 7–12.

27. Moore A, McQuay H. Single-patient data meta-analysis of 3453 postoperative patients: oral tramadol versus placebo, codeine, and combination analgesics. Pain 1997; 67: 287–294.

28. Sunshine A, Olson NZ, Zighelboim I, DeCastro A, Minn FL. Analgesic oral efficacy of tramadol hydrochloride in postoperative pain. Clin Pharmacol Ther 1992; 51: 740–746.

29. Putland AJ, McCluskey A. The analgesic efficacy of tramadol versus ketorolac in day-case laparoscopic sterilisation. Anaesthesia 1999; 54: 382–385.

30. Lehmann KA. Update of patient controlled analgesia. Curr Opin Anaesthesiol 1997; 10: 374–379.

31. Sidebotham D, Dijkhuizen MR, Schug SA. The safety and utilisation of patient controlled analgesia. J Pain Symptom Manage 1997; 14: 202–209.

32. Woodhouse A, Hobbes AF, Mather AE et al. A comparison of morphine, pethidine and fentanyl in the postsurgical patient controlled analgesia environment. Pain 1996; 64: 115–121.

33. Peng WH, Sandler AN. A review of the use of fentanyl analgesia in the management of pain in adults. Anesthesiology 1990; 90: 576–599.

34. Hopkins D, Shipton EA, Potgieter D et al. Comparison of tramadol and morphine via subcutaneous PCA following orthopaedic surgery. Can J Anaesth 1998; 45: 435–442.

35. Stamer UM, Maier C, Grond S, Veh-Schmidt B, Klaschik E, Lehmann KA. Tramadol in the management of postoperative pain: a double-blind, placebo- and active drug controlled study. Eur J Anaesthesiol 1997; 14: 646–654.

36. Schug SA, Fry RA. Continuous regional analgesia in comparison with intravenous opioid administration for routine postoperative pain control. Anaesthesia 1994; 49: 528–532.

37. Schug SA, Sidebotham DA, McGuinnety M, Thomas J, Fox L. Acetaminophen as an adjunct to morphine by patient controlled analgesia in the management of acute postoperative pain. Anesth Analg 1998; 87: 368–372.

38. Park J, Forrest J, Kolesar R, Bhola D, Beattie S, Chu C. Oral clonidine reduces postoperative PCA morphine requirements. Can J Anaesth 1996; 43: 900–906.

39. Gilliland HEM, Prasad BK, Mirakur RK, Fee JPH. An investigation into the potential morphine sparing effects of midazolam. Anaesthesia 1996; 51: 808–811.

40. Roytblat L, Korotkoruchko A, Katz J, Glazer M, Greemberg L, Fisher A. Postoperative pain: the effect of low dose ketamine in addition to general anaesthesia. Anesth Analg 1993; 77: 1161–1165.

41. Fu ES, Miguel R, Scharf JE. Pre-emptive ketamine decreases postoperative narcotic requirements in patients under going abdominal surgery. Anesth Analg 1997; 84: 1088–1090.

42. Javery KB, Ussery TW, Steger HG, Colclough GW. Comparison of morphine and morphine with ketamine for postoperative analgesia. Am J Anesth 1996; 43: 212–215.

43. Gan TJ, Ginsberg B, Gass PS, Fortney J, Jhaveri R, Perno R. Opioid sparing effects of low dose naloxone, in patient administered morphine sulphate. Anesthesiology 1997; 87: 1075–1081.

44. Klahsen AJ, O'Reilly D, McBride J, Ballentyne M, Parlow JL. Reduction in postoperative nausea and vomiting with combination of morphine and droperidol in patient controlled analgesia. Can J Anaesth 1996; 43: 1100–1107.

45. Shen Q, Schug SA, Ritchie J, Thomas JM, Sidebotham DA. Dose finding study on droperidol as an adjunct to morphine via PCA to reduce postoperative nausea and vomiting. In: Abstracts 9th World Congress on Pain. Seattle: IASP Publications, 1999; 78.

46. Liu SS, Allen HW, Olsson GL. Patient controlled epidural analgesia with bupivacaine and fentanyl on hospital wards. Prospective experience with 1030 surgical patients. Anesthesiology 1998; 88: 688–695.

47. Brodner G, Podgatzki E, Wempe H, Van Aken H. Patientenkontrollierte post-operative Epiduralanalgesie. Prospektiver Befund in 1799 Patienten. Anaesthesist 1997; 46 (Suppl 3): S165–S171.

48. Zaric D, Nydahl PA, Philipson L, Samuelsson L, Heierson A, Axelsson K. The effect of continuous infusions of ropivacaine (0.1%, 0.2%, and 0.3%) and 0.25% bupivacaine on sensory and motor block in volunteers: a double blind study. Reg Anesth 1996; 21: 14–25.

49. Muldoon T, Milligan K, Quinn P, Connolly DC, Nilsson K. Comparison between extradural infusion of ropivacaine or bupivacaine for the prevention of postoperative pain after total knee arthroplasty. Br J Anaesth 1998; 80: 680–681.

50. Reiz S, Haggmark S, Johansson G, Nath S. Cardiotoxicity of ropivacaine – a new amide local anaesthetic. Acta Anaesthesiol Scand 1989; 33: 93–98.

51. Scott DA, Emanuelsson B-M, Mooney PH, Cook RJ. Pharmacokinetics and efficacy of long-term epidural ropivacaine infusion for postoperative analgesia. Anesth Analg 1997; 85: 1322–1330.

52. Sidebotham DA, Russell K, Dijkhuizen MR, Tester P, Schug SA. Low dose fentanyl improves continuous bupivacaine epidural analgesia following orthopaedic, urological or general surgery. Acute Pain 1997; 1: 27–32.

53. de Leon-Casasola OA, Lema MJ. Postoperative epidural opioid analgesia: what are the choices? Anesth Analg 1996; 83: 867–875.

54. Samso E, Valles J, Pol O, Gallert L, Puig MM. Comparative assessment of the anesthetic and analgesic effects of intramuscular and epidural clonidine in humans. Can J Anaesth 1996; 43: 1195–1202.

55. De Kock M, Wiederkher P, Laghmiche A, Scholtes JL. Epidural clonidine used as the sole analgesic agent during and after abdominal surgery. Anesthesiology 1997; 86: 285–292.

56. Paech MJ, Pavy TJ, Orlikowski CE, Lim W, Evans SF. Postoperative epidural infusion: a randomised, double-blind, dose-finding trial of clonidine in combination with bupivacaine and fentanyl. Anesth Analg 1997; 84: 1323–1328.

57. Malinovsky JM, Cozian A, Lepage JY, Mussini JM, Pinaud M, Souron R. Ketamine and midazolam neurotoxicity in the rabbit. Anesthesiology 1991; 79: 105–111.

58. Bjorgberg FM, Svensson BA, Frigast C, Gordh Jr T. Histopathology after repeated intrathecal injections of preservative-free ketamine in the rabbit: a light and electron microscope examination. Anesth Analg 1994; 79: 105–111.

59. Wong CS, Liaw WJ, Tung CS, Su YF, Ho ST. Ketamine potentiates analgesic effect of morphine in postoperative epidural pain control. Reg Anesth 1996; 21: 534–541.

60. Shigihara A, Suzuki M, Kumada Y, Akama Y, Tase C, Okuaki A. Use of ketamine combined with local anesthetics in epidural anesthesia. Masui 1995; 44: 538–587.

61. Choe H, Choi YS, Kim YM et al. Epidural morphine plus ketamine for upper abdominal surgery: improved analgesia from preincisional versus postincisional administration. Anesth Analg 1997; 84: 560–563.

62. Rawal N. Spinal opioids. Curr Opin Anaesthesiol 1997; 10: 350–355.

63. Milner AR, Bogod DG, Harwood RJ. Intrathecal administration of morphine for elective Caesarean section: a comparison between 0.1 mg and 0.2 mg. Anaesthesia 1996; 51: 871–873.

64. Gwirtz K, Young JV, Byers RS et al. The safety and efficacy of intrathecal opioid analgesia for acute postoperative pain: seven years' experience with 5969 surgical patients at Indiana University Hospital. Anesth Analg 1999; 88: 599–604.

65. Goodchild CS, Noble J. The effects of intrathecal midazolam on sympathetic nervous system reflexes in man – a pilot study. Br J Clin Pharmacol 1987; 23: 279–285.

66. Svensson BA, Welin M, Gordh Jr T, Westman J. Chronic subarachnoid midazolam in the rat. Morphologic evidence of spinal cord neurotoxicity. Reg Anesth 1995; 20: 426–434.

67. Collins JG, Spinally administered neostigmine – something to celebrate. Anesthesiology 1995; 82: 327–328.

68. Buerkle H, Yang LC. The novel analgesic neostigmine and the morning after: nothing more than sedation, nausea and vomiting. Acute Pain 1999; 2: 41–46.

69. Klamt JG, Garcia LV, Prado WA. Analgesic and adverse effects of a low dose of intrathecally administered hyperbaric neostigmine alone or combined with morphine in patients submitted to spinal anaesthesia: a pilot study. Anaesthesia 1999; 54: 27–31.

70. Neuraxial Anesthesia and Anticoagulation. Reg Anesth Pain Med 1998; 23 (Suppl. 2): 129–193.

71. Horlocker TT, Wedel DJ. Neuroaxial block and low-molecular-weight-heparin: balancing perioperative analgesia and thromboprophylaxis. Reg Anesth Pain Med 1998; 23 (Suppl. 2): 164–177.

72. Tryba M. European practice guidelines: thromboembolism prophylaxis and regional anesthesia. Reg Anesth Pain Med 1998; 23 (Suppl. 2): 178–182.

73. Rawal N. Acute pain services should be nurse-based. Acute Pain 1997; 1: 50–52.

74. Practice guidelines for the management of acute pain. Task force on acute pain management of the German Societies of Anaesthesiologists and Surgeons. Stuttgart: Thième 1997.

75. Neugebauer E, Hemple K, Sauerland S, Lempa M, Koch G. The status of perioperative pain therapy in Germany. Results of a representative, anonymous survey of 1000 surgical clinics. Chirurg 1998; 69: 461–466.

76. Ferguson J. The development of a postoperative pain service (1): an overview. Br J Theatre Nurs 1995; 5: 28–31.

77. Field L. Are nurses still underestimating patients' pain postoperatively? Br J Nurs 1996; 5: 778–784.

78. Hamer M, Davies KA. The effect of education, assessment and a standardised prescription on postoperative pain management. Anaesthesia 1998; 53: 424–430.

79. Coleman SA, Booker-Milburn J. Audit of postoperative pain control. Influence of a dedicated acute pain nurse. Anaesthesia 1996; 51: 1093–1096.

80. Schug SA. Intramuscular opioids – the slow extinction of a dinosaur. Acute Pain 1999; 2: 56–58.

81. Gould TH, Upton PM, Collins P. A survey of the intended management of acute postoperative pain by newly qualified doctors in the South West region of England in August 1992. Anaesthesia 1994; 49: 807–810.

82. Wulf H, Schug SA, Allvin R, Kehlet H. Postoperative patient management – how can we make progress? Acute Pain 1998; 1: 32–44.

Christian Werner Kristin Engelhard

CHAPTER 5

Cerebral resuscitation: current concepts and perspectives

Cerebral ischaemia and/or hypoxia may occur as a consequence of shock, vascular stenosis or occlusion, vasospasm, neurotrauma, and cardiac arrest. The ischaemic/hypoxic insult evokes a cascade of pathophysiological processes which will result in neuronal death. The first level of the ischaemic cascade is the accumulation of lactic acid due to anaerobic glycolysis. This leads to increased membrane permeability and consecutive oedema formation. Since anaerobic metabolism is inadequate to maintain cellular energy states, the ATP stores deplete and failure of energy-dependent membrane ion pumps occurs. At the second stage of the ischaemic cascade, terminal membrane depolarization along with excessive release of excitatory neurotransmitters (i.e. glutamate, aspartate), activation of NMDA- (N-methyl-D-aspartate), AMPA- (α-amino-3-hydroxy-5-methyl-4-isoxazolpropionate), and voltage-dependent Ca^{2+}- and Na^+-channels. The consequent Ca^{2+} and Na^+ influx leads to catabolic intracellular processes. Ca^{2+} activates lipid peroxidases, proteases, and phospholipases which in turn increase the intracellular concentration of free fatty acids (FFA) and free radicals. Additionally, activation of caspases (ICE-like proteins), translocases, and endonucleases initiate progressive structural changes to biological membranes and the nucleosomal DNA (DNA fragmentation, inhibition of DNA repair). Together, these events lead to membrane degeneration of vascular and cellular structures and consequent necrosis or programmed cell death (apoptosis).

The strategies to protect the brain from ischaemic/hypoxic insults are based on the understanding of these pathophysiological processes. Maintenance of normal to high cerebral perfusion pressure, normoxia, and surgical decompression are by far the most important and effective neuroprotective

Professor Christian Werner, Professor of Anaesthesiology, Klinikum rechts der Isar, Klinik für Anaesthesiologie, Technische Universität München, Ismaninger Strasse 22, D-81675 München, Germany (for correspondence)
Dr Kristin Engelhard, Resident in Anaesthesiology, Klinikum rechts der Isar, Klinik für Anaesthesiologie, Technische Universität München, Ismaninger Strasse 22, D-81675 München, Germany

interventions. Besides these treatment modalities, concepts of physical and pharmacological brain protection include interventions to increase cerebral blood flow (CBF) in the ischaemic territory, reduction of cerebral metabolism and intracranial pressure (ICP), inhibition of lactic acid accumulation and excitatory neurotransmitter activity, prevention of Ca^{2+}-influx, inhibition of lipid peroxidation, and free radical scavenging.

PHYSICAL NEUROPROTECTION

MANAGEMENT OF CEREBRAL PERFUSION PRESSURE (CPP)

Two different approaches in the management of CPP attempt to maintain cerebral perfusion at a level adequate to fuel cerebral metabolic needs. Although both of these concepts differ with respect to the level of CPP, either of them may be appropriate depending of the individual status of CBF autoregulation and the blood–brain barrier.

Cascade of cerebral vasodilation and vasoconstriction ('Rosner concept', 'Edinburgh concept')

Studies in patients with severe head injury have shown that hypotension and low CPP are important factors in the generation of secondary insults. For example, the incidence, severity, and duration of arterial hypotension or CPP < 80 mmHg significantly increased morbidity and mortality in these patients. The CPP approach requires intact cerebrovascular autoregulation in order to induce autoregulatory vasoconstriction for ICP control (i.e. as autoregulation is intact, elevations in CPP will produce autoregulatory vasoconstriction to maintain CBF normal while reducing intracranial blood volume and thus ICP; 'Rosner concept'). This concept also applies to patients with a shift of the autoregulatory curve towards higher pressures (i.e. with 'normal' CPP these patients present pressure-passive perfusion while elevations in CPP return their pressure-flow relationship into the autoregulatory range; 'Edinburgh concept'). These considerations are consistent with data in head injured patients showing fewer events with critical intracranial hypertension (plateau waves) as long a CPP was maintained with the range of 75–95 mmHg.[1]

Treatment of post-traumatic brain oedema formation ('Lund concept')

This approach assumes defective blood–brain barrier and cerebrovascular autoregulation. As a consequence, the Lund concept targets at low precapillary hydrostatic pressures and cerebral venous constriction to reduce oedema formation and elevated cerebral blood volume by infusion of: (i) dihydro-ergotamine (DHE); (ii) the α_2-agonist clonidine and the β_1-antagonist metoprolol; and (iii) normalization of colloidosmotic pressure (plasma albumin concentration >40 g/l). Although there may be subgroups of patients that benefit from a reduction in precapillary hydrostatic pressure along with cerebral venous constriction, there are currently no convincing data that support improved outcome with the 'Lund concept'.[2,3]

Based on this analysis, it is currently believed that stabilization of CPP within the range of 65–70 mmHg by means of sedation, osmodiuretics (*see below*), normovolaemia, and vasopressors will improve neurological outcome following cerebral ischaemia.

HYPERVENTILATION

Therapeutic hyperventilation is part of the traditional concept to reduce intracranial pressure in mechanically ventilated patients. Hyperventilation is supposed to reduce secondary brain injury by the following mechanisms: (i) increasing the extracellular and intracellular pH; (ii) increasing perfusion to ischaemic territories by redistribution of blood (inverse steal effect); and (iii) reduction of cerebral blood volume and intracranial pressure.

During ischaemia, neuronal acidosis occurs as a function of anaerobic glycolysis with accumulation of lactic acid. Hyperventilation produces respiratory compensation of ischaemic acidosis. However, respiratory alkalosis is only effective for a period of less than 24 h due to compensatory loss of bicarbonate ions.[4] Additionally, hyperventilation to $PaCO_2$ values < 25 mmHg (3.3 kPa) increases the extent of ischaemia. Together, there is no experimental or clinical evidence which supports the use of hyperventilation to decrease infarct size and improve neurological outcome by this mechanism.

Hyperventilation may theoretically improve perfusion in ischaemic territories by hypocapnic vasoconstriction in non-ischaemic tissues (inverse steal effect). This hypothesis is based on observational reports indicating recovery of the EEG or cerebral perfusion with hyperventilation.[5] In contrast, controlled experimental and clinical studies suggest that hypocapnic vasoconstriction increases, rather than decreases, the degree of cerebral ischaemia.[4,6] This indicates that hypocapnic cerebrovascular constriction is ineffective in redistributing perfusion in favour of ischaemic territories and may even aggravate neuronal injury.

In patients with transient but critical elevations of intracranial pressure (e.g. plateau waves), acute hyperventilation ($PaCO_2$ = 30–34 mmHg [4.0–4.5 kPa]) still represents a life-saving treatment until more specific interventions will reduce the intracranial hypertension. With recovery of intracranial pressure, hyperventilation must be carefully reversed to maintain normocapnia ($PaCO_2$ = 36–40 mmHg [4.8–.5.3 kPa]). In contrast, prophylactic hyperventilation has adverse effects on outcome in patients with head injury as hypocapnic vasoconstriction further reduces CBF and worsens outcome despite decreases in ICP. However, hyperventilation may be beneficial in patients with relative or absolute hyperaemia.[7,8] As a consequence, monitoring of the CBF or the balance between O_2 demand and O_2 supply is necessary to identify the proper ventilation pattern in the individual patient. Chronic hyperventilation to $PaCO_2$ values <30 mmHg (4.0 kPa) is never indicated even in the presence of permanent intracranial hypertension, as this concept does not reduce intracranial pressure over time but may worsen neurological outcome in patients with head injury.[8]

HYPOTHERMIA

Recent interest in thermal interventions is related to the cerebral effects of moderate (29–32°C) and mild hypothermia (33–36°C). This is due to observations in laboratory animals and humans showing neuronal protection with small reductions in brain temperature during increased ICP and cerebral ischaemia. It has been suggested that hypothermic protection is related to suppression of major biochemical processes such as decreases in cerebral metabolism, reduction of excitatory neurotransmitter release, and inhibition of accumulation of lipid peroxidation products and free radical generation. Other studies indicate that small changes in temperature economize CBF and prevent postischaemic hyper- and hypoperfusion and formation of brain oedema.

HYPOTHERMIA AND EXPERIMENTAL NEUROPROTECTION

In rats, hypothermia (33–30°C) induced during focal or global cerebral ischaemia with reperfusion produced decreases in infarct size and improved neurological outcome in a temperature-dependent fashion. In contrast, hypothermia was not protective during permanent focal ischaemia.[9]

In a cardiac resuscitation model, histopathological damage was reduced with mild (34°C) or moderate hypothermia (32–30°C); however, deep hypothermia (28–15°C) did not improve neurological outcome due to the generation of toxic metabolites and myocardial depression.[10] This suggests a temperature threshold below which there will be no beneficial effect of hypothermia in the setting of cerebral ischaemia.

In rats subjected to focal cerebral ischaemia, postischaemic hypothermia (34°C) reduced infarct size and improved neurological outcome.[11] Similarly, hypothermia (34°C) induced immediately following cardiopulmonary resuscitation and maintained for 1 h effectively reduced histopathological and functional damage. In rats and dogs subjected to a fluid percussion injury or epidural compression, post-traumatic moderate hypothermia (31–30°C) reduced mortality and improved neurofunctional behaviour in surviving animals.[12] However, neuroprotection occurred only if hypothermia was initiated within a time window of 15–90 min after the insult.

HYPOTHERMIA AND CLINICAL NEUROPROTECTION

Between 1958 and 1962, several studies in patients with severe head injury investigated the effects of mild to moderate hypothermia (28–34°C within the first 12–24 h following trauma for a period of 2–10 days). In these studies, mortality was 43–72% and the majority of deaths occurred during rewarming. Despite the subjective impression of neuronal protection by hypothermia, no conclusion could be drawn from these investigations due to the lack of control patients. More recently, phase I and II studies in patients following head injury, cardiac arrest, and stroke suggest that neurological deficit and mortality are significantly reduced when mild to moderate hypothermia is induced within 6–24 h following the insult and maintained for 24–48 h.[13–17] While multicentre trials on the effects of therapeutic hypothermia following stroke, cardiac arrest, and during cerebral aneurysm surgery are currently in process, the promising phase II results in head injured patients were not confirmed by a prospective, controlled, randomized phase III investigation. In that study, neurological outcome was not improved by mild or moderate hypothermia irrespective of Glasgow coma scale on admission.[18] In order to use therapeutic hypothermia properly in patients with acute cerebrovascular disorders, the following factors need to be defined: (i) timing of initiation of hypothermia; (ii) optimal temperature; (iii) duration of hypothermia; and (iv) the optimal regimen of rewarming. While the beneficial effects of hypothermia remain unclear in humans, hyperthermia must be treated aggressively in patients with cerebral ischaemia.[19]

SURGICAL DECOMPRESSION

Rapid evacuation of epidural, subdural, or parenchymal mass lesions is an effective and causal intervention in the treatment of secondary insults. Additionally, decompressive craniectomy for refractory intracranial hypertension following head injury, cardiopulmonary resuscitation, or stroke may be considered as an option. Observational studies using historical controls from the Traumatic Coma Data Bank suggest that wide bilateral decompressive frontotemporoparietal craniectomy combined with dura patch–plasty reduces mortality and improves neurological outcome, particularly in younger patients. While surgical decompression is currently ranked as a second tier treatment, along with forced hyperventilation or hypothermia, protagonists of this technique suggest surgery at an early stage in order to avoid ischaemic neuronal injury from sustained intracranial hypertension.[20,21]

PHARMACOLOGICAL BRAIN PROTECTION

ANAESTHETICS

The proposed mechanisms of anaesthetic protection include reduction of cerebral metabolism, and ICP, suppression of seizures and sympathetic discharge, and a reset of thermoregulatory threshold. Additionally, anaesthetics may reduce intracellular Ca^{2+} and free radical accumulation. However, the clinical and experimental data remain controversial.

VOLATILE ANAESTHETICS

Isoflurane, sevoflurane and desflurane produce maximum cerebral metabolic suppression in parallel at concentrations >2 MAC end-tidal. This effect suggests that volatile anaesthetics may correct for the imbalance between oxygen supply and demand during focal cerebral ischaemia. Animal studies with focal or incomplete hemispheric ischaemia have shown that isoflurane, sevoflurane, and desflurane may decrease infarct size and improve neurological outcome when given prior to the ischaemic challenge.[22,23] These experimental data are consistent with studies in sevoflurane anaesthetized patients undergoing carotid endarterectomy showing increased tolerance to lower levels of cerebral blood flow with preserved neuronal function during carotid cross clamping when compared to halothane, enflurane or isoflurane background anaesthesia.[24] In contrast, volatile anaesthetics have no neuroprotective properties in the setting of global cerebral ischaemia and when given after the insult.

HYPNOTICS

Studies in laboratory animals have shown that barbiturates as well as propofol reduce infarct size and improve neurological outcome following focal or incomplete global cerebral ischaemia as long as physiological variables were controlled during the experiments.[25] While experimental data support the preventive neuroprotective effects of hypnotic agents, the clinical evidence is less convincing. In patients undergoing cardiac surgery with normothermic cardiopulmonary bypass, the infusion of thiopentone (total dose during extra-corporeal circulation (ECC) = 39.5 ± 8.4 mg/kg, i.v.) was able to reduce postoperative neuropsychological deficits.[26] In contrast, barbiturates infused to comatose patients within the first hour following cardiopulmonary resuscitation were ineffective in reducing mortality as well as neurological deficits in survivors compared to standard ICU treatment.[27] These data are consistent with the view that the infusion of hypnotics prior to focal, but not global, ischaemic insults may increase the ischaemic tolerance of neurones. Barbiturates may be also beneficial in patients with severe head injury and refractory intracranial hypertension. This conclusion is related to a series of clinical studies where infusion of barbiturates was effective in reducing intracranial pressure, and likely the mortality rate, following brain trauma as long as systemic haemodynamic stability was maintained.[28] More recently, propofol was suggested as an alternative to barbiturates in patients undergoing cardiac surgery or for sedation following head injury due to a favourable context-sensitive half-time. While propofol did not reduce neuropsychological deficits following cardiac valve surgery compared to sufentanil anaesthetised patients, it turned out to be more effective in treating elevated ICP with a similar neurological outcome following head injury when compared to an opioid-based sedative regimen.[29,30]

OSMODIURETICS

Mannitol is an osmodiuretic agent which decreases ICP, increases CPP, and improves CBF in laboratory animals and humans. These effects are related to plasma expansion with consequent reduction in haematocrit, plasma viscosity, and cerebral blood volume as well as mobilization of extracellular fluids along the osmotic gradient. Treatment of intracranial hypertension using mannitol in concentrations of 0.25–1 g/kg (maximum = 4 g/kg/day) is more effective than the infusion of barbiturates. Likewise, bolus administration, rather than continuous or prophylactic infusion as part of a rigid algorithm, is recommended to control ICP.[31,32] Since acute tubular necrosis may occur in response to rapid changes in the osmotic gradient, plasma osmolarity must be monitored and should not exceed 320 mOsmol/l. Any concern with respect to rebound effects of mannitol (i.e. accumulation of mannitol within the extracellular space) appear to be relevant only with a defective blood–brain barrier or duration of treatment > 4 days. Nevertheless, mannitol can be used beyond these end-points as long as critical elevations of ICP remain osmosensitive.

As an alternative, hypertonic saline (7.5%) may be used to control ICP. In patients with multiple injuries, hypertonic saline used as 'small volume resuscitation' increases arterial blood pressure in parallel to decreases in ICP.[33] Currently, hypertonic saline represents an option, rather than a standard, in the treatment of elevated ICP due to lack of convincing clinical data showing superiority over mannitol.

PLASMA GLUCOSE CONCENTRATION

Studies in laboratory animals and humans have shown that hyperglycaemia is associated with worsened outcome following stroke or neurotrauma. The mechanisms by which normoglycaemia may protect neuronal tissue include decreases in intracellular lactic acidosis along with decreases in membrane permeability and reduced oedema of endothelial cells, neuroglia, and neurones.[34] As a consequence, plasma glucose concentrations should be assayed every 2 h and maintained within the range of 100–150 mg/dl.

Ca^{2+} CHANNEL BLOCKERS

Ca^{2+} may enter the intracellular space by action of agonist controlled Ca^{2+} channels (e.g. glutamate, NMDA) or by activation of presynaptic voltage-dependent L-, T-, N-, P-, and Q-type Ca^{2+} channels with consequent release of excitatory neurotransmitters, nitric oxide, and activation of intracellular catabolic processes. The proposed mechanisms of neuronal protection by Ca^{2+} channel blockers include cerebral vasodilation, prevention of vasospasm, reduced Ca^{2+} influx and modulation of free fatty acid metabolism. Unfortunately, the results in animal models are rather contradictory. While several studies found decreases in neuronal injury and improved outcome following focal ischaemia, others have failed to produce protection with Ca^{2+} channel blockers. Only the N-type Ca^{2+} antagonist, SNX-111, an ω-conopeptide, was neuroprotective in animal models of focal and global cerebral ischaemia even when infused within 24 h following the insult.[35]

Clinical trials have tested the neuroprotective effects of the L-type Ca^{2+} channel blocker nimodipine in patients with acute ischaemic stroke and aneurysmatic or traumatic subarachnoid haemorrhage. According to a meta-analysis of 9 placebo-controlled trials with a total of 3700 patients with acute stroke, oral administration of nimodipine appears to be associated with a favourable outcome as long as the treatment commences within the first 12 h following the onset of the symptoms.[36] This is consistent with the results from a meta-analysis of 8 placebo-controlled studies in 1202 patients with aneurysmatic subarachnoid haemorrhage demonstrating a better chance to develop a favourable outcome with the prophylactic administration of nimodipine and reduced incidence of cerebral vasospasm.[37] Patients with traumatic subarachnoid haemorrhage may also benefit from the infusion of nimodipine.[38] However, Ca^{2+} channel blockers may induce arterial hypotension below the individual ischaemic threshold of the patients and any relevant decrease in arterial blood pressure will reverse any potentially neuroprotective effects of the intended treatment.

NMDA RECEPTOR ANTAGONISTS

Glutamate and aspartate are known as excitatory neurotransmitters which stimulate N-methyl-D-aspartate receptors (NMDA; Ca^{2+} and Na^+ influx). Since the activation of these receptors initiates catabolic intracellular processes, blockade of NMDA-receptors may protect cerebral tissue.

Ketamine, MK-801 (dizocilpine), aptiganel, dextromethorphan, dextrorphan, and Mg^{2+} represent non-competitive NMDA receptor antagonists. In animal models of focal (but not global) cerebral ischaemia and head injury, ketamine as well as MK-801 reduced neuronal injury and improved outcome.[39] Likewise, infusion of the competitive NMDA receptor antagonist CGS 19755 (selfotel) reduced infarct size following focal and global ischaemia. Clinical trials using MK-801 were terminated due to toxic side-effects and the induction of mitochondrial vacuolization. The clinical development of the antitussive agents, dextromethorphan and dextrorphan, was also terminated because of side-effects such as hallucination, agitation, and sedation. Clinical phase III trials in patients with acute stroke and head injury using aptiganel (Cerestat, CNS-1102) are currently in process, but the safety committee has indicated major concern because of the induction of severe hallucinations with this NMDA receptor blocker. Four clinical trials in patients with acute stroke or head injury were also prematurely terminated because of adverse effects with the competitive NMDA receptor antagonist CGS 19755 (selfotel).[40] The anti-epileptic drug, remacemide, is the only NMDA receptor antagonist with proven neuroprotective efficacy. In patients undergoing coronary artery bypass surgery, the peri-operative administration of remacemide significantly reduced postoperative neuropsychological deficits along with some dizziness as the only relevant side-effect.[41]

GLUCOCORTICOIDS

The proposed mechanisms by which glucocorticoids reduce neuronal injury include increased order of lipid bilayers, free radical scavenging, and prevention of free fatty acid accumulation by inhibition of lipid peroxidation. Studies in patients with acute stroke or following cardiac arrest could not demonstrate a significant reduction in infarct size or improvement in neuro-logical outcome with the infusion of glucocorticoids (e.g. dexamethasone or methylprednisolone) despite some positive effects in experimental prepar-ations. Likewise, controlled clinical trials could not exclude moderate bene-ficial nor moderate harmful effects in patients with head injury receiving either dexamethasone or methylprednisolone.[42] However, rather than generally banning these agents, it is likely that subgroups among patients with acute ischaemic or traumatic brain lesions exist who may improve from lipid peroxidase inhibition. In contrast to stroke or head injury, infusion of methyl-prednisolone (30 mg/kg bolus; 5.4 mg/kg/day within 3 h from injury or 30 mg/kg bolus; 5.4 mg/kg/2 days within 3–8 h from injury) following spinal cord injury may reduce motor deficit and improve function of sensory tracts.[43,44]

21-AMINOSTEROIDS

Tirilazad mesylat (U-74006F) is a potent inhibitor of oxygen free radical-induced lipid peroxidation. Most of the laboratory investigations have shown that tirilazad reduces infarct size and improves neurological outcome in models of transient or permanent focal or global cerebral ischaemia even when infused after the insult.[45] In contrast, phase III clinical trials in patients with acute stroke, subarachnoid haemorrhage, and head injury failed to confirm the experimental neuroprotective evidence.[46–48]

FREE RADICAL SCAVENGERS

During ischaemia and reperfusion, molecular oxygen is reduced to the following oxidants: superoxide radicals, hydrogen peroxides, and hydroxyl radicals. Oxygen free radicals represent a highly reactive species which rapidly interact with cellular membranes, nuclear acids, receptors, and enzymes and induce lysis in these structures. Superoxide dismutase (SOD) is a physiological free radical scavenger which exists in two isoforms: cytosolic copper-zinc-SOD and mitochondrial manganese-SOD. Studies in cell cultures and transgenic mice overexpressing SOD have shown that SOD produces a maximum reduction in cellular oxidative stress. Unfortunately, SOD has an extremely low penetration through the blood–brain barrier and cellular membranes. Consequently, SOD was conjugated with polyethylene-glycol (PEG) to enhance its bioavailability. In patients with severe head injury (phase II trial), PEG-SOD reduced mortality when given in high concentrations. However, a subsequent phase III trial in 463 head-injured patients failed to confirm the neuroprotective effects of PEG-SOD.[49] In patients with aneurysmatic subarachnoid haemorrhage (phase III trial), the hydroxyl-scavenger AVS (nicaraven) reduced neurological deficits.[50]

FUTURE CONCEPTS

NITRIC OXIDE

Nitric oxide (NO) is a molecular messenger contributing to a variety of intra-, extra-, and intercellular processes.[51,52] NO occurs as a by-product during the conversion of L-arginine to citrulline by the enzyme NO-synthase (NOS). Three isoforms of NOS have been identified: constitutive NOS-isoforms I (neuronal NOS, nNOS) and III (endothelial NOS, eNOS) are present in neurones, astrocytes, perivascular nerve fibres, and endothelial cells. The inducible isoform NOS II (immunological NOS, iNOS) is present at least in macrophages. NO is a diffusible, highly reactive molecule with a half-life in the order of few seconds. During hypoxic ischaemic conditions, NO exerts positive as well as negative effects on neuronal functions and structure. NO increases CBF and inhibits platelet and neutrophil aggregation, and the release of glutamate. However, NO is cytotoxic by inhibition of mitochondrial enzymes, DNA trauma, and formation of peroxynitrites, hydroxyl radicals and nitrogen dioxide. Experiments in nNO knock-out mice found a substantial reduction in infarct size following focal cerebral ischaemia compared to wild-type mice. In contrast, infarct size was increased in eNOS knock-out animals. As a consequence, designing drugs that selectively stimulate eNOS while inhibiting nNOS should increase the ischaemic tolerance of neuronal tissue.[52]

POLYMORPHONUCLEAR LEUKOCYTES

Cerebral ischaemia and reperfusion are associated with inflammatory responses, such as chemotaxis of polymorphonuclear leukocytes, with mechanical obstruction of the microcirculation and direct toxic effects to the endothelial cells and neurones. Adhesion of polymorphonuclear leukocytes is triggered by vascular (VCAM) and intercellular (ICAM) adhesion molecules secondary to an increase in the concentration of tumour necrosis factor, interleukins and exotoxins. Inhibition of VCAM and ICAM reduced infarct size in animals subjected to focal ischaemia and reperfusion.[53] Therefore, selective inhibition of mechanisms known to trigger the activity of polymorphonuclear leukocytes may produce clinically relevant neuroprotection in the future.

PROGRAMMED CELL DEATH (APOPTOSIS)

Following severe hypoxia and ischaemia, neurones may die from necrosis (cellular swelling, loss of mitochondrial membrane potential and ATP production, lysis of biological membranes with consequent uptake of cellular debris by macrophages). If the tissue is exposed to a lesser degree of hypoxia and ischaemia, initiation of a cellular suicide programme may occur leading to delayed neuronal death (apoptosis).[54] In the initial stage of programmed cell death, apoptotic neurones do not show histopathological evidence for neuronal disintegration and provide adequate ATP production and a physiological membrane potential. It may take several days for these neurones to develop the characteristic apoptotic pattern: progressive degradation of the nuclear membrane, chromatin condensation and DNA fragmentation ('DNA laddering'), and production of small particles consisting of cell debris (apoptotic bodies). The initiation of apoptosis is related to activation of a death signalling complex involving calpain and caspases with consequent activation of translocases and endonucleases. Caspases represent proteases related to the family of interleukin converting enzymes (ICE).[54] Consequently, the ICE inhibitor z-VAK.FMK (N-benzyloxycarbonyl-val-ala-asp-fluoromethylketone) and the protein synthase inhibitor cycloheximide were able to inhibit apoptosis in vitro and in vivo. It is, therefore, possible that an anti-apoptotic approach will increase the therapeutic window in patients following head injury or acute stroke.

CONCLUSIONS

Normal to high cerebral perfusion pressure, normoxia, and surgical decompression are by far the most important and effective neuroprotective treatments. Interventions to increase CBF in the ischaemic territory, reduction of cerebral metabolism, lactic acidosis and excitatory neurotransmitter activity, prevention of Ca^{2+} influx, inhibition of lipid peroxidation, and free radical scavenging have been proposed to be protective in cerebral ischaemia. However, only a few of these treatments have been proven to be efficacious for of experimental or clinical ischaemia. With currently available knowledge, the following physical and pharmacological interventions seem to be protective in a variety of different pathophysiological states.

1. Normoventilation ($PaCO_2$ = 36–40 mmHg [4.8–5.3 kPa]) is permissible in patients with normal or moderately elevated ICP. Avoid prophylactic hyperventilation but transiently hyperventilate ($PaCO_2$ = 30–34 mmHg [4.0–4.5 kPa]) during episodes of acute intracranial hypertension (plateau waves) until other interventions can reduce ICP.

2. Mild to moderate hypothermia prevents experimental neuronal necrosis and improves neurological outcome when induced before, during, or after cerebral ischaemia. Mild to moderate hypothermia may also improve neurological outcome following stroke and cardiopulmonary resuscitation. In patients following head injury, mild hypothermia cannot be recommended as a standard procedure, but rather as an option when other treatment strategies fail to reduce ICP. In any case, the precise degree of hypothermia, the duration and the rewarming technique still have to be defined.

3. Anaesthetics given prior to ischaemic challenges appear to extend the ischaemic tolerance of neurones. Barbiturates may decrease elevated ICP and improve neurological outcome.

4. Hyperglycaemia is associated with worsened outcome following stroke or neurotrauma and plasma glucose concentrations should be assayed every 2 h and maintained within the range of 100–150 mg/dl.

5. In patients with acute stroke or subarachnoid haemorrhage from ruptured aneurysms, nimodipine improves neurological outcome, reduces the incidence of cerebral vasospasm, and appears to decrease the occurrence of delayed neurological deficits. Patients with traumatic subarachnoid haemorrhage may also benefit from the infusion of nimodipine. However, nimodipine may worsen neurological outcome in any of these patients if CPP decreases with drug administration.

6. In general, glucocorticoids have no significant positive or negative effect in patients with head injury or acute stroke. High-dose methylprednisolone slightly improves sensory and motor function following spinal cord injury.

Key points for clinical practice

- *Management of cerebral perfusion pressure (CPP)*: it is currently believed that stabilization of CPP within the range 8.5–9.5 kPa (65–70 mmHg) by means of sedation, osmodiuretics, normovolaemia and vasopressors will improve neurological outcome following cerebral ischaemia.

- *Hyperventilation*: short-term interventional hyperventilation ($PaCO_2$ = 4–4.45 kPa, 30–34 mmHg) is justified in situations with critical elevations in intracranial pressure (ICP), e.g. cerebral protrusions during neurological craniotomy or plateau waves. In contrast, prophylactic (chronic) hyperventilation will increase cerebral ischaemia and worsen neurological outcome.

- *Hypothermia*: multicentre trials on the effects of therapeutic hypothermia following stroke, cardiac arrest, and during cerebral aneurysm surgery are currently in process based on promising phase II results. In head injured patients, neurological outcome was not improved by mild or moderate hypothermia.

- *Surgical decompression*: decompressive craniectomy for refractory intracranial hypertension following head injury, cardiopulmonary resuscitation, or stroke may be considered as a second tier treatment along with forced hyperventilation or hypothermia.

- *Anaesthetics*: barbiturates appear to be neuroprotective when infused prior to cerebral ischaemia. In head injured patients, barbiturates decrease ICP and may improve outcome.

- *Osmodiuretics*: bolus administration of mannitol decreases ICP, increases CPP, and improves cerebral blood flow in laboratory animals.

- *Plasma glucose*: plasma glucose concentrations should be assayed every 2 h and maintained within the range of 100–150 mg/dl.

- *Ca^{2+} channel blockers*: in patients with acute ischaemic stroke and aneurysmatic or traumatic subarachnoid haemorrhage, nimodipine appears to be associated with a favourable outcome as long as the treatment commences within the first 12 h following the onset of the symptoms and arterial hypotension is strictly avoided.

- *Glucocorticoids*: they have no significant positive or negative effect in patients with head injury or acute stroke. High dose methylprednisolone slightly improves sensory and motor function following spinal cord injury.

REFERENCES

1. Rosner MJ, Rosner SD, Johnson AH. Cerebral perfusion pressure: management protocol and clinical results. J Neurosurg 1995; 83: 949–962.
2. Asgeirsson B, Grände P-O, Nordström C-H. A new therapy of post-trauma brain oedema based on haemodynamic principles for brain volume regulation. Intensive Care Med 1994; 20: 260–267.
3. Asgeirsson B, Grände P-O, Nordström C-H, Berntman L, Messeter K, Ryding E. Effects of hypotensive treatment with alpha-2-agonist and beta-1-antagonist on cerebral haemo-dynamics in severely head injured patients. Acta Anaesthesiol Scand 1995; 39: 347–351.
4. Ruta TS, Drummond JC, Cole DJ. The effect of acute hypocapnia on local cerebral blood flow during middle cerebral artery occlusion in isoflurane anesthetized rats. Anesthesiology 1993; 78: 134–140.
5. Artru AA, Merriman HG. Hypocapnia added to hypertension to reverse EEG changes during carotid endarterectomy. Anesthesiology 1989; 70: 1016–1018.
6. Cold GE. Does acute hyperventilation provoke cerebral oligaemia in comatose patients after acute head injury. Acta Neurochir (Wien) 1989; 96: 100–106.
7. Obrist WD, Langfitt TW, Jaggi JL, Cruz J, Gennarelli TA. Cerebral blood flow and metabolism in comatose patients with acute head injury. J Neurosurg 1984; 61: 241–253.
8. Muizelaar JP, Marmarou A, Ward JD et al. Adverse effects of prolonged hyperventilation in patients with severe head injury: a randomized clinical trial. J Neurosurg 1991; 75: 731–739.
9. Morikawa E, Ginsberg MD, Dietrich WD et al. The significance of brain temperature in focal cerebral ischemia: histopathological consequences of middle cerebral artery occlusion in the rat. J Cereb Blood Flow Metab 1992; 12: 380–389.
10. Weinrauch V, Safar P, Tisherman S, Kuboyama K, Radovsky A. Beneficial effect of mild hypothermia and detrimental effect of deep hypothermia after cardiac arrest in dogs. Stroke 1992; 23: 1454–1462.
11. Hoffman WE, Werner C, Baughman VL, Thomas C, Miletich DJ, Albrecht RF. Postischemic treatment with hypothermia improves outcome from incomplete cerebral

ischemia in rats. J Neurosurg Anesth 1991; 3: 34–38.

12. Clifton GL, Jiang JY, Lyeth BG, Jenkins LW, Hamm RJ, Hayes RL. Marked protection by moderate hypothermia after experimental traumatic brain injury. J Cereb Blood Flow Metab 1991; 11: 114–121.

13. Clifton GL, Allen S, Barrodale P et al. A phase II study of moderate hypothermia in severe brain injury. J Neurotrauma 1993; 10: 263–271.

14. Marion DW, Penrod LE, Kelsey SF et al. Treatment of traumatic brain injury with moderate hypothermia. N Engl J Med 1997; 336: 540–546.

15. Shiozaki T, Sugimoto H, Taneda M et al. Effect of mild hypothermia on uncontrollable intracranial hypertension after severe head injury. J Neurosurg 1993; 79: 363–368.

16. Bernard SA, Jones BM, Horne MK. Clinical trial of induced hypothermia in comatose survivors of out-of-hospital cardiac arrest. Ann Emerg Med 1997; 30: 146–153.

17. Schwab S, Schwarz S, Spranger M, Keller E, Bertram M, Hacke W. Moderate hypothermia in the treatment of patients with severe middle cerebral artery infarction. Stroke 1998; 29: 2461–2466.

18. Clifton GL. First results of the North American multicenter trial on the usage of hypothermia in head injury patients. Update in therapeutic hypothermia. Vienna: Proceedings of the 2nd International Symposium on Therapeutic Hypothermia, 1999.

19. Reith J, Jørgensen HS, Pedersen PM et al. Body temperature in acute stroke: relation to stroke severity, infarct size, mortality, and outcome. Lancet 1996; 347: 422–425.

20. Polin RS, Shaffrey ME, Bogaev CA et al. Decompressive bifrontal craniectomy in the treatment of severe refractory posttraumatic cerebral edema. Neurosurgery 1997; 41: 84–94.

21. Kleist-Welch Guerra W, Gabb MR, Dietz H, Mueller J-U, Piek J, Fritsch MJ. Surgical decompression for traumatic brain swelling: indications and results. J Neurosurg 1999; 90: 187–196.

22. Werner C, Möllenberg O, Kochs E, Schulte am Esch J. Sevoflurane improves neurological outcome following incomplete cerebral ischaemia in rats. Br J Anaesth 1995; 75: 756–760.

23. Engelhard K, Werner C, Reeker W et al. Desflurane and isoflurane improve neurological outcome after incomplete cerebral ischaemia in rats. Br J Anaesth 1999; 83: 415–421.

24. Grady RE, Weglinski MR, Sharbrough FW, Perkins WL. Correlation of regional cerebral blood flow with ischemic electroencephalographic changes during sevoflurane-nitrous oxide anesthesia for carotid endarterectomy. Anesthesiology 1998; 88: 892–897.

25. Warner DS, Takaoda S, Wu B et al. Electroencephalographic burst suppression is not required to elicit maximal neuroprotection from pentobarbital in a rat model of focal cerebral ischemia. Anesthesiology 1996; 84: 1475–1484.

26. Nussmeier NA, Arlund C, Slogoff S. Neuropsychiatric complications after cardiopulmonary bypass: cerebral protection by a barbiturate. Anesthesiology 1986; 64: 165–170.

27. Brain Resuscitation Clinical Trial I Study Group. Randomized clinical study of thiopental loading in comatose survivors of cardiac arrest. N Engl J Med 1986; 314: 397–403.

28. Bullock R, Chesnut RM, Clifton G et al. The use of barbiturates in the control of intracranial hypertension. J Neurotrauma 1996; 13: 711–714.

29. Kelly DF, Goodale DB, Williams J et al. Propofol in the treatment of moderate and severe head injury: a randomized, prospective double-blinded pilot trial. J Neurosurg 1999; 90: 1042–1052.

30. Roach GW, Newman MF, Murkin JM et al. Ineffectiveness of burst suppression therapy in mitigating perioperative cerebrovascular dysfunction. Anesthesiology 1999; 90; 1255–1264.

31. Schwartz ML, Tator CH, Rowed DW. The University of Toronto Treatment Study. A prospective randomized comparison of pentobarbital and mannitol. Can J Neurol Sci 1984; 11: 434–440.

32. Smith HP, Kelly DL, McWorther JM et al. Comparison of mannitol regimens in patients with severe head injury undergoing intracranial monitoring. J Neurosurg 1986; 65: 820–824.

33. Freshman SP, Battistella FD, Matteucci M, Wiesner DH. Hypertonic saline (7.5%) versus mannitol: a comparison for treatment of acute head injuries. J Trauma 1993; 35: 344–348..

34. Woo J, Lam C, Kay R, Wong A, Teoh R, Nicholls M. The influence of hyperglycemia and diabetes mellitus on immediate and 3-month morbidity and mortality after acute stroke. Arch Neurol 1990; 47: 1174–1177.

35. Buchan AM, Gertler SZ, Li H et al. A selective N-type Ca^{++}-channel blocker prevents CA1 injury 24 h following severe forebrain ischemia and reduces infarction following focal ischemia. J Cereb Blood Flow Metab 1994; 14: 903–910.

36. Mohr JP, Orgogozo JM, Harrison MJG et al. Meta-analysis of oral nimodipine trial in acute ischemic stroke. Cerebrovasc Dis 1994; 4: 197–203.

37. Barker FG, Ogilvy CS. Efficacy of prophylactic nimodipine for delayed ischemic deficit after subarachnoid hemorrhage: a metaanalysis. J Neurosurg 1996; 84: 405–414.

38. Harders A, Kakarieka A, Braakman R et al. Traumatic subarachnoid hemorrhage and its treatment with nimodipine. J Neurosurg 1996; 85: 82–89.

39. Hoffman WE, Pelligrino D, Werner C, Kochs E, Albrecht RF, Schulte am Esch J. Ketamine decreases plasma catecholamines and improves neurologic outcome from incomplete cerebral ischemia in rats. Anesthesiology 1992; 76: 755–762.

40. Grotta J, Clark W, Coull B et al. Safety and tolerability of the glutamate antagonist CGS 19755 (selfotel) in patients with acute ischemic stroke. Stroke 1995; 26: 602–605.

41. Arrowsmith JE, Harrison MJG, Newman SP, Stygall J, Timberlake N, Pugsley WB. Neuroprotection of the brain during cardiopulmonary bypass: a randomized trial of remacemide during coronary artery bypass in 171 patients. Stroke 1998; 29: 2357–2362.

42. Alderson P, Roberts I. Corticosteroids in acute traumatic brain injury: systematic review of randomised controlled trials. BMJ 1997; 314: 1855–1859.

43. Bracken MB, Shepard MJ, Collins WF et al. A randomized, controlled trial of methylprednisolone or naloxone in the treatment of acute spinal-cord injury. N Engl J Med 1990; 322: 1405–1411.

44. Bracken MB, Shepard MJ, Holford TR et al. Administration of methylprednisolone for 24 or 48 hours or tirilazat mesylate for 48 hours in the treatment of acute spinal-cord injury. Results from the third national acute spinal cord injury randomized controlled trial. National acute spinal cord injury study. JAMA 1997; 277: 1597–1604.

45. Smith SL, Scherch HM, Hall ED. Protective effects of tirilazad mesylate and metabolite U-89678 against blood brain barrier damage after subarachnoid hemorrhage and lipid peroxidative neuronal injury. J Neurosurg 1996; 84: 229–233.

46. Haley EC, Kassell NF, Apperson-Hansen C et al. A randomized double-blind, vehicle controlled trial of tirilazad mesylate in patients with aneurysmal subarachnoid hemorrhage: a cooperative study in North America. J Neurosurg 1997; 86: 467–474.

47. Kassell NF, Haley EC, Apperson-Hansen C et al. A randomized double-blind, vehicle controlled trial of tirilazad mesylate in patients with aneurysmal subarachnoid hemorrhage: a cooperative study in Europe, Australia, and New Zealand. J Neurosurg 1996; 84: 221–228.

48. Marshall LF, Maas AI, Marshall SB et al. A multicenter trial on the efficacy of using tirilazad mesylate in cases of head injury. J Neurosurg 1998; 89: 519–525.

49. Young B, Runge JW, Waxman KS et al. Effects of pegorgotein on neurologic outcome of patients with severe head injury. JAMA 1996; 276: 538–543.

50. Asano T, Takakura K, Sano K et al. Effects of a hydroxyl radical scavenger on delayed ischemic neurological deficits following aneurysmal subarachnoid hemorrhage: results of a multicenter, placebo-controlled double-blind trial. J Neurosurg 1996; 84: 792–800.

51. Garthwaite J, Boulton CL. Nitric oxide signaling in the central nervous system. Annu Rev Physiol 1995; 57: 683–706.

52. Samdani AF, Dawson TM, Dawson VL. Nitric oxide synthase in models of focal ischemia. Stroke 1997; 28: 1283–1288.

53. Zhang RL, Chopp M, Jiang N et al. Anti-intercellular adhesion molecule-1 antibody reduces ischemic cell damage after transient but not permanent middle cerebral artery occlusion in the Wistar rat. Stroke 1995; 26: 1438–1443.

54. McConkey DJ, Zhivotovsky B, Orrenius S. Apoptosis – molecular mechanisms and biomedical implications. Mol Aspects Med 1996; 17: 1–110.

Bernard Riley

CHAPTER 6

Permissive hypotension

The treatment of the hypotensive trauma patient involves an immediate assessment of airway, breathing and circulation with simultaneous resuscitation of any life-threatening injury found. Of all the life-threatening injuries likely to be encountered during the ABC component of the primary survey, haemorrhage producing hypovolaemic shock is the most common. The treatment of hypovolaemic shock has two basic requirements, haemorrhage control and volume replacement.[1] The goal of therapy is to restore tissue perfusion and oxygen delivery by correcting the reduced intravascular volume. Classically, this has involved early and rapid infusion of crystalloid or colloid fluids in volumes suitable to replace the volume of blood lost. This approach developed largely as the result of experiments in animals during which they were bled until they showed the clinical signs of hypovolaemic shock.[2,3] The animals were bled from in-dwelling vascular catheters which allowed a specific volume of blood, or percentage of the animal's blood volume to be removed and then further bleeding from the catheter was stopped. Fluid replacement with various replacement regimens was then commenced with on-going monitoring of vital signs. These experiments suggested that prompt, efficient fluid replacement improved survival. Such animal experiments using these controlled haemorrhage models do not accurately reflect bleeding in real trauma since the bleeding is not arrested after a specific volume has been lost, but continues unabated towards exsanguination unless surgical control, or the body's normal haemostatic mechanisms supervene to stop further haemorrhage. The administration of large volumes of intravenous fluids prior to surgical control of bleeding is felt by some to be potentially deleterious since increasing blood pressure and vessel diameter, decreasing blood viscosity, diluting platelets and clotting factors could all increase uncontrolled haemorrhage actually

Dr Bernard Riley, Consultant in Adult Intensive Care, University Hospital, Nottingham NG7 2UH, UK

promoting further blood loss.[4–6] The hypothesis that fluid resuscitation should be delayed until surgical control of haemorrhage has taken place, has been termed permissive hypotension.[7] The concept that fluid replacement prior to surgical control of bleeding may do more harm than good is not new and can be traced to military surgeons' experiences during the first and second World Wars,[8,9] although by the 1980s military medical doctrine in both the US and UK concerning intravenous fluid replacement was that rapid high volume fluid replacement was an important factor in the early treatment of hypovolaemic shock.[10,11] This chapter aims to explain the development of the hypothesis of permissive hypotension and to assess its place in current practice.

ANIMAL RESEARCH

Newer animal models of haemorrhage are of the 'uncontrolled' type in that they include an on-going vascular leak which simulates the continued bleeding that occurs during trauma. The haemorrhage rate and volumes lost then depend on the size of the hole in the vessel, the pressure gradient across it and factors relating to vessel contractility, platelet aggregation, clot formation and stabilisation as in real life. Such models have been used to study the effect of simultaneous fluid resuscitation on the haemorrhagic process and the mortality outcome with a range of different fluids and volume replacement regimens. The swine aortotomy model developed by Bickell and colleagues is of uncontrolled haemorrhagic shock. In anaesthetised pigs, one end of a surgical wire is passed through the anterior wall of the abdominal aorta into its lumen and is brought out again in the same plane 5 mm cephallically and externalised to the surface of the abdomen. After recovery from this procedure, the pigs can be re-anaesthetised a few days later, monitoring lines inserted and the wire pulled out from the surface of the abdomen resulting in a 5 mm tear of the abdominal aorta and uncontrolled haemorrhage. Using this model, the haemodynamic responses to aortotomy and fluid replacement can be monitored and haematoma volumes determined after death or euthanasia.[12] Using this model, intravenous crystalloid fluid replacement in 'standard' volumes at 80 ml/kg in 8 pigs resulted in mean haematoma volume of 2142 ± 178 ml; no animal survived. In a further 8 pigs, no volume was replaced; all the pigs survived aortotomy and the mean haematoma volume after euthanasia was 783 ± 85 ml. This initial experiment lead Bickell to suggest that normal volume resuscitation was detrimental.[13]

One of the objections to this model was that the haemorrhage produced by aortotomy was not severe enough to mimic reality, was non-lethal and the volume losses of only 20–25 ml/kg would not normally require large volume crystalloid resuscitation. The model was modified in subsequent experiments to include controlled haemorrhage of 40–50 ml/kg to produce clinical hypovolaemic shock prior to aortotomy. Such methods produce uncontrolled severe haemorrhagic shock with a high 1 h mortality. Kowalenko and co-workers used such a model to examine the effects of fluid resuscitation to various mean arterial pressure (MAP) end points.[14] Anaesthetised miniature swine, each with an aortotomy wire in place, were bled via a femoral catheter and blood pump to a MAP of 30 mmHg. At that point, the aortotomy wire was pulled producing a 4 mm aortic tear and free intraperitoneal bleeding. When the pulse pressure fell to 5 mmHg, resuscitation was commenced. The animals were randomly allocated to one of three resuscitation end-point groups, each with 8 animals per group: group 1 MAP = 40 mmHg; group 2 MAP = 80 mmHg; and group 3 no resuscitation. Measurements were made for 60 min or until death. Physiological saline was used up to a maximum of 90 ml/kg; thereafter the shed blood was re-infused at 2 ml/kg/min. Survival at 1 h was 87.5%, 37.5% and 12.5% for groups 1, 2 and 3, respectively. The difference in survival between groups 1 and 2 was statistically significant, but there was no significance to the survival difference between groups 2 and 3. Only 1 of the non-resuscitated animals survived indicating that the model was near fatal unless resuscitation was undertaken. There was no significant difference in the haematoma volume at postmortem between groups 1 and 3, but the haematoma volume in group 2 (resuscitated to the 80 mmHg end point) was significantly greater than groups 1 and 3. It was concluded that large volume saline resuscitation increased haemorrhage volumes and failed to improve survival in the setting of severe uncontrolled haemorrhage.[14]

The same group further hypothesised that increasingly aggressive fluid resuscitation to reach stepwise increments in blood pressure end-points would be matched by increased death rates and haemorrhage volumes. They also investigated the relationship of better perfusion to oxygen delivery and tissue oxygenation. The same animal model was used and the effect of fluid resuscitation to MAP end-points of 40, 60 or 80 mmHg was investigated. Mean survival time was least and mortality greatest in the group given highest volumes of fluid to attain the 80 mmHg MAP end-point. Survival rate was highest in the 40 mmHg MAP group and survival in the 60 mmHg group was intermediate; this group had the best tissue oxygenation delivery and the lowest serum lactate levels. It was suggested that resuscitation to normotension in the presence of on-going bleeding worsened outcome as a result of increasing MAP at a time when clot was not mature, haemodilution reduced blood viscosity and that too much fluid caused a decrease in the oxygen carrying capacity beyond which the animal's compromised cardiovascular system could compensate. Resuscitation with fluid to normotension was not considered desirable in the presence of non-compressible vascular injury.[15]

ABDOMINAL AORTIC ANEURYSMS

Not surprisingly, the findings of the above and similar animal studies stimulated debate and a search for evidence in man as to whether delayed fluid resuscitation and permissive hypotension had any advantages or disadvantages in clinical practice. One source of indirect evidence in support of restricting fluid replacement until after haemorrhage control came from reviews of clinical practice in the repair of ruptured abdominal aortic aneurysms. In 1991, Johansen reported an operative mortality of 70% for ruptured abdominal aortic aneurysm despite rapid prehospital fluid replacement, transport to hospital, diagnosis, surgical repair and postoperative intensive care.[16] The accompanying editorial in the *Journal of Vascular Surgery* by Crawford described a personal retrospective mortality rate of only 23%.[17] This difference was suggested to be due to the practice of avoiding vigorous fluid replacement prior to the application of the vascular clamp, thus substantially arresting haemorrhage before fluid replacement. He suggested that systolic blood pressure be maintained at 50–70 mmHg prior to clamping, although no details of the methods and consequences of induction of anaesthesia were given.[17] Similar retrospective series with pre-clamping fluid restriction are available. Lawrie quoted a mortality rate of 15% and suggested that this low mortality rate was due to early diagnosis and immediate transfer to the operating theatre for surgery even before blood was available.[18] He considered that any elevation of blood pressure by fluid administration or vasopressors was futile prior to arresting haemorrhage as it would simply lead to further blood loss and hypotension. He suggested that small volumes of fluid, and vasopressor therapy, should be reserved for those patients with severe hypovolaemic shock with systolic blood pressures of 70–80 mmHg. This permissive hypotension regimen may not entirely explain the improved mortality figures: less than 30% of these patients had a systolic blood pressure below 100 mmHg on admission as opposed to about 60% of patients in most other series.[18] Fluid restriction is opposed by others on the basis that the systolic blood pressure at presentation is a good predictor of mortality. A pressure of less than 90 mmHg is associated with a mortality in excess of 60% in most series with the development of multi-system organ dysfunction, ARDS and renal failure which correlates with the severity and duration of shock.[19–22] Not all retrospective series have shown permissive hypotension to be effective, even when no blood or fluid was administered until the abdomen was opened. Gayliss reported a mortality rate of 58%.[23] In Martin's series,[24] fluid resuscitation was started early and his mortality rate of 28% contrasts with the 23% rate of Crawford, the advocate of permissive hypotension. Brimacombe and Berry concluded that a policy of minimal fluid resuscitation was compatible with improved survival if it was combined with early surgery, rapid aortic clamping and meticulous control of bleeding; but that if hypotension produced any myocardial or cerebral underperfusion, then it should be treated provided that this did not delay surgery. They suggested that the precise level of blood pressure at which fluids should be given was difficult to define and considered Crawford's recommendation of 50–70 mmHg systolic to be too low and recommended a mean arterial pressure of 65 mmHg, although they stated that this figure is also unsubstantiated.[25]

Formulating fluid resuscitation protocols on the basis of several retrospective studies carried out in different centres at different times is never satisfactory. There are numerous confounding variables, such as age of patient, size of aneurysm, hospital transfer times, patients' pre-operative condition, initial investigation and diagnostic tests used, time to surgery, competence of surgeon and anaesthetist, postoperative management and the case-load and experience of the hospitals involved. Taking all of these into account, it is difficult to conclude that permissive hypotension alone is responsible for any given improvement in hospital mortality rate for the management of ruptured abdominal aortic aneurysm. As yet there have been no published randomised prospective trials of preclamping fluid resuscitation protocols in ruptured abdominal aortic aneurysm.

PENETRATING TRUNCAL INJURY

Two prospective trials have considered immediate versus delayed fluid resuscitation in penetrating truncal injury.[26,27] Both are from the same team, in the same urban setting, where a single pre-hospital emergency medical system exists and triage of all major trauma is to a single level 1 trauma hospital. The group's initial study looked at 300 consecutive patients with gunshot or stab wounds to the trunk who had a systolic blood pressure of 90 mmHg or less.[26] Patients less than 16-years-old, pregnant patients or patients with additional injuries outside the trunk were excluded. One group received fluid resuscitation during transit and in the emergency room (ER) in accordance to existing paramedic and Advanced Trauma Life Support protocols (immediate resuscitation group). The patients in this group had 2 or more 14 gauge cannulae placed in arm veins and were given crystalloid and packed red blood cells if necessary to attain a pre-operative blood pressure of 100 mmHg. The other group (delayed resuscitation group) also had 14 gauge cannulae placed but these were then flushed with 1 ml of heparinised saline and then capped. Any further lines inserted on arrival in the ER were either flushed and capped or kept open with infusion rates at 10 ml/h or less. The aim in this group was to delay intravenous fluid resuscitation until either thoracotomy (including resuscitative thoracotomy in the ER) or laparotomy was commenced. Patients were allocated to groups according to the day of the month being either an odd or even date; the 24 h periods of delayed or immediate resuscitation corresponded to the 24 h shifts of the paramedics and ER trauma teams. Informed consent was not obtained; the investigators considered that consent for appropriate emergency treatment was implied if a patient or someone acting on their behalf called the paramedics. They further considered that a hypotensive patient could not give informed consent and that, since a relative was often not available, then the concept of 'implied consent' could be applied to the study.

During the 1 year study, 300 patients were entered of whom 161 were placed in the immediate resuscitation group and 139 in the delayed resuscitation group. The others were excluded from the study because they were lifeless at the scene ($n = 62$), had minor chest or abdominal wounds that did not require surgery ($n = 52$) or were found to be pregnant or too young ($n = 6$). There were no statistically significant differences between groups in terms of: demographics, Revised Trauma Score, Injury Severity Score, paramedic response times to scene, time on scene, time for transfer to ER or time in the ER prior to surgery. There were 9 documented protocol violations in the delayed resuscitation group who were given fluids instead of having them restricted. There were no statistically significant differences in survival, pre-operative death rates, length of stay in Intensive Care Units or in hospital, nor in the incidence of renal failure, ARDS, coagualopathy, sepsis, multiple organ failure, pneumonia or wound infection between the 2 groups. The authors were surprised to have found no difference between the groups and offered various possible explanations. The mean pre-operative fluid volume in the delayed resuscitation group was 771 ± 1238 ml. The investigators seem to have considered that the protocol was not being followed since they state 'the logistics of absolute control of fluid restriction in the ambulance, emergency centre, and pre-incision in the operating room are extremely difficult'. To try to eliminate any influence of protocol violations, they conducted a separate *post-hoc* analysis on a non-random sample in which patients in the delayed resuscitation group who had received more than 250 ml of fluid pre-operatively, and patients in the immediate resuscitation group who received less than 250 ml of fluid pre-operatively were eliminated. There were 90 patients in the immediate resuscitation group and 49 in the delayed resuscitation group; the sub-set appeared to be matched for injury severity scores and TRISS probability of survival. There was no significant difference in survival between the groups. The number of protocol violations in the delayed resuscitation group highlights the problem of ensuring strict compliance by over 400 people involved in carrying out the study at the 'shop-floor' level.

Undaunted, the same group repeated the study, using the same methodology; over a 3 year period, 1069 hypotensive patients with gunshot or stab wounds to the torso were admitted.[27] Of these, 172 had revised trauma scores of zero, and 299 patients had minor injuries not requiring operative intervention so were excluded from the study. Among the remaining 598 patients, 289 patients were randomised to the delayed resuscitation group and 309 patients to the immediate resuscitation group. The groups were well matched for demographic and clinical characteristics. Seventy patients died before they reached the operating room, 41 in the immediate resuscitation group and 29 in the delayed resuscitation group. On arrival in the operating room, the groups were similar in respect of systolic and diastolic blood pressures, pH and venous bicarbonate values. Those patients in the delayed resuscitation group had significantly lower haemoglobin concentrations and fluid volumes than those in the immediate resuscitation group. During the prehospital phase, the average crystalloid volumes given to the immediate and delayed resuscitation groups were 870 ml and 92 ml, respectively. Prior to surgery, but after arrival in the emergency room, the average volumes for the groups were 1608 ml and 283 ml, respectively – a significant difference. In the delayed resuscitation group, rapid infusions were instigated in error in 10 patients before admission to hospital and in 12 other patients after their arrival in the trauma centre. These 22 patients constitute protocol violations, but, since the rapid infusions were stopped, the investigators did not exclude them from the final analysis. The overall survival rate was significantly higher in the delayed resuscitation group than in the immediate resuscitation group (70% versus 62%, $P = 0.04$). The total stay in hospital was longer for the immediate resuscitation group, but the length of stay in intensive care was not. There was no statistically significant difference in the incidence of ARDS, sepsis-SIRS, acute renal failure, pneumonia, coagulopathy or wound infection between the 2 groups. The authors concluded that for hypotensive patients with penetrating torso injuries, delay of aggressive fluid resuscitation until operative intervention improves the outcome. They pointed out that this conclusion should not be extrapolated to all age groups, to hypotensive patients with blunt trauma, severe head injuries or to rural trauma care settings (which often have long point-of-injury to point-of-treatment times) and that similar studies in these groups need to be undertaken. Such studies have not been reported.

Not surprisingly, this study stimulated much comment and an accompanying editorial in the *New England Journal of Medicine* was not entirely supportive.[28] It pointed out that the time from wounding to operation was remarkably short in both groups (averages of 74 min and 77 min for the immediate and delayed groups, respectively) and cautioned this approach if the delay to operative treatment was such that exsanguination could occur. The severity of the haemorrhage was questioned. In the delayed group, the mean systolic blood pressure quoted for patients on arrival in the emergency room was 72 mmHg, but those who survived to reach the operating room had a mean systolic blood pressure of 113 mmHg. This could be partly explained by the fact that those patients who died were more shocked and did not have comparable blood pressures in the operating room. The conclusion was that further studies were needed to stratify the severity of haemorrhage, the corresponding degrees of hypotension, organ damage and cause of death. The degree of shock in the immediate resuscitation group would also seem to be minor; the mean volume of fluid administered from point-of-wounding to surgery being 2500 ml given over a mean time of 74 min. This hardly suggests massive on-going bleeding. The relatively short times to surgery probably make the differences in volume administered of little physiological importance, particularly when the intra-operative fluid volumes show no significant difference between the 2 groups. The paper has also been criticised for its randomisation by odd or even date since this is not true random allocation, and also for the statistical analysis of the mortality in both groups.[29] The authors chose to analyse survival-to-hospital discharge in the 2 groups but the deaths occurred in 2 distinct time periods; pre-operatively, and those who died intra- or postoperatively. Pre-operative deaths occurred in 21 of the 309 immediate resuscitation patients (13%) and 29 of the 289 delayed resuscitation patients (10%). Intra- or postoperative deaths occurred in 75 of the remaining 268 immediate resuscitation patients (28%) and in 57 of the remaining 260 delayed resuscitation patients (22%). Neither difference is significant and if this approach is taken then, together with the lack of any difference in the incidence of ARDS, SIRS/sepsis, renal failure, coagualopathy, wound infection or pneumonia, the authors' conclusion is not justified.

WHERE NEXT?

Since these two attempts at managing prospective randomised trials of permissive hypotension, no such further investigations have been published; but Bickell and his colleagues' work has been widely quoted as providing hard evidence for the utility of delayed fluid resuscitation. Some have suggested that the application of the principles should be more widely adopted.[30] Others have suggested that, before permissive hypotension is extended to all trauma patients, one should reconsider both the animal experimental methodology for producing uncontrolled haemorrhage and the source of bleeding. In reality, unlike the swine aortotomy model, bleeding is unlikely to be stopped spontaneously by vasoconstriction, clot formation and haematoma tamponade. Others suspect that, while the delayed fluid resuscitation approach may be advantageous in patients with short wounding to surgery times, there may be a critical point at which the duration of low perfusion starts to produce irreversible ischaemia within poorly perfused organs. This would mean that death caused by on-going haemorrhage is delayed until multiple organ failure as a result of inadequate organ perfusion has occurred. They suggest that perhaps the best approach is not 'no volume' as in permissive hypotension, nor 'high volume' as in classical fluid resuscitation. Rather 'enough volume' to maintain organ perfusion at a level that does not promote further bleeding but, at the same time, preserves organ perfusion at a minimal level sufficient to pre-empt organ failure. Various investigators have returned to laboratory studies in animal models to attempt to answer these questions and those raised in Bickell and colleagues' first paper concerning blunt trauma, non-vascular injury and head injury.

The question regarding the relevance of large vessel injury as an appropriate model for the majority of trauma-induced haemorrhage has largely been investigated by 2 models of either the unstoppable haemorrhage or parenchymal injury types.[31,32] A porcine model of uncontrolled haemorrhage, where bleeding is induced from a flow monitored shunt placed between the femoral artery and the peritoneal cavity, simulates a situation where cessation of bleeding is unlikely until either surgical intervention or exsanguination occurs. If such animals are randomised to receive either no fluid or traditional fluid resuscitation, then there is no significant survival advantage in either group. There were only 5 animals in each group, but the investigators postulated that much of the benefit from permissive hypotension may depend on an injury that ceases to bleed.[31] Parenchymal injury models are suggested to closely mimic the type of haemorrhage occurring in the majority of blunt trauma patients who have not had a large vessel injury. One such rat model of liver injury has been used to investigate the role of no volume, small volume (4 ml/kg) high volume (24 ml/kg) Ringer's lactate versus a small volume of hypertonic saline (4 ml/kg). Mortality rates were reduced in the group resuscitated with hypertonic saline (10%) compared to those resuscitated with no volume, small volume or high volume Ringer's lactate (47–50%). These authors demonstrated that large volume isotonic crystalloid resuscitation increased bleeding and transiently expanded intravascular volume after solid abdominal visceral injury compared with no volume or small volume isotonic resuscitation. There was no difference in the mortality rate between the no volume and large volume groups. They suggested that conclusions drawn from large vessel injury models may not equate to injury of visceral organs and that results of clinical trials of penetrating torso trauma may not generalise to other types of trauma. They thus conclude that low volume is better than no volume but only if hypertonic saline is used![32]

The question of no volume, low volume and high volume and the potential effects on organ perfusion in non-large vessel injury has been investigated in rats using an uncontrolled venous haemorrhage model in an attempt to simulate the level of vascular injury seen in blunt trauma.[33] Anaesthetised rats had both lumbar veins severed at the point of entry to the vena cava. When MAP fell to 40 mmHg and was stable for 45 min, the rats were resuscitated with 0, 10 or 30 ml of Ringer's lactate over a period of 60 min. Cardiac output and regional blood flow by radioactive microsphere injection was determined at a fixed time. Fluid resuscitation with 10 or 30 ml of Ringer's increased MAP, cardiac output and hepatic blood flow. It was concluded that fluid resuscitation after uncontrolled venous haemorrhage was better than no volume in terms of increased MAP, cardiac output and hepatic blood flow. Nevertheless, increasing volume loading from low volume to high volume did not improve haemodynamic parameters or regional perfusion. They recommended moderate rather than no fluid resuscitation in this uncontrolled model of venous haemorrhage.[33]

These and other animal experiments investigate the role of 'controlled resuscitation' to balance the potential risk of low organ perfusion against the risk of provoking bleeding by giving more fluid than is absolutely necessary. The US military remain, predictably, very interested in finding the right balance in penetrating injury and their most recently published work has returned to the animal aortotomy model in rats using a 25 gauge needle stab through either side of the aorta.[34] Resuscitation 5 min after injury was continued for 2 h with either lactated Ringer's (LR), hypertonic saline/hetastarch (HH) or no fluids (NF).

Key points for clinical practice

- Regardless of the resuscitation regimen, haemorrhage control or limitation is the goal; 'operative' resuscitation turns off the tap of haemorrhage that allows fluid replacement to restore organ perfusion.

- The evidence for permissive hypotension, the concept of delayed fluid resuscitation and the acceptance of lower than normal mean arterial pressures until surgical control of haemorrhage is achieved, suggests it is only appropriate for penetrating truncal trauma in urban settings with wounding to definitive care times of around 1 h maximum.

- In observational cohort studies of ruptured abdominal aortic aneurysm surgery, permissive hypotension may confer a survival advantage.

- Where permissive hypotension is employed, adequate vascular access must be established prior to induction of anaesthesia with appropriate techniques and drug dosage together with rapid, effective surgical haemorrhage control which must be followed by rapid warmed fluid loading to restore organ perfusion.

- Permissive hypotension is not an option in shocked multiple trauma patients with head injury. Preservation of cerebral perfusion pressure to prevent secondary brain injury by ischaemia is a vital goal and early operative intervention to stop haemorrhage coupled with simultaneous volume replacement to achieve normovolaemia and normotension is required.

- In blunt trauma with parenchymal haemorrhage, animal evidence suggests that 'controlled resuscitation' to a mean arterial pressure end-point of 70–80 mmHg may be the best compromise between provocation of further bleeding by over-enthusiastic volume loading and low organ perfusion and ischaemia by no volume loading.

- The difficulties of constructing a prospective randomised controlled trial of various resuscitation regimens versus each other under reproducible conditions makes solid evidence for one particular regimen unlikely in the near future.

Those rats randomised to receive fluid had infusion rates adjusted to achieve MAP of 40, 80 or 100 mmHg in six groups: NF, LR 40, LR 80, LR 100, HH 40 and HH 80. Blood loss was measured after 1 h of resuscitation. The NF rats did not survive 4 h. After 72 h, the survival rate for LR 80 rats was 80% and for HH 40 rats 67%, a statistically significant improvement over the 0% survival of the no fluid rats. Re-bleeding and death were also associated with attempts to restore normal MAP as in the LR 100 group (30% survival).[34] This would seem to suggest that where time is a factor, then controlled resuscitation may be advantageous to maintain a compromise MAP. The group did not study regional organ perfusion but serum lactate was normal in all survivors at 24, 48 and 72 h.

CONCLUSIONS

The best regimen of fluid resuscitation before surgery for haemorrhage control remains controversial. The question is not only 'what volume', but 'what fluid', 'what resuscitation end-point' and 'what body temperature'. The difficulty of performing prospective randomised controlled trials in patients for all the various modalities of treatment and mechanisms of haemorrhage, obtaining informed consent and being able to control for emergency medical systems, environment and surgical technique are probably insurmountable. Solid evidence for the use of permissive hypotension in its pure form, i.e. no volume, is only available for one very particular circumstance. Otherwise, it is only possible to emphasise general principles based on a range of clinical cohort studies and animal experiments. There will always be proponents for each extreme and it seems likely that the truth will probably lie somewhere in between, with all the various regimens having advantages or disadvantages depending on the patient, the injury, the time factor and the ability to provide definitive surgical treatment.

REFERENCES

1. Anon. Shock. In: American College of Surgeons, Committee on Trauma. Advanced Trauma Life Support program for doctors: Instructor Course Manual. Chicago: American College of Surgeons, 1997; 97–117.
2. Wiggers CJ. Physiology of Shock. New York: Commonwealth Fund, 1950; 121–146.
3. Shires T, Coln D, Carrico J, Lightfoot S. Fluid therapy in hemorrhagic shock. Arch Surg 1964; 88: 688–693.
4. Shaftan GW, Chiu C, Dennis C. Fundamentals of physiological control of arterial haemorrhage. Surgery 1965; 58: 851–853.
5. Gross D, Landau EH, Kiln B. Quantitative measurement of bleeding following hypertonic saline therapy in 'uncontrolled' hemorrhagic shock. J Trauma 1989; 29: 79–82.
6. Bickell WH. Are victims of injury sometimes victimised by attempts at fluid resuscitation? Ann Emerg Med 1993; 22: 225–226.
7. Oakley PA, Morrison PJ. Resuscitation and monitoring of hypovolaemic shock. Curr Opin Anesthesiol 1994; 7: 177–183.
8. Cannon WB, Fraser J, Cowell EM. The preventative treatment of wound shock. JAMA 1918; 70: 618–621.
9. Office of the Surgeon General, Department of the Army. Surgery in World War II: General Surgery. Washington DC: Government Printing Office, 1952; 6–17.
10. Shock and resuscitation. In: United States Department of Defence, Emergency War Surgery. Washington DC: Government Printing Office, 1988; 133–148.

11. Kirby NG, Blackburn G. (eds) Field Surgery Pocket Book. London: HMSO; 1981; 34–49.
12. Bickell WH, Bruting SP, Wade CE. Haemodynamic response to aortotomy in anaesthetised swine. Circ Shock 1989; 28: 332–333.
13. Bickell WH, Bruting SP, Wade CE, Millanmow GA. The detrimental effects of iv crystalloid after aortotomy in the swine. Ann Emerg Med 1989; 18: 476.
14. Kowalenko T, Stern S, Dronen S, Wang W. Improved outcome with hypotensive resuscitation of uncontrolled hemorrhagic shock in a swine model. J Trauma 1992; 33: 349–351.
15. Stern SA, Dronen SC, Birrer P, Wang X. Effect of blood pressure on haemorrhage volume and survival in a near fatal model incorporating a vascular injury. Ann Emerg Med 1993; 22: 155–163.
16. Johansen KJ, Kohler TR, Nicholls SC, Zierler RE, Clowes AW, Karmers A. Ruptured abdominal aortic aneurysm; the Harbourview experience. J Vasc Surg 1991; 13: 220–247.
17. Crawford ES. Ruptured abdominal aortic aneurysm: an editorial. J Vasc Surg 1991; 13: 348–350.
18. Lawrie GM, Crawford ES, Morris GC. Progress in the treatment of ruptured abdominal aortic aneurysm. World J Surg 1980; 4: 653–660.
19. Wakefield TW, Whitehouse WM, Wu S. Abdominal aortic aneurysm rupture: statistical analysis of factors affecting outcome of surgical treatment. Surgery 1982; 91: 586–589.
20. Ouriel K, Geary K, Green RM, Fiore W, Geary JE, DeWeese JA. Factors determining survival after ruptured aortic aneurysm: the surgeon, the hospital and the patient. J Vasc Surg 1990; 11: 493–496.
21. Halpern VJ, Kline RG, D'Angelo AJ, Cohen JR. Factors that affect the survival rate of patients with ruptured abdominal aortic aneurysms. J Vasc Surg 1997; 26: 939–945.
22. Glovieski P, Pairolero PC, Mucha P. Ruptured abdominal aortic aneurysm: repair should not be denied. J Vasc Surg 1992; 15: 851–859.
23. Gayliss H, Kessler E. Ruptured aortic aneurysms. Surgery 1980; 87: 300–304.
24. Martin RS, Edwards WH, Jenkins JM, Mulherin JL. Ruptured abdominal aortic aneurysm: a 25 year experience. Am Surg 1988; 54: 539–543.
25. Brimacombe J, Berry A. A review of anaesthesia for ruptured abdominal aortic aneurysm with special emphasis on preclamping fluid resuscitation. Anaesth Intensive Care 1993; 21: 311–323.
26. Martin RR, Bickell WH, Pepe PE, Burch JM, Mattox KL. Prospective evaluation of preoperative fluid resuscitation in hypotensive patients with penetrating truncal injury: a preliminary report. J Trauma 1992; 33: 354–362.
27. Bickell WH, Wall MJ, Pepe PE et al. Immediate versus delayed fluid resuscitation for hypotensive patients with penetrating torso injuries. N Engl J Med 1994; 331: 1105–1109.
28. Lenworth MJ. Timing of fluid resuscitation in trauma. N Engl J Med 1994; 331: 1153–1154.
29. Siegel JH. Immediate versus delayed resuscitation in patients with trauma. N Engl J Med 1995; 332: 681–683.
30. Myers C. Fluid resuscitation. Eur J Emerg Med 1997; 4: 224–232.
31. Silbergleit R, Satz W, McNamara RM, Lee DC, Schoffstall JM. Effect of permissive hypotension in continuous uncontrolled intra-abdominal haemorrhage. Acad Emerg Med 1996; 10: 922–926.
32. Matsuoka T, Hildreth J, Wisner DH. Uncontrolled haemorrhage from parenchymal injury: is resuscitation helpful? J Trauma 1996; 40: 915–921.
33. Smail N, Wang P, Cioffi WG, Bland KI, Chaudry IH. Resuscitation after uncontrolled venous haemorrhage: does increased resuscitation volume improve regional perfusion? J Trauma 1998; 44: 701–707.
34. Burris D, Rhee P, Kaufmann C et al. Controlled resuscitation for uncontrolled haemorrhagic shock. J Trauma 1999; 46: 216–223.

Thomas Frietsch Christian Lenz Klaus F. Waschke

Artificial blood

Driven by a possible shortage of human donor blood and other limitations of homologous blood transfusion,[1,2] artificial blood was developed during the last decades as either cell-free haemoglobin solutions, encapsulated haemoglobin cells or perfluorocarbon emulsions. This process provided additional knowledge about oxygen transport and release.[3] Major functions of red blood cells are not only restricted to oxygen transport but are also involved in the regulation of vascular tone in dependence of oxygen demand.[4] Several haemoglobin- and perfluorocarbon-based oxygen carriers are under current clinical investigation as alternatives to the transfusion of homologous red cells. However, artificial blood substitutes are not confined only to their use as oxygen carriers. They may find a wide and further divergent spectrum of interdisciplinary applications. Beside an improved oxygen delivery to ischaemic tissues which cannot be reached by cellular blood components, they may deliver drugs in the future.[5]

This review covers the introduction of these new treatments into clinical practice, reports early pitfalls in the development and recent improvements in the area of artificial oxygen carriers (AOC), and provides future perspectives in this field.

Dr med Thomas Frietsch, Research Assistant and Staff Anaesthetist, Institut für Anästhesiologie und Operative Intensivmedizin, Fakultät für Klinische Medizin Mannheim der Ruprecht-Karls-Universität Heidelberg, Universitäts-Klinikum Mannheim, Theodor-Kutzer-Ufer, D-68167 Mannheim, Germany (for correspondence)

Dr med Christian Lenz, Staff Anaesthetist, Institut für Anästhesiologie und Operative Intensivmedizin, Fakultät für Klinische Medizin Mannheim der Ruprecht-Karls-Universität Heidelberg, Universitäts-Klinikum Mannheim, Theodor-Kutzer-Ufer, D-68167 Mannheim, Germany

Dr med Klaus F. Waschke, Assistant Professor, Institut für Anästhesiologie und Operative Intensivmedizin, Fakultät für Klinische Medizin Mannheim der Ruprecht-Karls-Universität Heidelberg, Universitäts-Klinikum Mannheim, Theodor-Kutzer-Ufer, D-68167 Mannheim, Germany

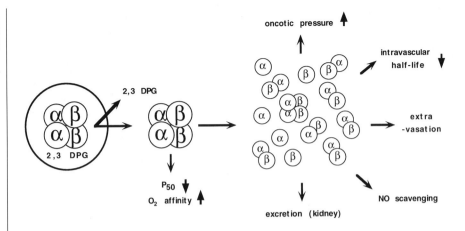

Figure 1 Isolation of haemoglobin from its natural environment. Haemoglobin outside the red cells dissociates into dimers and monomers. The loss of 2,3-diphosphoglycerate (DPG) and the reduction of the P_{50} changes its O_2-binding properties. The removal of the red cell membrane from tetrameric haemoglobin increases the intravascular oncotic pressure by monomers and dimers. Extravasation and NO scavenging occurs, and the dimers are renally excreted rapidly.

HAEMOGLOBIN-BASED OXYGEN CARRIERS (HBOC)

ALTERATIONS OF HAEMOGLOBIN CHARACTERISTICS OUTSIDE THE RED BLOOD CELL

Free haemoglobin derived from haemolysed blood has been used as red blood cell substitute for decades. Early investigations have described many adverse effects and problems after the use of haemoglobin solutions as AOC in humans. Increases in blood pressure, bradycardia, renal dysfunction occurred, and a short intravascular retention time was observed. Most of these limitations are induced by the necessary isolation of haemoglobin from its natural environment (Fig. 1). Inside the red blood cell, haemoglobin is a tetrameric protein formed by two dimers of αβ-subunits which quickly dissociate into dimers and monomers outside the red cell. Dimers, especially, undergo capillary filtration and are rapidly excreted by the kidneys resulting in the known short intravascular half-life of free haemoglobin (1–2 h).

The loss of 2,3-diphosphoglycerate (2,3-DPG) and other allosteric modulators of oxygen affinity induce an increase in oxygen affinity of haemoglobin outside the red blood cells. In comparison with intracellular haemoglobin, the P_{50} (partial pressure of oxygen at which half of all haem groups are saturated with oxygen) of free haemoglobin is reduced from 26–28 mmHg (3.5–3.7 kPa) to 12–15 mmHg (1.6–2.0 kPa). Another reason for the increased oxygen affinity of free haemoglobin is the pH-dependency of oxygen binding (Bohr effect) since pH inside the red blood cell is lower than in plasma. The reduced P_{50} of free haemoglobin impairs the release of oxygen to the tissues.

Due to the strong increase in oncotically active molecules in solution, the osmotic pressure of free haemoglobin is about 3 times that of whole blood at an equal haemoglobin concentration. Thus, in order to achieve an iso-oncotic solution, the concentration of free haemoglobin has to be limited to approximately 5–7 g/dl. Higher concentrations increase the risk of volume overload in the recipient.

A further problem with the use of haemoglobin solutions resulted from the contamination of such solutions with erythrocytic detritus. The removal of red blood cell membrane fragments in ultrapurified haemoglobin solutions could reduce the incidence of renal insufficiency and interference with blood coagulation as described in previous studies.[6,7]

Bovine haemoglobin offers several advantages over human blood as a haemoglobin source. Apart from its unlimited availability, the oxygen affinity of bovine haemoglobin is not modulated by 2,3-DPG but primarily by chloride ions. The chloride concentration in human plasma results in a physiological P_{50} of bovine haemoglobin of about 28–33 mmHg (3.7–4.4 kPa). In addition, a pronounced Bohr effect in bovine haemoglobin augments oxygen delivery to tissues with low pH. Thus, in bovine haemoglobin, chemical modifications are only required to prevent the dissociation of the haemoglobin molecule outside the red blood cells. However, the use of bovine haemoglobin as AOC has to be weighed against the uncertainties regarding the questions of animal-to-human transmission of diseases such as bovine spongiform encephalitis (BSE). As long as scientific and medical knowledge about interspecies transmission of diseases is in its infancy, caution is advised. In addition, the public BSE discussion might impede the development of these kinds of AOC. However, the risk of infection by both animal and human haemoglobin-based blood substitutes can be minimised by selection of blood tested for viruses, radiation, ultrafiltration or heat pasteurisation.[8–10]

Modern biotechnology offers promising perspectives in the field of AOC. Using recombinant DNA technology, functional human haemoglobin could be produced in bacteria (Escherichia coli[11]) and yeast (Saccharomyces cerevisiae[12]), and also in plants.[13,14] By splicing human haemoglobin genes into mice,[15] pigs[16] and tobacco[13] adequate amounts of human haemoglobin could be expressed by transgenic techniques. Genetic engineering offers the advantage that certain functional characteristics of the resulting haemoglobin molecule can be achieved by specific amino acid substitutions that occur naturally in other species or known human haemoglobin mutants. Recent studies have demonstrated impressively the potential of biotechnology. For example, in crocodiles, oxygen affinity is modulated by bicarbonate ions instead of 2,3-DPG. The accumulation of bicarbonate ions as metabolic end products reduces oxygen affinity and increases the fraction of oxygen off-loaded to tissues. This effect allows crocodiles to stay under water for a long time without breathing. The bicarbonate ion binding site in crocodile haemoglobin could be located. After isolation of the corresponding amino acids, this sequence could be successfully transplanted into human haemoglobin. It could be shown that oxygen binding characteristics of the resulting haemoglobin 'Scuba' did not differ from those of native crocodile haemoglobin.[17,18] Furthermore, genetic engineering of the haemoglobin molecule resulted in an improved solution stability.[19]

P_{50} values are known to be adjusted by altering electrostatic and steric interactions between the bound ligand and residues at the Leu (B10), His (E7) and Val (E11) positions modifying the 2,3-DPG pocket. Nitric oxide (NO)-induced oxidation and auto-oxidation could be modulated by large apolar residues (Leu, Phe, Trp) at the B10 and E11 positions of the molecule. Efforts to obtain an enhanced oxygen transport capacity by this approach have been successful.[20-22]

Modifications of haemoglobin

To overcome the difficulties associated with the use of haemoglobin outside red blood cells, haemoglobin has to be modified. A variety of haemoglobin modifications have been described in the literature.[23]

1. Pyridoxylation by derivatives of pyridoxal-5-phosphate, or *bis*-pyridoxal-4-phosphate, carboxymethylation of the amino terminal haemoglobin residues, and fumaryl-acylation decrease the oxygen affinity.

2. Intramolecular cross-linking of the α-subunits by di-bromosalicyl-*bis*-fumarate or of the β-subunits by *bis*(N-maleimidomethyl)ether reduces the tetramer–dimer dissociation and increases the intravascular retention time.

3. Polymerisation of haemoglobin molecules by glutaraldehyde results in polymeric haemoglobins, reduces the oncotic pressure of haemoglobin solutions and prolongs intravascular half-life. Furthermore, the extravasation of tetramers and NO scavenging is reduced by an increased particle size. Residual vasopressor effects depend on the solution purity.[24,25]

4. Conjugation of haemoglobin to macromolecules such as dextran, polyvinyl-pyrrolidone and polyethylene glycol increases intravascular retention time by prevention of the rapid dissociation of haemoglobin tetramers.

HBOC are under evaluation in a variety of clinical investigations (Table 1, Appendix).

ARTIFICIAL BLOOD CELLS (ABC)

The cumbersome imitation of nature by introducing haemoglobin into cell-like structures offers a variety of advantages. The oxygen dissociation curve of encapsulated haemoglobin is similar to that of red blood cells. In addition, an artificial membrane protects endothelial cells during circulation from enzymatic activity and released haem. However, intravascular oxygen transport could be optimized by a combination of encapsulated haemoglobin in artificial cells with a pure haemoglobin solution.[26] Aside from combinations, the potential of artificial cells in medicine seems to be unlimited.[27] Even the oral application of artificial cells containing genetically engineered micro-organisms has been evaluated.[28] The release of encapsulated proteins can be tailored by co-encapsulation of enzymes.[29] To illustrate their exciting potential, basic properties of these new kinds of artificial blood and therapeutics are mentioned below. However, these products have not been investigated in humans and their availability to clinicians and patients is still years away.

LIPOSOMES

Micro-encapsulation of haemoglobin in bilayered phospholipids and sterols, so-called liposomes,[30-32] results in the formation of artificial red blood cells

Table 1 Haemoglobin solutions

Company	Product	Source/ origin	Trademark	Study phase
Enzon Corp. (USA)	Polyoxyethylene glycol conjugated haemoglobin	Bovine	No	I/II[a]
Hemosol Inc. (Canada)	o-Raffinose cross-linked and poly-merised haemoglobin	Human	HemoLink™	III
BioPure Corp. (USA)	Glutaraldehyde polymerised haemoglobin	Bovine	Hemopure™	II
Somatogen Inc. (USA)	Recombinant human haemoglobin	Protein engineering (*E. coli*)	Optro™	II
Apex Bioscience Inc. (USA)	Polyoxyethylene glycol conjugated haemoglobin	Human	No	II[a,b]
Northfield Laboratories Inc.(USA)	Pyridoxylated and glutaraldehyde polymerised haemoglobin	Human	PolyHeme™	III
Baxter Healthcare Corp. (USA)	Diaspirin cross-linked haemoglobin	Human	HemAssist™	Production stopped

[a]Under clinical investigation as an adjunct to radiation in human cancer therapy.
[b]Under clinical investigation as a nitric oxide scavenger for the treatment of refractory, pressor-dependent shock.

('neohaemocytes' or 'pseudo-erythrocytes'). However, this approach also results in a rapid removal of the liposomes from circulation by reticulo-endothelial system (RES) uptake if the lipid vesicles have diameters greater than 0.2 μm.[24] Improvement of vascular retention time, up to an average half-time of more than 24 h, was achieved by modification of the surface properties of the liposomes including surface charge and the use of sialic acid analogues.[33,34] The inclusion of allosteric effectors such as pyridoxal 5'-phosphate varies the oxygen affinity (P_{50}), thus influencing microvascular responses to haemodilution.[35] Studies in Japan and in the US have shown substantial progress in the development of micro-encapsulated HBOC and large scale industrial production now seems feasible.[33,34]

Incorporation of an enzymatic reduction system of methaemoglobin[36,37] or an artificial reduction system[38] may solve problems related to methaemoglobin formation in HBOC. As inside the erythrocyte, methaemoglobin can be reduced to haemoglobin if a reducing enzymatic system is present.

NANOCAPSULES

Micro-encapsulation of polymer haemoglobin and enzymes in biodegradable nanocapsules decreases effects of lipids on the RES, avoids peroxidation of lipids and increases stability during storage and after infusion.[39] The polymer materials are polyglycolides and polylactides, degraded to lactic acid, and further metabolised to carbon dioxide and water. The rate of degradation depends on molecular weight, particle size and on the type of polymer or co-polymer. Normally, the metabolisation of nanocapsules takes about 7 days and the body load of lactic acid produced by degradation of a 500 ml solution is below 0.2% of the body's break-down capacity for lactic acid.[40] The diameters of the nanocapsules are between 80–200 nm. In contrast to lipid vesicles, the content of haemoglobin can be increased to an amount known from red cells (35 g/dl). In addition, with porous membranes, nanocapsules can be made permeable for external molecules like glucose. Enzymes reducing methaemoglobin and radical scavenger formation, such as superoxide dismutase and catalase, can be included in these nanocapsules.[38,41] Furthermore, the inclusion of glycoproteins such as erythropoietin[42] in HBOC unifies acute and chronic treatment of anaemia. Nanoencapsulated HBOC does not seem to induce vasoconstriction.[43]

ADVERSE EFFECTS OF HBOC AND ABC

Although most of the problems associated with the use of haemoglobin solutions as AOC have been overcome by the introduction of new products, questions of toxicity and possible adverse effects still remain. Furthermore, the biodistribution and metabolism of modified haemoglobin solutions are complex and not completely understood. Therefore, uncertainties exist about the maximum dose that can be administered without harming tissues and organs involved in uptake and metabolism of modified haemoglobin.

IMMUNE SUPPRESSION

The immunological consequences of modifying the haemoglobin molecule and the use of animal haemoglobin as AOC are points to consider when evaluating the safety of haemoglobin solutions, especially after repeated administrations in humans. Infusions of heterologous haemoglobin have led to higher antibody titres than do homologous infusions.[44] Anaphylactic reactions have been reported after repeated exposures to heterologous HBOC.[45]

Sepsis and endotoxaemia may contribute to mortality in haemorrhagic shock.[46] The ability of involved fixed macrophages to phagocytise micro-organisms could be impaired by HBOC. Furthermore, haptoglobin and transferrin availability are important in fighting infection by sequestering iron and prohibiting its use by invading bacteria. Saturation of haemoglobin-binding and iron-binding capacities with HBOC could further impede host defences.

NEPHROTOXICITY

Purification and removal of erythrocytic membrane fragments from haemo-globin solutions could reduce acute renal failure and coagulation impairment. Cross-linked tetrameric HBOC are prevented from urinary excretion but are deposited in lymph nodes, liver, spleen and in renal tubules.[47] Due to a delay of renal elimination, infusion of a polymerised HBOC is associated with elevated serum Fe^{2+} and ferritin levels peaking within 8 h and 48 h, respectively.[48]

Increased erythropoietin plasma levels within the first 24 h after infusion of a HBOC seem to be caused by hindrance of renal elimination capacities.[49]

FREE RADICAL PRODUCTION

Once stored in different tissues, haemoglobin becomes vacuolated and degraded by, among other mechanisms, hydrogen peroxide oxidation, leading to the production of toxic free oxygen radicals.[50] Furthermore, superoxide ion production, which is minimised inside red blood cells by methaemoglobin reductase, could occur in the absence of reducing enzymes. In ischaemia during haemorrhagic shock or inadequate organ perfusion, accumulated ATP breakdown products induce conversion of hypoxanthine dehydrogenase to xanthine oxidase. Re-supplied with oxygen and in the presence of a molecule which can donate an electron (e.g. iron), xanthine oxidase converts hypoxanthine into superoxide. This results in a number of mechanisms for the formation of oxygen radicals which can cause tissue damage, the 'reperfusion injury'. The lack of erythrocyte enzymes and radical scavengers such as catalase and superoxide dismutase in HBOC may result in a higher risk of reperfusion injury.

Haem and free iron derived from haemoglobin breakdown are also known to be involved in free radical generation. Oxidation products resulting from reperfusion injury have been observed in experimental models of haemorrhagic shock resuscitated with unmodified haemoglobin solutions.[51] To overcome these problems, current research uses haemoglobin conjugated to free radical scavengers (superoxide dismutase, desferroxamine) and antioxidants (selenium, catalase).[52,53] The clinical relevance of this phenomenon has to be established, but the inclusion of radical scavengers into nanoglobules with HBOC have been shown to be advantageous.[54]

VASOCONSTRICTION

Mechanisms by which HBOC induce vasoconstriction include the uptake of haemoglobin by endothelial cells resulting in the direct interaction with NO.[4] Haemoglobin itself serves to regulate NO bioactivity and chemistry. Simultaneously, this has been shown to regulate vasomotor activity.[55] Current research efforts[55,56] aim at a modification of the NO binding site of tetrameric haemoglobin by changing specific amino acids in the molecule. Steric alterations adjust the affinity of oxyhaemoglobin for s-nitrothiols (SNO) or the affinity of desoxyhaemoglobin for NO. Under physiological conditions, NO preferentially binds to the vacant haem with a greater affinity in the oxygenated state. When haemoglobin picks up oxygen in the lung, it preserves NO bioactivity by converting it into s-nitroso-haemoglobin and nitrosylated haems. Additional reactive pathways are the formation of SNO and dinitrosyl iron complexes. When oxygen saturation is low in peripheral tissues, it unloads oxygen and converts to desoxyhaemoglobin. Consequently, controlled by the allosteric state of haemoglobin, the inactivation of NO by haemoglobin nitrosyl derivatives is reversed. If this cycle is implicated in the present design of HBOC, a reduction of haemodynamic haemoglobin effects by purified or encapsulated solutions without considerable amounts of tetrameric haemoglobin would result. Therefore, the vasopressor effect seems to be variable for different HBOC.[57]

Artificial blood

In animal studies, the effect was dose-dependent[58] but independent in humans.[59] Since overproduction of NO seems to be involved in the haemodynamic effects of hypotensive septic shock,[60] tetrameric haemoglobin solutions have been proposed as a possible treatment modality under these conditions.[61,62] However, since the quantitative amount of NO scavenging by HBOC and its contribution to the regulation of haemodynamics are unknown, other factors, such as blood volume and cardiac index (depending on the oncotic pressure of an AOC), may also be of clinical relevance.[63] Furthermore, vasoconstriction by HBOC in haemorrhage might be dominated by elevated plasma levels of the vasoconstrictor peptide endothelin.[64] Other plausible explanations of vasoconstriction by haemoglobin involve the interaction with phagocytes, white blood cells, or platelets. Thromboxane A_2 is a potent vasoconstrictor released from platelets and activated macrophages. In rats, infusion of liposome encapsulated haemoglobin caused an immediate decrease in platelet count and increase in serum thromboxane levels, mean arterial pressure, and heart rate.[65] However, all parameters returned to pre-infusion values within hours.

NEUROTOXICITY

The role of NO in the brain remains controversial since recent data suggest both neurotoxic and neuroprotective actions of NO in the scenario of cerebral ischaemia.[66] There is evidence of considerable reduction of hippocampal cell density after induction of transient forebrain ischaemia and partial blood replacement with HBOC.[67] Nevertheless, in the study by Cole and colleagues,[68] haemodilution was performed with different doses of a diaspirin cross-linked HBOC with known NO binding properties. Infarct size and neurological outcome were found to be decreased in a dose-dependent manner. This effect might have been induced by an increase in mean arterial blood pressure (MAP) which is known to augment cerebral blood flow and thereby to reduce ischaemia. Since the MAP did not differ significantly between the different groups of the Cole and co-workers study, the reduction in infarct size does not seem to be caused only by an elevated cerebral blood flow.[68] Further studies to delineate the potential role of molecular haemoglobin solutions in decreasing brain NO levels during ischaemia are in progress.

INTERFERENCE WITH LABORATORY CHEMISTRY

Standard colorimetric laboratory assays for many plasma constituents are impaired in the presence of high concentrations of HBOC. These include bilirubin, liver enzymes, amylase, some electrolytes, and optical methods for coagulation times. Since haemoglobin content measurement is performed in haemolysed samples, this value is reliable. Essential analysis in the perioperative or critical care setting such as important electrolytes, blood gases, prothrombin and partial thromboplastin time are unaffected. Plasma glucose and creatinine also are valuable if measured enzymatically.[69] Thus, water and electrolyte homeostasis, acid–base status, renal function, and cardiac damage can be monitored adequately in recipients of a HBOC. Furthermore, and important for recipient's safety, pulse oximetry is also unimpaired over the

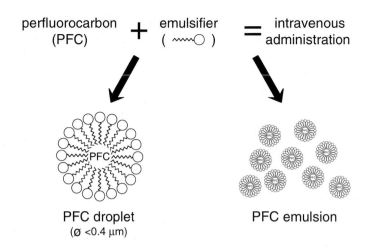

PFC droplet
(ø <0.4 µm)

PFC emulsion

Figure 2 Emulsification of perfluorocarbons. Perfluorocarbons are immiscible with water and plasma. Therefore, an emulsifier like lecithin is used to form small particles. The PFC emulsion can be infused intravenously after emulsification. This procedure is not necessary when PFC are used for liquid ventilation, eye surgery or as gastrointestinal contrast agents.

whole range of saturations.[70] However, elevated potassium concentrations in true haemolysis of the recipient's own red cells might be undetected.[69]

PERFLUOROCARBON EMULSIONS

CHARACTERISTICS OF PERFLUOROCARBONS

Perfluorocarbons (PFCs) are synthetic carbon-fluorine compounds derived from fluorination of cyclic or straight-chain hydrocarbons. PFCs are able to dissolve large quantities of gases including oxygen and carbon dioxide. Gas solubility depends on the molecular volume of the specific gas and ranks in the order $CO_2 > O_2 > N_2$. The strong carbon–fluorine bond (504 kJ/mol) prevents metabolism or breakdown of PFCs in biological systems.

EMULSIFICATION

Since PFCs are immiscible in aqueous systems, they have to be emulsified prior to intravenous administration. This emulsification results in a dispersion of droplets with average diameters of about 0.1–0.2 µm (Fig. 2). Older emulsions, such as Fluosol-DA™, were limited by their low concentration of PFCs (20% w/v). With respect to the high density of PFCs (1.8–2.0 g/ml) only 10% of the final emulsion volume administered to patients had oxygen carrying capacities. At room air, this resulted in an oxygen content of only 1.0–1.5 vol% (for comparison, under physiological conditions blood releases approximately 5 vol% oxygen). In addition, these older emulsions could only be stored and shipped in the frozen state and had to be mixed immediately before infusion. The stability of these preparations was limited to several hours. In recent years, progress in emulsification techniques has lead to the development of so-called 'second generation' PFC emulsions. The surfactants used in these newer emulsions are egg yolk phospholipids which are safely and extensively used for fat emulsions in routine parenteral nutrition. To date, ready-for-use emulsions with prolonged shelf stability and minimal adverse effects after intravascular use are available. These emulsions contain up to 90% w/v of the specific PFC with an increase in oxygen content at lower partial pressures of oxygen.

METABOLISM AND EXCRETION

PFCs are mainly excreted unmetabolised by exhalation, either primarily or after passage through the reticulo-endothelial system. The dose-dependent intravascular half-life ranges from 2–18 h depending on the RES activity. The rate and time of elimination primarily depends on the molecular weight of each PFC, influencing the specific boiling point.

ADVERSE EFFECTS

Although PFCs are biologically inert, this does not hold for the emulsifiers. Fluosol-DA™ uses a polyoxyethylene–polypropylene block polymer as surfactant. This Pluronic F-68™ is able to induce anaphylactic reactions in patients receiving Fluosol-DA™. Interference with neutrophil chemotaxis, activation of the complement system, and induction of platelet aggregation has also been described.[71,72]

Although the use of egg yolk lecithin instead of Pluronic F-68™ as surfactant has minimised complement activation, adverse side-effects at higher dosage of 'second generation' PFC emulsions could be observed. Transient moderate reductions in platelet counts were associated with a dose-dependent elevation of fibrin degradation products and fibrinogen concentration, a prolonged prothrombin time, and a modest rise in bleeding time. Elevated liver enzymes and febrile responses were caused by the clearance of PFC particles from circulation into the Kupffer cells. Therefore, the use of newer PFC-based AOC in patients is still limited to lower dosages.

OXYGEN TRANSPORT AND DELIVERY

In contrast to oxygen transport in blood or in haemoglobin solutions, there is no chemical interaction in PFC gas transport. In comparison to water and plasma with an oxygen solubility of about 3%, typical PFCs dissolve 40–50% oxygen when equilibrated with 100% oxygen at atmospheric pressure and at 37°C. Due to the dependence of dissolved oxygen in PFC emulsions on oxygen partial pressure, the extraction ratio of oxygen from PFC emulsions is much higher than the oxygen extraction in blood or haemoglobin solutions (Fig. 3). In early clinical studies with Fluosol-DA™ 20% as well as in recent investigations it could be shown that, when both PFC and blood are present in the circulation simultaneously, most of the oxygen consumed is delivered by the PFC before the oxygen bound to haemoglobin is released.[73] Thus, the use of PFC as AOC serves as a buffer for oxygen consumption and protects the endogenous haemoglobin from early extraction and desaturation. It has also

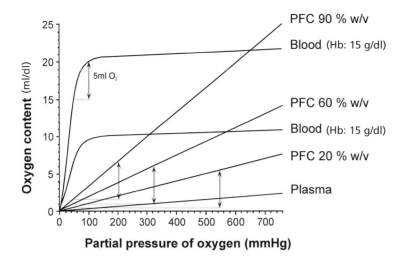

Figure 3 Solubility of oxygen in blood and perfluorocarbon emulsions. Dependency of oxygen content on partial pressure of oxygen in whole blood, in perfluorocarbon emulsions and in plasma. Arrows indicate the necessary partial pressure of oxygen required for a specific perfluorocarbon emulsion to achieve a release of oxygen comparable to the amount of oxygen released under physiological conditions from whole blood.

been suggested that PFC might improve oxygen passage through endothelial barriers by facilitating oxygen diffusion even in the absence of an increased inspiratory oxygen concentration.[74]

CLINICAL CHEMISTRY

Coming closer to clinical practice, the necessity of PFC plasma level measurements becomes evident. However, this is still not available as an immediate bedside test, but requires quantitative detection by chromatography. The interference of PFOB with standard laboratory analyses has been examined at 3 times the current clinical dosages.[69] At this concentration, the majority of tests (except ammonia, amylase and iron) were not impaired. Phosphorus was increased by the emulsion buffer of PFOB itself.[69]

PFC emulsions under clinical investigation are outlined in Table 2 and in the Appendix.

BIOMEDICAL APPLICATIONS OF AOC

AOCs under current clinical investigation mainly aim at approval as oxygen carriers or as blood substitutes during peri-operative haemodilution. The primary goal in this context is a reduction of patient's exposure to homologous blood transfusion.

In a variety of pre-clinical animal studies, AOCs have been used successfully as red blood cell substitutes in the treatment of haemorrhagic shock and extreme haemodilution. Whether these promising results can be transferred to the clinical situation of patients has to be proven by the ongoing phase I–III

Table 2 Perfluorocarbon emulsions

Company	Product	Indication	Trademark	Study phase
Green Cross Corp. (Japan)	Perfluorodecaline and perfluorotripropylamine	High risk coronary angioplasty Adjunct to chemo/radiotherapy	Fluosol DA™	Approved 1989, Production discontinued
Alliance Pharmaceutical Corp. (USA)	Perfluorooctylbromide	Peri-operative haemodilution/anaemia Adjunct to chemo/radiotherapy Contrast agent	Oxygent™ Oxygent CA™ Imagent BP™	III II III
HemaGenPFC Inc. (USA)	Perfluorodichlorooctane	Cardiac bypass surgery	Oxyfluor™	I/II
Sierra Ventures (USA)	Perfluorphenanthrene	Adjunct to chemo/radiotherapy	Oncosol™	I
Sonus Pharmaceuticals (USA)	Do-deca-fluoropentane	Echocardiographic contrast agent	EchoGen™	Approved 1998 (in Europe)

trials in humans (Tables 1 & 2). Since uncertainties regarding toxicity issues of AOCs remain, a careful evaluation of the risk-versus-benefit ratio seems to be necessary, especially in patients with co-existing diseases. Furthermore, the lack of interference with specific laboratory chemistry tests, particularly immunoassays and dry-chemistry methods, has to be shown. Moreover, the blood samples of recipients have to be identified by the laboratory to avoid analyses with known interference.

In addition to the initially proposed use of AOC as alternatives to red blood cell transfusion in fluid resuscitation or peri-operative blood loss, many further applications will appear in the near future (Table 3). It can be expected that microcirculatory support and perfusion of ischaemic tissues will be one of the major additional applications of AOCs due to their low viscosity and small particle size (Fig. 4). It is known that microcirculatory disturbances occur under different pathophysiological conditions. Global ischaemia, induced by haemorrhagic shock, or focal ischaemia, by arterial vessel obstruction, result in microcirculatory alterations such as leukocyte adhesion and activation, endothelial cell swelling, and capillary plugging by red blood cells and other cellular blood components. These changes are likely to increase vascular resistance at the capillary level. PFC emulsions are known to decrease leukocyte adhesion and activation in ischaemic tissue. Since acellular oxygen carriers are much smaller than erythrocytes, they are able to pass such microcirculatory obstructions and re-oxygenate ischaemic tissues (Fig. 4). In animal experiments, the beneficial effects of AOC have been reported for global as well as for focal ischaemia of different organs.[68,75–78] Detrimental effects on ischaemic tissue when reperfused with both, PFC and HBOC due to the enhanced generation of free oxygen radicals have been discussed. However, animal studies in myocardial or temporary cerebral ischaemia have shown beneficial effects of PFC and HBOC.[68,79–83]

In acute ischaemia of the limbs by embolism or thrombosis or during ischaemia induced by surgical occlusion of endarteries, the microparticles and micromolecules of AOC could reduce ischaemic tissue damage. However, until now, the efficacy of AOC in anti-ischaemic protection has been limited by restriction of the dose[84] or by use of low concentrated first generation PFCs.[85] Due to the increased gas solubility of PFCs, air embolism during extracorporal circulation might be reduced and neurological outcome of patients improved.[86,87]

Table 3 Possible biomedical applications for artificial oxygen carriers

Fluid resuscitation and peri-operative blood loss
Peri-operative haemodilution
Oxygen delivery to ischaemic tissues
Organ preservation for transplantation
Cell culture
Cancer therapy
Imaging and diagnostics*
Prevention of air embolism*
Liquid ventilation*
Ophthalmic surgery*
Wound healing

*Perfluorocarbons only

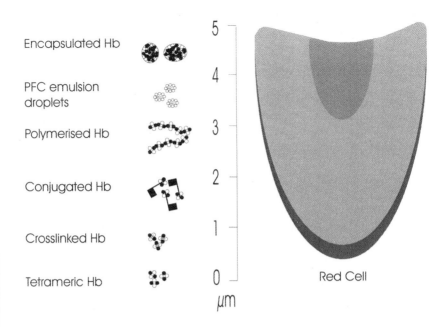

Figure 4 Size of intravascular oxygen carriers. Artificial oxygen carriers are much smaller than red cells. Oxygen carried outside the red cell does not have to pass the erythrocyte membrane. Furthermore, the distribution of smaller particles at the vessel wall decreases the distance for oxygen diffusion to the cell. These properties may reduce ischaemic damage and improve outcome after vessel obstruction.

Organs awaiting transplantation have been successfully preserved by perfusion with AOC.[88] Even in humans, successful transplantations have been performed after a prolonged time of organ perfusion with AOC.[89]

Oxygen supply in different kinds of cell cultures can be achieved in a more sophisticated way by AOC than by conventional approaches, thus reducing the potential of cell damage. In the same way, wound healing could be improved by external application of PFCs by enhanced cellular repair, improved wound closure, minimised hypertrophic scarring, or avoided scar contracture.[90]

In cancer therapy, it is known that hypoxic tumour cells are relatively resistant to radiation and chemotherapy. Tumour susceptibility to chemo- and radiotherapy is selectively improved by oxygen delivery to cells otherwise insensitive to cancer treatment. Perfusion of solid tumours with PFCs as well as with haemoglobin solutions has been shown to re-oxygenate hypoxic tumour cells thus increasing their sensitivity to ionizing radiation and anti-cancer drugs.[91] The development of artificial cells carrying both oxygen and drugs[5] possibly could increase the efficacy of such therapy.

In contrast to haemoglobin solutions, specific characteristics of PFCs will offer additional biomedical applications. Since the magnetic properties of [^{19}F]-fluorocarbons correlate with organ oxygen partial pressure, PFC tagged with ^{19}F can be used as diagnostic tools to assess tissue oxygenation by magnetic resonance imaging. Some PFCs can also be used as contrast agents in sonography, computed tomography and conventional radiology.

Key points for clinical practice

- Oxygen transport by existing blood substitutes differs from bondage of oxygen in haemoglobin solutions (HBOC) to physical solution of oxygen in perfluorocarbon emulsions (PFCs).

- Characteristics of all cell-free haemoglobin solutions outside the red cells include: dissociation of the tetrameric haemoglobin molecule, short intravascular half-life, vasoconstriction due to interference with nitric oxide, higher oxygen affinity due to the lack of 2,3-diphosphoglycerate, and a shifted oxygen binding curve (impaired oxygen delivery to tissues).

- Modifications to overcome these changes include: use of bovine or recombinant haemoglobin with lower oxygen affinity, decreasing oxygen affinity by linkage to molecules like pyridoxal-5-phosphate, intramolecular cross-linking with or without conjugation to other macromolecules, polymerisation of the haemoglobin tetramers, and encapsulation into artificial cells.

- Artificial blood cells (ABC) containing haemoglobin, enzymes and drugs provide similar properties to red blood cells but are smaller in size. However, their introduction into clinical practice cannot be expected in the near future.

- Adverse effects of HBOC and ABC are known and differ for each solution. They include vasoconstriction due to nitric oxide scavenging, nephro- and neurotoxicity, immunogenicity, free radical production and the disturbance of laboratory tests.

- Perfluorocarbons have to be emulsified prior to intravascular use. PFCs are not metabolised in biological systems, temporarily stored in the RES and exhaled completely unchanged. Adverse effects (fever and liver enzyme elevation, anaphylaxis to the emulsifier, modest coagulation impairment) are mild and transient in humans in clinical doses, but limit the use of PFC emulsions.

- To improve their oxygen transport capacity, PFC emulsions require artificial ventilation with a high fraction of inspired oxygen. Used as an adjunct to peri-operative isovolaemic haemodilution, they may reduce homologous blood transfusions during high blood loss surgery.

- Oxygen carriers are in phase III trials as blood substitutes, but current investigations indicate their potency in a variety of other clinical applications. This includes the reduction of gaseous microemboli during extracorporal circulation, improved oxygen delivery to ischaemic tissues, enhancing tumour sensitivity to cancer therapy, organ preservation in transplantation medicine and more.

In eye surgery, an approved liquid PFC (perfluoron, perfluoro-*n*-octane, Vitreon™)[92] has been used successfully for retinal detachments complicated by proliferative vitreoretinopathy, giant retinal tears and trauma.[93]

Recent data reveal that liquid ventilation with PFC might improve pulmonary gas exchange in animal models of severe lung failure. Human trials are in phase IIc, most of them suggesting that partial liquid ventilation with PFCs is also beneficial for paediatric and adult patients with severe respiratory failure.[94] Although the exact underlying mechanisms of these beneficial effects are not completely known, liquid ventilation in severe lung failure will undergo intense clinical investigation.

CONCLUSIONS

The research area of artificial blood, artificial cells and oxygen carriers unifies an amazing diversity of suggestions, results, future applications. Every month, a new piece of an overwhelming puzzle is added. Even new modes of application appear, such as intra-abdominal injections of PFCs[95] for oxygenation or vaporisation of PFC during respiratory failure.[96] Although this indicates the potency of AOC, the clinical applicability has to be proven by ongoing research.

ACKNOWLEDGEMENT

Part of this work has been previously published in the *European Journal of Anaesthesiology* (1998; 15: 571–584). The authors would like to thank Blackwell Science Ltd for permission to reproduce Figures 1 and 2 and Tables 3, 4 and 5 from this publication.

REFERENCES

1. Vamvakas EC, Taswell HF. Epidemiology of blood transfusion. Transfusion 1994; 34: 464–470.
2. Goodnough LT, Scott MG, Monk TG. Oxygen carriers as blood substitutes. Past, present, and future. Clin Orthop 1998; 357: 89–100.
3. Kawai N, Ohkawa H, Maejima H et al. Oxygen releasing from cellular hemoglobin. Artif Cells Blood Substit Immobil Biotechnol 1998; 26: 507–517.
4. Gow AJ, Luchsinger BP, Pawloski JR, Singel DJ, Stamler JS. The oxyhemoglobin reaction of nitric oxide. Proc Natl Acad Sci USA 1999; 96: 9027–9032.
5. Working PK, Newman MS, Sullivan T et al. Comparative intravenous toxicity of cisplatin solution and cisplatin encapsulated in long-circulating, pegylated liposomes in cynomolgus monkeys. Toxicol Sci 1998; 46: 155–165.
6. Rabiner SF, Helbert JR, Lopas H, Friedman LH. Evaluation of a stroma-free hemoglobin solution for use as a plasma expander. J Exp Med 1967; 126: 1127–1142.
7. Birndorf NI, Lopas H, Robboy SJ. Disseminated intravascular coagulation and renal failure: production in the monkey with autologous red blood cell stroma. Lab Invest 1971; 25: 314–319.
8. Bechtel MK, Bagdasarian A, Olson WP, Estep TN. Virus removal or inactivation in hemoglobin solutions by ultrafiltration or detergent/solvent treatment. Biomater Artif Cells Artif Organs 1988; 16: 123–128.
9. Estep TN, Bechtel MK, Miller TJ, Bagdasarian A. Virus inactivation in hemoglobin solutions by heat. Biomater Artif Cells Artif Organs 1988; 16: 129–134.
10. Ehrlich J, Zietlow J. Diaspirin crosslinked hemoglobin (DCLHb). Development status and perspectives. In: Mempel W, Mempel M, Endres W. (eds) Aktuelles zur Eigenbluttransfusion. München: Sympomed, 1997; 80–88.
11. Hoffman SJ, Looker DL, Roehrich JM et al. Expression of fully functional tetrameric human hemoglobin in *Escherichia coli*. Proc Natl Acad Sci USA 1990; 87: 8521–8525.
12. Wagenbach M, O'Rourke K, Vitez L et al. Synthesis of wild type and mutant human hemoglobins in *Saccharomyces cerevisiae*. Biotechnology (NY) 1991; 9: 57–61.
13. Dieryck W, Pagnier J, Poyart C et al. Human haemoglobin from transgenic tobacco. Nature 1997; 386: 29–30.

14. Dieryck W, Gruber V, Baudino S et al. Expression of recombinant human hemoglobin in plants. Transfus Clin Biol 1995; 2: 441–447.

15. Behringer RR, Ryan TM, Reilly MP et al. Synthesis of functional human hemoglobin in transgenic mice. Science 1989; 245: 971–973.

16. Swanson ME, Martin MJ, O'Donnell JK et al. Production of functional human hemoglobin in transgenic swine. Biotechnology 1992; 10: 557–559.

17. Komiyama N, Tame J, Nagai K. A hemoglobin-based blood substitute: transplanting a novel allosteric effect of crocodile Hb. Biol Chem 1996; 377: 543–548.

18. Komiyama NH, Miyazaki G, Tame J, Nagai K. Transplanting a unique allosteric effect from crocodile into human haemoglobin. Nature 1995; 373: 244–246.

19. Olson JS, Eich RF, Smith LP, Warren JJ, Knowles BC. Protein engineering strategies for designing more stable hemoglobin-based blood substitutes. Artif Cells Blood Substit Immobil Biotechnol 1997; 25: 227–241.

20. Fronticelli C, Sanna MT, Perez-Alvarado GC et al. Allosteric modulation by tertiary structure in mammalian hemoglobins. Introduction of the functional characteristics of bovine hemoglobin into human hemoglobin by five amino acid substitutions. J Biol Chem 1995; 270: 30588–30592.

21. Kavanaugh JS, Chafin DR, Arnone A et al. Structure and oxygen affinity of crystalline desArg141 alpha human hemoglobin A in the T state. J Mol Biol 1995; 248: 136–150.

22. Mathews AJ, Olson JS. Assignment of rate constants for O_2 and CO binding to alpha and beta subunits within R- and T-state human hemoglobin. Methods Enzymol 1994; 232: 363–386.

23. Chang TM. Modified hemoglobin blood substitutes: present status and future perspectives. Biotechnol Annu Rev 1998; 4: 75–112.

24. Chang TM. Recent and future developments in modified hemoglobin and microencapsulated hemoglobin as red blood cell substitutes. Artif Cells Blood Substit Immobil Biotechnol 1997; 25: 1–24.

25. Johnson JL, Moore EE, Offner PJ et al. Resuscitation of the injured patient with polymerized stroma-free hemoglobin does not produce systemic or pulmonary hypertension. Am J Surg 1998; 176: 612–617.

26. Page TC, Light WR, McKay CB, Hellums JD. Oxygen transport by erythrocyte/hemoglobin solution mixtures in an in vitro capillary as a model of hemoglobin-based oxygen carrier performance. Microvasc Res 1998; 55: 54–64.

27. Chang TM, Prakash S. Therapeutic uses of microencapsulated genetically engineered cells. Mol Med Today 1998; 4: 221–227.

28. Prakash S, Chang TM. Growth and survival of renal failure rats that received oral microencapsulated genetically engineered E. coli DH5 cells for urea removal. Artif Cells Blood Substit Immobil Biotechnol 1998; 26: 35–51.

29. Franssen O, Stenekes RJ, Hennink WE. Controlled release of a model protein from enzymatically degrading dextran microspheres. J Controlled Release 1999; 59: 219–228.

30. Rabinovici R, Neville LF, Rudolph AS, Feuerstein G. Hemoglobin-based oxygen-carrying resuscitation fluids. Crit Care Med 1995; 23: 801–804.

31. Rudolph AS. Biomaterial biotechnology using self-assembled lipid microstructures. J Cell Biochem 1994; 56: 183–187.

32. Chang TM. Artificial red blood cells. Trans Am Soc Artif Intern Organs 1980; 26: 254–257.

33. Rudolph AS, Cliff RO, Klipper R, Goins B, Phillips WT. Circulation persistence and biodistribution of lyophilized liposome-encapsulated hemoglobin: an oxygen-carrying resuscitative fluid. Crit Care Med 1994; 22: 142–150.

34. Sakai H, Takeoka S, Park SI et al. Surface modification of hemoglobin vesicles with poly(ethylene glycol) and effects on aggregation, viscosity, and blood flow during 90% exchange transfusion in anesthetized rats. Bioconjug Chem 1997; 8: 23–30.

35. Sakai H, Tsai AG, Rohlfs RJ et al. Microvascular responses to hemodilution with Hb vesicles as red blood cell substitutes: influence of O_2 affinity. Am J Physiol 1999; 276: H553–H562.

36. Ogata Y, Goto H, Kimura T, Fukui H. Development of Neo Red Cells (NRC) with the enyzmatic reduction system of methemoglobin. Artif Cells Blood Substit Immobil Biotechnol 1997; 25: 417–427.

37. Ohki N, Kimura T, Ogata Y. The reduction of methemoglobin in Neo Red Cell. Artif Cells Blood Substit Immobil Biotechnol 1998; 26: 477–485.

38. Takeoka S, Ohgushi T, Sakai H et al. Construction of artificial methemoglobin reduction systems in Hb vesicles. Artif Cells Blood Substit Immobil Biotechnol 1997; 25: 31–41.

39. Yu WP, Chang TM. Submicron biodegradable polymer membrane hemoglobin nanocapsules as potential blood substitutes: a preliminary report. Artif Cells Blood Substit Immobil Biotechnol 1994; 22: 889–893.

40. Chang TMS, Yu WP. Nanoencapsulation of hemoglobin and red blood cell enzymes based on nanotechnology and biodegradable polymer. In: Chang TMS. (ed) Blood Substitutes: Principles, Methods, Products and Clinical Trials. Basel: Karger Landes Systems, 1998; 216–231.

41. Yu WP, Chang TM. Submicron polymer membrane hemoglobin nanocapsules as potential blood substitutes: preparation and characterization. Artif Cells Blood Substit Immobil Biotechnol 1996; 24: 169–183.

42. Pistel KF, Bittner B, Koll H, Winter G, Kissel T. Biodegradable recombinant human erythropoietin loaded microspheres prepared from linear and star-branched block copolymers: influence of encapsulation technique and polymer composition on particle characteristics. J Controlled Release 1999; 59: 309–325.

43. Rudolph AS, Cliff R, Kwasiborski V et al. Liposome-encapsulated hemoglobin modulates lipopolysaccharide-induced tumor necrosis factor-alpha production in mice. Crit Care Med 1997; 25: 460–468.

44. Marks DH, Brown DR, Ottinger WE, Atassi MZ. Antibody response to transfusion with pyridoxylated polymerized hemoglobin solution. Mil Med 1987; 152: 473–477.

45. Chang TM, Varma R. Immunological and systemic effects of transfusions in rats using pyridoxylated hemoglobin and polyhemoglobin from homologous and heterogeneous sources. Biomater Artif Cells Artif Organs 1988; 16: 205–215.

46. Wiessner WH, Casey LC, Zbilut JP. Treatment of sepsis and septic shock: a review. Heart Lung 1995; 24: 380–392.

47. Bleeker WK, van der Plas J, Feitsma RI et al. In vivo distribution and elimination of hemoglobin modified by intramolecular cross-linking with 2-nor-2-formylpyridoxal 5'-phosphate. J Lab Clin Med 1989; 113: 151–161.

48. Hughes Jr GS, Francome SF, Antal EJ et al. Hematologic effects of a novel hemoglobin-based oxygen carrier in normal male and female subjects. J Lab Clin Med 1995; 126: 444–451.

49. Winslow RM. Blood substitutes – a moving target. Nat Med 1995; 1: 1212–1215.

50. Vincent SH, Grady RW, Shaklai N, Snider JM, Muller-Eberhard U. The influence of heme-binding proteins in heme-catalyzed oxidations. Arch Biochem Biophys 1988; 265: 539–550.

51. Tam SC, Blumenstein J, Wong JT. Soluble dextran-hemoglobin complex as a potential blood substitute. Proc Natl Acad Sci USA 1976; 73: 2128–2131.

52. Razack S, D'Agnillo F, Chang TM. Crosslinked hemoglobin-superoxide dismutase-catalase scavenges free radicals in a rat model of intestinal ischemia-reperfusion injury. Artif Cells Blood Substit Immobil Biotechnol 1997; 25: 181–192.

53. Simoni J, Simoni G, Garcia EL et al. Protective effect of selenium on hemoglobin mediated lipid peroxidation in vivo. Artif Cells Blood Substit Immobil Biotechnol 1995; 23: 469–486.

54. D'Agnillo F, Chang TM. Reduction of hydroxyl radical generation in a rat hindlimb model of ischemia-reperfusion injury using crosslinked hemoglobin-superoxide dismutase-catalase. Artif Cells Blood Substit Immobil Biotechnol 1997; 25: 163–180.

55. Stamler JS, Jia L, Eu JP et al. Blood flow regulation by S-nitrosohemoglobin in the physiological oxygen gradient. Science 1997; 276: 2034–2037.

56. Jia L, Bonaventura J, Stamler JS. S-nitrosohaemoglobin: a dynamic activity of blood involved in vascular control. Nature 1996; 380: 221–226.

57. Caron A, Menu P, Faivre-Fiorina B et al. Cardiovascular and hemorheological effects of three modified human hemoglobin solutions in hemodiluted rabbits. J Appl Physiol 1999; 86: 541–548.

58. Barve A, Sen AP, Saxena PR, Gulati A. Dose response effect of diaspirin crosslinked hemoglobin (DCLHb) on systemic hemodynamics and regional blood circulation in rats. Artif Cells Blood Substit Immobil Biotechnol 1997; 25: 75–84.

59. Saxena R, Wijnhoud AD, Carton H et al. Controlled safety study of a hemoglobin-based oxygen carrier, DCLHb, in acute ischemic stroke. Stroke 1999; 30: 993–996.

60. Evans T, Carpenter A, Kinderman H, Cohen J. Evidence of increased nitric oxide production in patients with the sepsis syndrome. Circ Shock 1993; 41: 77–81.

61. Kilbourn RG, Joly G, Cashon B, DeAngelo J, Bonaventura J. Cell-free hemoglobin reverses the endotoxin-mediated hyporesponsivity of rat aortic rings to alpha-adrenergic agents. Biochem Biophys Res Commun 1994; 199: 155–162.

62. Aranow JS, Wang H, Zhuang J, Fink MP. Effect of human hemoglobin on systemic and regional hemodynamics in a porcine model of endotoxemic shock. Crit Care Med 1996; 24: 807–814.

63. Migita R, Gonzales A, Gonzales ML, Vandegriff KD, Winslow RM. Blood volume and cardiac index in rats after exchange transfusion with hemoglobin-based oxygen carriers. J Appl Physiol 1997; 82: 1995–2002.

64. Gulati A, Sen AP, Sharma AC, Singh G. Role of ET and NO in resuscitative effect of diaspirin cross-linked hemoglobin after hemorrhage in rat. Am J Physiol 1997; 273: H827–H836.

65. Rabinovici R, Rudolph AS, Ligler FS, Smith EFI, Feuerstein G. Biological responses to exchange transfusion with liposome-encapsulated hemoglobin. Circ Shock 1992; 37: 124–133.

66. Dalkara T, Moskowitz MA. Neurotoxic and neuroprotective roles of nitric oxide in cerebral ischaemia. Int Rev Neurobiol 1997; 40: 319–336.

67. Hanzawa K, Ohzeki H, Moro H et al. Effects of partial blood replacement with pyridoxalated hemoglobin polyoxyethylene conjugate solution on transient cerebral ischemia in gerbil. Artif Cells Blood Substit Immobil Biotechnol 1997; 25: 105–114.

68. Cole DJ, Drummond JC, Patel PM, Reynolds LR. Hypervolemic-hemodilution during cerebral ischemia in rats: effect of diaspirin cross-linked hemoglobin (DCLHb) on neurologic outcome and infarct volume. J Neurosurg Anesthesiol 1997; 9: 44–50.

69. Ma Z, Monk TG, Goodnough LT et al. Effect of hemoglobin- and perflubron-based oxygen carriers on common clinical laboratory tests. Clin Chem 1997; 43: 1732–1737.

70. Hughes GS, Francom SF, Antal EJ et al. Effects of a novel hemoglobin-based oxygen carrier on percent oxygen saturation as determined with arterial blood gas analysis and pulse oximetry. Ann Emerg Med 1996; 27: 164–169.

71. Vercellotti GM, Hammerschmidt DE, Craddock PR, Jacob HS. Activation of plasma complement by perfluorocarbon artificial blood: probable mechanism of adverse pulmonary reactions in treated patients and rationale for corticosteroids prophylaxis. Blood 1982; 59: 1299–1304.

72. Virmani R, Warren D, Rees R, Fink LM, English D. Effects of perfluorochemical on phagocytic function of leukocytes. Transfusion 1983; 23: 512–515.

73. Tremper KK, Anderson ST. Perfluorochemical emulsion oxygen transport fluids: a clinical review. Annu Rev Med 1985; 36: 309–313.

74. Faithfull NS, Cain SM. Critical oxygen delivery levels during shock following normoxic and hyperoxic haemodilution with fluorocarbons or dextran. Adv Exp Med Biol 1987; 215: 79–87.

75. Oldham KT, Guice KS, Gore D, Gourley WK, Lobe TE. Treatment of intestinal ischemia with oxygenated intraluminal perfluorocarbons. Am J Surg 1987; 153: 291–294.

76. Peerless SJ, Nakamura R, Rodriguez-Salazar A, Hunter IG. Modification of cerebral ischemia with Fluosol. Stroke 1985; 16: 38–43.

77. Peerless SJ. The use of perfluorochemicals in the treatment of acute cerebral ischemia. Prog Clin Biol Res 1983; 122: 353–362.

78. Takahashi F, Tsai TM, Fleming PE, Ogden L. The ability of oxygenated fluorocarbon solution to minimize ischemic skeletal muscle injury. Plast Reconstr Surg 1987; 80: 582–590.

79. Cole DJ, Nary JC, Drummond JC, Patel PM, Jacobsen WK. Alpha-alpha diaspirin crosslinked hemoglobin, nitric oxide, and cerebral ischemic injury in rats. Artif Cells Blood Substit Immobil Biotechnol 1997; 25: 141–152.

80. Cole DJ, Drummond JC, Patel PM, Nary JC, Applegate RLN. Effect of oncotic pressure of diaspirin cross-linked hemoglobin (DCLHb) on brain injury after temporary focal cerebral ischemia in rats. Anesth Analg 1996; 83: 342–347.

81. Martin SM, Laks H, Drinkwater DC et al. Perfluorochemical reperfusion yields improved myocardial recovery after global ischemia. Ann Thorac Surg 1993; 55: 954–960.

82. Rice HE, Virmani R, Hart CL, Kolodgie FD, Farb A. Dose-dependent reduction of myocardial infarct size with the perfluorochemical Fluosol-DA. Am Heart J 1990; 120: 1039–1046.

83. Schaer GL, Karas SP, Santoian EC et al. Reduction in reperfusion injury by blood-free reperfusion after experimental myocardial infarction. J Am Coll Cardiol 1990; 15: 1385–1393.

84. Sakas DE, Whittaker KW, Crowell RM, Zervas NT. Perfluorocarbons: recent developments and implications for neurosurgery. J Neurosurg 1996; 85: 248–254.

85. Geyer RP. Perfluorochemicals as oxygen transport vehicles. Biomater Artif Cells Artif Organs 1988; 16: 31–49.

86. Spiess BD, Cochran RP. Perfluorocarbon emulsions and cardiopulmonary bypass: a technique for the future. J Cardiothorac Vasc Anesth 1996; 10: 83–89.

87. Menasche P, Fleury JP, Piwnica A. Fluorocarbons: a potential treatment of cerebral air embolism in open-heart surgery. 1992 update. Ann Thorac Surg 1992; 54: 392–393.

88. Skibba JL, Sonsalla J, Petroff Jr RJ, Denor P. Canine liver isolation-perfusion at normo- and hyperthermic temperatures with perfluorochemical emulsion (Fluosol-43). Eur Surg Res 1985; 17: 301–309.

89. Funakoshi Y, Fujita S, Fuchinoue S, Agishi T, Ota K. Neo red cell as an organ preservation solution. Artif Cells Blood Substit Immobil Biotechnol 1997; 25: 407–416.

90. http://www.fluoros.co.uk/f2chemicals/flutec/medical/

91. Teicher BA. An overview on oxygen carriers in cancer therapy. Artif Cells Blood Substit Immobil Biotechnol 1995; 23: 395–405.

92. http://www.infinitec.com/index.html

93. Peyman GA, Schulman JA, Sullivan B. Perfluorocarbon liquids in ophthalmology. Surv Ophthalmol 1995; 39: 375–395.

94. Hirschl RB, Pranikoff T, Gauger P et al. Liquid ventilation in adults, children, and full-term neonates. Lancet 1995; 346: 1201–1202.

95. Chiba T, Harrison MR, Ohkubo T et al. Transabdominal oxygenation using perfluorocarbons. J Pediatr Surg 1999; 34: 895–900.

96. Bleyl JU, Ragaller M, Tscho U et al. Vaporized perfluorocarbon improves oxygenation and pulmonary function in an ovine model of acute respiratory distress syndrome. Anesthesiology 1999; 91: 461–469.

APPENDIX

HBOC UNDER CURRENT CLINICAL INVESTIGATION

Pyridoxylated, polyoxyethylene glycol conjugated human haemoglobin (Apex Bioscience)

An analogue of 2-3 DPG, pyridoxal-5-phosphate is used in this HBOC stabilised with maltose to prevent methaemoglobin formation. Making use of its NO binding properties, it is intended to achieve beneficial effects in patients with pressor-refractory arterial hypotension in septic shock by single bolus and continuous infusion of this product. After the demonstration of successful restoration of blood pressure and the reduction of vasopressor drugs in spring 1997, further progress to phase III trials has been announced by the company for the end of year 1999.[1]

Diaspirin cross-linked human haemoglobin DCLHB (Baxter Healthcare, HemAssist™)

Products of cross-linked alpha chains of the haemoglobin molecule with *bis*-3,5-dibromosalicyl fumarate are manufactured under rigorous protein purification and viral inactivation procedures. This HBOC can be stored for at least 6 months. Clinical trials aim at a reduction of patient's exposure to homologous blood transfusion. An efficacy trial in cardiac surgery and peri-operative haemodilution has been completed.[2] This concept reduced the frequency of allogenic transfusion by 39% and 19% within 1 and 7 days, respectively. Unfortunately, another American and European phase III multicentre trial failed to reduce morbidity and mortality in patients with haemorrhagic shock due to trauma and was interrupted. As a further setback, in a phase II safety and efficacy clinical trial in 85 patients with stroke, the treatment with DCLHB was associated with worse outcome and more frequent serious adverse events.[3] Unfavourable outcomes at 3 months were associated with treatment of stroke by any dose of DCLHB in 85% of included patients (compared to 51% bad outcomes in the control group). Severe hypertension occurred in 3.5% only in the treatment group. The magnitude of the observed rise in mean arterial pressure was the same at all doses (25, 50, and 100 mg/kg) but the duration was dose-dependent. The results are questionable for a number of reasons, such as the very inhomogeneous severity score of strokes, the small number of included patients, the wide window until therapy was started (treatment was delayed up to 18 h). As a consequence and despite a lot of investigations of HBOC were done with DCLHB and a lot of money, effort and work was spent to reach the level of product safety, the producing company decided to stop the development and to shift the resources to recombinant haemoglobin technologies without further comments.[4]

Glutaraldehyde polymerised bovine haemoglobin (BioPure Corporation, Hemopure™)

Purified bovine haemoglobin reacts with glutaraldehyde giving a mixture of polymers and unreacted, haemoglobin dimers and tetramers. The latter have to be removed by postreaction processing resulting in a purity above 99%.[5] This HBOC combines a high haemoglobin content with a long storage capacity at room temperature. In clinical research trials evaluating isovolaemic haemodilution, this HBOC acted similarly to hydroxyethylated starches with respect to volume expansion, but improved tissue oxygenation better than stored packed red cells and fresh whole blood.[6] Compared to human red blood cell haemoglobin, a 3-fold enhanced oxygenation potency of this HBOC was explained by an improved P_{50} and enhanced diffusion capacity.[5] However, despite an improved purity, preliminary studies suggested a limited efficacy to increase oxygen delivery in clinical doses due to increases in vascular resistance and decreased cardiac output.[7] The results of its actual evaluation for human use in a pivotal phase III clinical trial in the US are expected.

Polyoxyethylene glycol conjugated bovine haemoglobin (Enzon)

Clinical trials with this HBOC focus on an enhanced radiosensitivity of tumours in carcinoma patients. This HBOC has a longer half-life and is intended for a weekly dosing combined with radiation therapy.

Raffinose cross-linked and polymerised human haemoglobin (Hemosol, HemoLink™)

Modified with ring-opened oxidised raffinose (o-raffinose) polymers of β-cross-linked human haemoglobin A_0 of various sizes (32–600 kDa) have been processed. Preclinical studies demonstrated no interference with the immune and coagulation system, unimpaired renal function, but minor gastrointestinal discomfort and haemodynamic effects. However, increases in blood pressure and decreases in heart rate were only slight and transient.[8] Thus, further phase III clinical trials to prevent and treat ischaemia in cardiac surgery patients with this HBOC have been initiated in Canada, the UK and the US.

Pyridoxylated and glutaraldehyde polymerised human haemoglobin (Northfield Laboratories, PolyHeme™)

After pyridoxylation with pyridoxal-5-phosphate, many properties of this AOC have been described to be similar to those of human blood, including oxygen affinity and colloid osmotic pressure. In a clinical phase II efficacy and safety trial, this HBOC could be administered safely in large volumes. A lost blood volume up to 3000 ml could be replaced without the occurrence of vasoconstriction. Since further clinical trials increased the maximum dose to 5000 ml, the intended indication for FDA approval is major traumatic blood loss.

Recombinant human haemoglobin (Somatogen, Optro™)

This human di-alpha haemoglobin is expressed in *E. coli* and consists of two α-globulin chains fused head-to-tail. Problems regarding achievement of high yield production, sufficient levels of gene expression, proper protein folding and assembly, purification from other *E. coli* products seem to be solved in the manufacturing process of this HBOC. However, whether costs of genetically engineered HBOC can be restricted to reasonable levels remains to be shown.

HBOC IN VETERINARY USE

Bovine polymerised haemoglobin (Biopure Corporation, Oxyglobin™)

Since the end of January 1998, this new HBOC has been approved by the FDA for use in anaemic dogs by licensed veterinarians. It contains a remarkably high haemoglobin content of 13 g/dl in polymerised form and is stable at room temperature for up to 24 months. Treatment of anaemia by a dose of 30 ml/kg was found to increase plasma haemoglobin concentration, to improve anaemia associated symptoms and to avoid additional blood transfusion in 95% of the Oxyglobin™ treated group compared with 32% in the control group. At that dose, the half-life of Oxyglobin™ in plasma was 30–40 days.

PERFLUOROCARBON EMULSIONS

Fluosol DA™ 20%

Clinical studies have shown that the oxygen carrying capacity of Fluosol-DA™ is not sufficient to serve as a blood substitute. However, Fluosol-DA™ was approved by the FDA in 1989 for use during percutaneous transluminal coronary angioplasty (PTCA) to prevent and treat distal myocardial ischaemia.[9] In a large clinical trial (TAMI-9, thrombosis and angioplasty in myocardial infarction trial), 430 patients were treated with Fluosol DA™ to reduce reperfusion injury in myocardial infarction. However, infarct size was significantly reduced only in the group with an anterior infarction. There were no differences in regional wall motion, ejection fraction or clinical outcome.[10] There have been three clinical trials which used Fluosol DA™ as an adjunct to radiation therapy and another three as an adjunct to chemotherapy. Fluosol DA™ finally reached clinical phase III trials as an adjunct to chemotherapy in high-grade glioma patients.[11] However, the production of Fluosol DA™ 20% has been discontinued.

Oxygent™

A 60% w/v emulsion of a primary PFC, perflubron (perfluorooctyl bromide), and a small quantity of a secondary PFC, perfluorodecyl bromide, is now under clinical evaluation during peri-operative haemodilution.[12] A current multicentre trial in clinical phase III is presently evaluating this PFC emulsion in patients during high-blood-loss surgery. By supplementing acute normovolaemic haemodilution with PFC and increased inspired oxygen concentration, surgery can be performed at lower haemoglobin levels. The autologous blood of the patient collected during the pre-blood loss phase of surgery can be re-transfused after haemeostasis has been achieved. The combination of acute normovolaemic haemodilution and PFC infusion might reduce the patient's exposure to homologous blood transfusion while maintaining tissue oxygenation at low haemoglobin levels during surgery. As an 90% w/v emulsion, Oxygent CA™ has been effective in animal studies of cancer therapy.[13]

Imagent™

The company producing Oxygent™ uses the same perfluorocarbon PFOB to process contrast agents. Actually Imagent™ BP, the one for ultrasound and echocardiography is evaluated in clinical phase III trials. Intended mainly for the early detection of primary and metastatic cancer, it is used either with CT scanning for liver tumours or to improve vascular imaging with ultrasound techniques. Impressive differences compared to conventional practice allow the differentiation of tumours 3–5 mm in size from same shaped blood vessels. It stays visible for several hours. Another product consisting of PFOB, Imagent™ LN is in clinical trial for improvement of tumour staging by subcutaneous injection. Now, the diagnosis of metastatic infiltration of lymph nodes by invasive lymphangiography could be substituted by CT scanning of contrasted lymph nodes several days after injection of Imagent™ LN14. Imagent™ MR had already been approved by the FDA for gastrointestinal imaging with MRI in 1993. However, the marketing of this preparation was suspended by the company in 1994 for financial reasons.[11]

Oxyfluor™

A 40% v/v PFC emulsion, Oxyfluor™ (perfluorodichlorooctane, PFDCO) has to be mixed with 23.4% saline to obtain isotonicity of the final product. As supplied in two parts, it can be stored for 6 months at 4–30°C. The mixture is under clinical investigation (phase Ic) for elimination of gaseous microemboli during cardiopulmonary bypass (CPB) surgery. Neurological (61%) or neuropsychological (79%) deficits are known to be a severe medical problem after CPB.[15] One year after CPB, these deficits have been found to persist (17% of the patients showing neurological and 38% neuropsychological disorders). Deficits are attributed to microemboli, generated during cannulation, hypothermia and extracorporal oxygenation of the blood.[16,17] Oxyfluor™ was investigated in dogs and it was able to reduce microemboli to a tenth.[18]

EchoGen™

Since July 1999, a 2% emulsion containing perflenapent (do-deca-fluoro-pentane (DDFP)) has been approved in Europe as an echocardiographic contrast agent. Due to hypobaric activation prior to use, this emulsion with a droplet size of 0.3 μm contains microbubbles of 6–8 μm in diameter. In real time echocardiography, EchoGen™ effectively opacifies the left ventricle, enhances markedly endocardial contrasts, and offers assessment of myocardial perfusion echocardiographically for up to 20 min intravascular stay.[19] Therefore, it improves non-invasive detection of shunts, valvular lesions, functional disorders.

REFERENCES

1. http://www.apexbioscience.com/products.htm
2. Baron F, Berridge J, Demeyere R et al. A randomized trial to assess the efficacy of diaspirin crosslinked hemoglobin (DCLHb) solution as an alternative to blood transfusion following cardiac surgery. Anesthesiology 1997; 87: A217.
3. Saxena R, Wijnhoud AD, Carton H et al. Controlled safety study of a hemoglobin-based oxygen carrier, DCLHb, in acute ischemic stroke. Stroke 1999; 30: 993–996.
4. http://www.baxter.com/patients/blood_therapies/hemo_therapeutics/index.html
5. Pearce LB, Gawryl MS. Overview of preclinical and clinical efficacy of Biopure's HBOCs. In: Chang TMS. (ed) Blood Substitutes: Principles, Methods, Products and Clinical Trials. Basel: Karger Landes Systems, 1998; 82–100.
6. Standl T, Horn P, Wilhelm S et al. Bovine haemoglobin is more potent than autologous red blood cells in restoring muscular tissue oxygenation after profound isovolaemic haemodilution in dogs. Can J Anaesth 1996; 43: 714–723.
7. Kasper SM, Grune F, Walter M et al. The effects of increased doses of bovine hemoglobin on hemodynamics and oxygen transport in patients undergoing preoperative hemodilution for elective abdominal aortic surgery. Anesth Analg 1998; 87: 284–291.
8. Adamson JG, Moore C. Hemolink™, an o-raffinose crosslinked hemoglobin-based oxygen carrier. In: Chang TMS. (ed) Blood Substitutes: Principles, Methods, Products and Clinical Trials. Basel: Karger Landes Systems, 1998; 62–81.
9. Kerins DM. Role of the perfluorocarbon Fluosol-DA in coronary angioplasty. Am J Med Sci 1994; 307: 218–221.
10. Wall TC, Califf RM, Blankenship J et al. Intravenous Fluosol in the treatment of acute myocardial infarction. Results of the Thrombolysis and Angioplasty in Myocardial Infarction 9 Trial, TAMI 9 Research Group. Circulation 1994; 90: 114–120.
11. Kaufman RJ. Clinical development of perfluorocarbon-based emulsions as red cell substitutes. In: Winslow RM, Vandegriff KD, Intaglietta M. (eds) Blood Substitutes. Physiological Basis of Efficacy. Basel: Birkhäuser, 1995; 53–75.
12. Wahr JA, Trouwborst A, Spence RK et al. A pilot study of the effects of a perflubron emulsion, AF 0104, on mixed venous oxygen tension in anesthetized surgical patients. Anesth Analg 1996; 82: 103–107.
13. Teicher BA. Use of perfluorochemical emulsions in cancer therapy. Biomater Artif Cells Immobil Biotechnol 1992; 20: 875–882.
14. http://pharminfo.com/pubs/msb/perflubron.html. Perflubrons. Medical Science Bulletin.
15. Shaw PJ, Bates D, Cartlidge NE et al. Neurologic and neuropsychological morbidity following major surgery: comparison of coronary artery bypass and peripheral vascular surgery. Stroke 1987; 18: 700–707.
16. Moody DM, Bell MA, Challa VR, Johnston WE, Prough DS. Brain microemboli during cardiac surgery or aortography. Ann Neurol 1990; 28: 477–486.
17. Blauth CI, Smith PL, Arnold JV et al. Influence of oxygenator type on the prevalence and extent of microembolic retinal ischemia during cardiopulmonary bypass. Assessment by digital image analysis. J Thorac Cardiovasc Surg 1990; 99: 61–69.
18. Taylor KM, Arnold JV, Fleming J et al. Cerebral protection during CPB using perfluorocarbon: a preliminary report. Key West (FL): Second International Conference on the Brain and Cardiac Surgery, 1992.
19. Main ML, Grayburn PA. Clinical applications of transpulmonary contrast echocardiography. Am Heart J 1999; 137: 144–153.

Neil Soni Michael Margarson

The human albumin controversy

Over the last decade, the subject of the use of albumin in clinical practice has become more and more controversial. Ten years ago, albumin was widely used in anaesthetic and intensive care practice for a range of indications. These included volume replacement, support of colloid oncotic pressure, supplementation of low serum albumin levels and even for nutritional support. Over the decade, the rationales underlying its use have been increasingly questioned. In mid-1998, two papers were published in the *British Medical Journal* under the auspices of the Cochrane Collaboration which seriously challenged the use of albumin and the role of colloids in general.[1,2] These papers were not clinical studies but rather systematic reviews, demonstrating not only no benefit but apparent detriment.

It should be emphasized that these papers were published under the auspices of the Cochrane Collaboration. The process of peer review and publication were the responsibility of the *British Medical Journal*. The combination of an authoritative source and an 'exacting' scientific journal implies heavily that the papers were credible and their conclusions both appropriate and noteworthy. The impact of these papers was magnified dramatically by the albumin review becoming a *cause célèbre* with the press.

Overnight, albumin became identified as a potentially hazardous agent. Current practice was threatened and both anaesthetists and intensivists were forced to re-evaluate their position and their practice. Whether or not these events have had an impact on practice still remains to be seen, but it has certainly generated debate which in its own right must be a 'good thing'. The systematic review was not the last word on the subject and already there are more publications relating to this topic; it is becoming apparent that this was just another twist in the tale of the use of albumin in clinical practice.

Dr Neil Soni, Consultant in Anaesthesia and Intensive Care Medicine, Chelsea and Westminster Hospital, 369 Fulham Road, London SW10 8NH, UK (for correspondence)
Dr Michael Margarson, Specialist Registrar in Anaesthesia and Intensive Care Medicine, Chelsea and Westminster Hospital, 369 Fulham Road, London SW10 8NH, UK

This episode provides an opportunity to look at the rationale behind albumin use: both the facts and the fiction.

ALBUMIN SOLUTIONS

Albumin is commercially available as 4.5% albumin and as 20% albumin, the latter being a hyperoncotic solution. Supposedly physiological solutions, the treatment of albumin requires fractionation in ethanol and heat treatment for several hours; it is, therefore, likely that the resultant solution may not possess exactly the same structure and function as the original compound. This may be particularly relevant in terms of both charge and binding sites. Nevertheless, the molecule is fundamentally the same and functions as a colloid. It has, therefore, been used for volume expansion and has the inherent advantage of being a relatively large molecule compared to, for example, the gelatins. It has always been assumed that it is, therefore, more likely to remain in the intravascular compartment.

The oncotic pressure of both solutions has been perceived to be of value in re-establishing and in maintaining the colloid oncotic pressure in plasma. The oncotic pressure of 4.5% albumin is closer to the normal range, but the 20% solution is considerably higher. The high oncotic pressure of the 20% albumin solution and the notion that the albumin remains intravascularly should in theory provide a method of manipulating the movement of fluids between spaces or compartments. This solution, although somewhat sodium deplete relative to the concentration of albumin (so-called 'salt poor'), still contains sodium.

PHYSIOLOGY OF ALBUMIN

Albumin has a molecular weight of about 66,000 Da and, compared with other proteins such as fibrinogen or immunoglobulin, is a relatively small molecule. The molecule is a single polypeptide made up of 585 amino acids with several minor variants in its actual configuration. It carries a strong negative charge.

It is synthesised in the polysomes bound to the endoplasmic reticulum of hepatocytes. Only 20–30% of hepatocytes seem to produce albumin at any one time, which implies that there is a considerable physiological reserve. In a healthy adult, it is probable that about 9–12 g of albumin is produced daily. There is no storage of albumin in the liver and, therefore, no reserve for release on demand. In states of maximal stimulus, the synthesis of albumin can only be increased 2–3-fold. Control of the rate of production is primarily mediated via changes in the colloid osmotic pressure and the osmolality of the extravascular liver space.[3,4] Other factors involved in the control of synthesis include raised levels of insulin, thyroxine and cortisol.[5,6] Growth hormone, despite its effects on reducing total urinary nitrogen loss, has no measurable effect on albumin synthesis in patients.

Amino acid deficiency, particularly of leucine, arginine, isoleucine and valine, can be rate limiting in the production of albumin, although this may only be of clinical significance in severe protein malnutrition states. The role of amino acid supplementation in enhancing synthesis of albumin in the absence of deficiency states remains unclear and in the setting of the critically ill patient unproved.

The catabolism of albumin is still poorly understood. It occurs in, or immediately adjacent to, the vascular endothelium of tissues, at a rate of some 9–12 g per day, which is of course very similar to the normal rate of production. Albumin is pinocytosed into cells at a rate which is related to atrial natriuretic peptide (ANP) levels.[7,8] It has been postulated that, because albumin is very low in tyrosine residues, it is a poor source of essential amino acids, and thus tends to be relatively spared in starvation and deficiency states.

The distribution of albumin, in man, is a source of considerable interest because it is predominantly an extravascular protein. There is more albumin outside the intravascular compartment than within. As the serum concentration of albumin is normally around 40 g/l, in an average adult with a 3 l plasma volume there will be an intravascular mass of ~120 g. The interstitial concentration is considerably lower, at around 14 g/l, and varies in different areas of the interstitium; but, with an interstitial volume of some 11–12 l, the total extravascular mass of albumin is ~160 g. Some of this albumin is easily mobilised from the loose interstitial tissues, whilst some is 'bound' particularly in the skin. These two 'compartments' are usually in a state of dynamic equilibrium which is influenced by any of the factors that increase or decrease the albumin pool. Changes in synthesis or catabolism will result in an altered total body albumin. The rate at which these changes can take place is fairly limited, even if synthesis decreases at the same time as catabolism increases. The time constant for these changes will be at a minimum hours and more usually days. In acute illness, protein catabolism increases dramatically particularly from muscle, but albumin is relatively spared. Loss of albumin from raw areas, the classic example being burns, will alter the dynamics of albumin homeostasis especially if the fluid is replaced by non-albumin containing solutions and these changes can occur relatively quickly. In contrast, the chronic losses seen in nephrotic syndrome may take longer to be seen, but result in significant depletion with time.[9,10]

Alteration of the distribution of albumin between compartments can result from changes in vascular permeability.[11] This, in company with alterations in lymphatic clearance and fluid replacement with non-albumin solutions, is a potent cause for rapid changes in albumin concentrations. All these mechanisms are functional, to a lesser or greater degree, following surgery trauma and in sepsis.

THE PHYSIOLOGICAL ROLES OF ALBUMIN

The key to the way in which albumin has been viewed in clinical practice are the perceived physiological roles that this molecule performs. It is a major component of the total protein in the intravascular compartment. It is a transport molecule which binds reversibly to ions and anions as well as a wide range of metabolites and drugs. The concentration of albumin will, therefore, influence the availability of albumin-bound drugs. It has a role as an oncotic agent and, in normal health, contributes a large component of the total intravascular colloid oncotic pressure (plasma oncotic pressure 25 mmHg). Indeed, the control of albumin synthesis is heavily influenced by the ambient colloid oncotic pressure. It is involved in the coagulation pathways and has an anticoagulant effect which is probably antithrombotic in nature, possibly mediated via inhibition of platelet aggregation.[12] It is a free radical scavenger and is a major source of reduced sulphydryl groups, the thiols.[13] These are in themselves involved in nitric oxide metabolism.[14] It has also been postulated that albumin plays a role in the maintenance of membrane permeability, although this is a subject of debate.[15,16]

It is clear that there are many mechanisms by which a change in the concentration of albumin in plasma can, at least in theory, influence physiological functions.

Furthermore, albumin can be and is measured relatively easily. It is measured routinely in hospital practice and both the absolute values and trend measurements are regularly used in clinical practice. The measurements provide a different perspective on this whole subject because knowledge of the values of albumin in a range of situations has led to clinical associations.

CLINICAL ASSOCIATIONS OF SERUM ALBUMIN

There are several well recognised associations. In surgical practice, a low serum albumin is associated with increased operative risk. In the critically ill patient and elsewhere in hospital patients, a low serum albumin is associated not only with higher morbidity from illness, and hence a longer hospital stay, but also with a higher mortality. In general, a low albumin is associated with a worse outcome or an exacerbated disease state. As a marker of morbidity, it has been of use in diseases in malignancy, in infection with human immunodeficiency virus (HIV) and even in acute problems such as community acquired pneumonia. It is a marker of debility.[17–26]

Low serum albumin is also associated with the formation of oedema. This has been observed classically not only in protein and calorie malnutrition but also in conditions associated with major protein loss, such as in nephrotic syndrome. There is an association between Starling's law and the formation of oedema and it is recognised that many patients with oedema do have low serum albumin concentrations. Albumin concentration is associated with colloid oncotic pressure and Starling's law describes the forces present across the capillary of which colloid oncotic pressure is a fundamental part. Therefore, there is an enticing association between a low serum albumin, colloid oncotic pressure and Starling's law.

While low albumin and surgery are associated with a poor outcome, it has been known since at least the 1930s, but almost certainly before then, that nutritional correction prior to surgery is associated with a far better outcome. One measure of nutritional correction is normalisation of serum albumin so that by default there is an association between normalising the serum albumin and a better outcome. Furthermore, there was an association between peripheral oedema and prolonged ileus.[27]

These are some of the associations and from these observations have derived some interesting assumptions.

ASSUMPTIONS

As a low serum albumin is associated with a poor outcome and a normal albumin with better outcome, increasing the serum albumin presumably may generate a better outcome. This has been applied in a range of circumstances but the most common is probably an observed low serum value in a critically ill patient leading to a simple reflex to correct the situation. In a nutritionally deplete patient, correction of the serum albumin implies nutritional repletion and this will come about faster if exogenous albumin is given. A basic assumption is made that a higher serum albumin will improve the patient's health.

ROLE AS AN ONCOTIC AGENT

Serum albumin constitutes a part of the colloid oncotic pressure (COP) and, therefore, a low serum albumin indicates a low COP. By invoking Starling's law, a low oncotic pressure implies a predisposition to oedema formation, or at least the threshold at which hydrostatic pressure will lead to oedema is reduced. Therefore, the use of albumin to return the COP towards normal will inevitably help the oedema which is a direct consequence of this pathophysiology.

Part of this assumption is based on the concept that albumin is a large molecule that stays within the intravascular compartment and cannot move anywhere else. It has a long half-life because it is trapped in the intravascular space and will sustain COP over prolonged periods.

There are also assumptions based on the idea that a decrease in the serum albumin is due either through loss or failure to synthesise, or a combination of both. That a low serum albumin is necessarily synonymous with a low total body albumin and as a consequence of this a low albumin means a deficiency of albumin.

There is a general assumption that, because albumin is a useful molecule with multiple physiological roles, a low serum value must be intrinsically damaging because those roles are all unfulfilled. In making these assumptions, a low serum albumin has evolved from an observed consequence of illness to a pathophysiological phenomenon responsible for morbidity in its own right.

USES OF ALBUMIN

The clinical uses of albumin are outlined in Table 1.

Table 1 Uses of albumin

Volume replacement
Support COP
Support serum albumin
     Transport molecule
     Membrane integrity
     Coagulation
     Prevent ileus
Free radical scavenging
Treating metabolic acidosis (neonates)
Fluid shifts (20%)
     Pull fluid back from interstitium
     Redistribute fluid during dialysis
     Improve oxygenation

CLINICAL RESPONSES

While clinical responses are changing slowly, it is not very long since the response to any of these problems was entirely predictable. If fluid resuscitation was needed, then albumin served multiple purposes and so should be and was the treatment of choice. If the serum albumin was low, then a better outcome could be sought by correcting the albumin concentration. A perceived low oncotic pressure could be corrected by albumin and, if there was any oedema, this could also be corrected by albumin administration. It would also be used to treat ileus postoperatively. If patients were septic the albumin would 'mop up' the free radicals. Problems with fluid distribution could be rectified by using concentrated albumin and this would improve oxygenation in the lung by reducing interstitial oedema.

In general, intensive care practice patients would progress better after treatment with albumin or at least would avoid the morbidity and mortality of allowing a low serum albumin to persist.

Thus, for a myriad of reasons, albumin was given.

PROBLEMS WITH THESE RATIONALES FOR ALBUMIN USE

There are both theoretical and observed problems with this approach. The fundamental problem with much of the theory relating to the use of albumin as a colloid, and in fact colloids in general, is the assumption that large molecules are effectively immobile. Albumin is in a dynamic equilibrium between the intravascular and extravascular spaces.[28] This equilibrium and the forces that govern it are often deranged in illness. The actual mechanisms in terms of membrane permeability, damaged membrane transport modalities, the influence of lymphatic drainage and others come under the loose classification of 'permeability changes'. The net result is that, in critically ill patients during some phases of their illness, intravascular volume is hard to sustain whatever fluid is used; the concept that large molecules sustain it better is only partially correct. The net flux of albumin between compartments increases and the extravascular component almost certainly also expands. In most patients admitted to an intensive care unit, the serum albumin value is already reduced at the time of admission. The rapid shifts in serum albumin concentration that are seen during resuscitation and in critical illness happen within minutes and hours rather than within hours and days, and cannot simply reflect changes in synthesis and catabolism no matter how large these are. Nevertheless, there is no doubt that these changes might contribute. The rapid fall in serum albumin must be largely due to redistribution. The net result to be gathered from these observations is that albumin, as with many other colloids, can be used to fill the intravascular space but in the sick patient may not be as efficient as hoped. It is important to emphasise that the vast majority of papers evaluating albumin as a colloid have focused specifically on these short-term effects relating to intravascular volume repletion and not its long-term effects, such as morbidity or mortality. From these papers it is quite clear, as might well be expected, that albumin is a colloid solution that is effective in intravascular volume repletion.[29–37] In this context, albumin solution was often considered as part of the 'crystalloid versus colloid' debate.

Redistribution of large molecules such as albumin and the fluid shifts that must occur in company with this will influence the colloid oncotic pressure. More importantly, it focuses attention on the fact that Starling's law is about gradients, not absolute pressures. If both large molecules and fluid move together, the impact on the gradient may be less profound than would be expected. There is also the observation that the range of proteins constituting total protein in the critically ill patient changes with an increase in acute phase proteins. Albumin may thus contribute less to plasma oncotic pressure in illness than in health. Certainly, the correlation between colloid oncotic pressure and total protein is far more impressive than that between albumin and colloid oncotic pressure. A low serum albumin does not always indicate a low colloid oncotic pressure. The role of albumin becomes less clear, as it can be postulated that movement of albumin out of the intravascular space with accompanying fluid will eventually increase the potential for a rising extravascular colloid component. It may then slow redistribution back towards the intravascular compartment as the insult subsides. Therefore, the role of albumin in sustaining colloid oncotic pressure is unclear.[38,39] But it is abundantly clear in critically ill patients that the oedema that is commonly seen is a consequence of an illness that leads to a reduction in the serum albumin concentration and that, in the greater part, the serum albumin value is an effect rather than a cause. This is supported by the simple observation that in postoperative patients the serum albumin improvement coincides with the diuretic phase of their recovery at a rate that cannot be accounted for by synthesis alone. In the critically ill patient, this improves as the patient improves, without intervention other than feeding.

High concentration albumin has been used to induce rapid changes in colloid oncotic pressure. Albumin (20%) given as a bolus increases the COP.[40–42] This can then encourage redistribution of extravascular fluid into the intravascular space; in the lung this could in theory enhance oxygenation. Because of the deranged physiology in the critically ill patient, the duration of such change is unpredictable, but may be quite short. Preliminary work looking at both fluid shift and oxygenation changes have to date been unconvincing (unpublished observations).

Albumin is a transport molecule and it would seem probable that there would be a major impact from altered drug binding. Information relating to this is sparse. Similarly, the role of albumin in coagulation is thought-provoking, but the only clinical relevance can be found in the priming of extracorporeal circuits where there is benefit. Membrane integrity has been a source of interest in physiology, but the data are contentious and has not yet found a documented clinical relevance; likewise oxygen radical scavenging.

However, if all of these factors have even a small relevance it might translate into changes in outcome. Most studies involving albumin have considered the short-term effects of its role as a colloid; very few have investigated the longer-term effects. Where these have been determined, several different approaches have been tried. Some studies have focused on the use of albumin to support COP with relation to outcome. Others have investigated its use as the main colloid while some have considered it as an adjunct to nutritional support. Historically, the perspective was usually taken from a viewpoint that albumin was certainly the best solution to use. Albumin has been used to support COP.[43] The studies to date are few, but suggest that albumin can be used to help maintain the COP; however, this has not translated into improvements in outcome.[44–46]

The value of adjunctive use of albumin in nutrition was assessed in a study of 61 patients suggesting a benefit in terms of reduced morbidity.[47] Supplementation in the critically ill patient has been reported and showed no benefit, albeit in a study of only 40 patients.[48] Two studies with 219 and 475 patients, respectively, did not show any benefit from the routine use of albumin in the critically ill patient.[49,50] In other scenarios, albumin is regularly used but it is again contentious and sadly lacking in focused outcome data. In cirrhotic liver disease, intravenous albumin infusions are regularly used. In specific circumstances, such as administration concurrent with paracentesis for ascites, this practice has no obvious benefit over infusion of synthetic colloids.[51] The time honoured treatment of oedema and attempts to promote a diuresis by the administration of 20% albumin in conjunction with a bolus of frusemide has not been shown to be of greater benefit than the use of diuretic alone.[52] The surgical claim of prolonged ileus resulting from hypoalbuminaemia, whilst not an outcome measure in its own right, has also been shown to be invalid.[53]

The great bastion of the clinical relevance of albumin use has been in paediatrics where it is still very popular. Again, the evidence is minimal and mainly from studies in burns. In one study, the benefits for the use of albumin in terms of maintenance fluid requirements, urine output, tube feedings received, days of antibiotic treatment, ventilatory requirements, complication rate, length of stay or mortality could not be shown. There were similar results in a second study.[54,55]

INTERIM CONCLUSIONS

These arguments outline the theoretical considerations behind the use of albumin in the context of the available information. The conclusion that albumin is not particularly beneficial derives from a very limited data pool. This is despite fluid administration being a fundamental part of patient management. The available information would suggest that there are no significant advantages or benefits from the routine use of albumin as a colloid replacement over other available colloids or indeed over crystalloids in any of the scenarios described.

It was in this context, in 1998, that two challenging systematic reviews were published. The first evaluated colloids versus crystalloids[1] and the second albumin versus crystalloids.[2] These two topics are to a significant degree inter-related and thus the combination of these two papers which were published in relatively rapid sequence has contributed to their impact.

THE SYSTEMATIC REVIEWS

Evidence-based medicine is 'de rigeur' and it is obvious from the previous discussion that the topic of fluid use is an area where there is limited evidence for common practice. As in other areas of medicine, systematic reviews are a means by which this might be addressed. A previous meta-analysis by Velanovich seemed to suggest colloids were better than crystalloids.[56] The conclusions of the two reviews were essentially that the use of colloids had a higher attributable mortality than the use of crystalloids, and that the use of albumin had a higher attributable mortality than the use of crystalloids. The reviews were based on 26 and 30 randomised control trials, respectively, and appeared to provide a definitive answer to two questions that had been controversial for so many years. This was in itself extraordinary. As can be seen from the preceding paragraphs, there are very few publications that address outcome following these fluids. However, as a result of publication in the *British Medical Journal* and being from the stable of the Cochrane Collaboration, these conclusions command respect and should be beyond reasonable doubt. The response both in practice and in the media was impressive especially following the albumin systematic review.

There are, in the authors' opinion, several problems with both of these controversial reviews. While they both obey the fundamental rules of systematic review, there are several areas that are contentious. To consider the positive aspects first. The literature search has been thorough, the trials selected were indeed randomised control trials and the authors were effectively 'blinded' to the outcome. On the negative side. in real terms neither of these reviews was very large in terms of total patient numbers and most of the trials were individually small. Furthermore, in the albumin study the reasons for administration were split across three domains: hypo-albuminaemia, burns and hypovolaemia. These are different populations with extremely variable anticipated mortality. The ages ranged from neonates to adults. The structure of most of the trials was quite different and the quantities of fluid and times of administration were variable. Most of the studies were not even outcome studies and when death was the outcome it was usually long after the end of the trial period. The heterogeneity in almost every aspect of these reviews is phenomenal and the methods used to 'eliminate' heterogeneity are not robust with the numbers involved. An interesting exercise with the earlier colloid/crystalloid review is to take out the three trials that have intrinsic weaknesses. These are the trials of Goodwin, and the two Vassar trials. When this is done, there remain 457 patients in one group and 456 in the other. The mortality figures are 86 and 84, respectively. If nothing else, it indicates the undue weight of three trials out of 26.

No matter what criticisms are levelled at these reviews, this was a serious attempt to answer some important questions and there are lessons to be learned both in terms of the problems intrinsic in systematic review but also the need for information about practice.

Since then, there has been a further systematic review by Choi and colleagues comparing crystalloids with colloids.[57] With carefully defined search parameters, 17 trials with 814 patients could be included. The results showed no difference in areas other than trauma resuscitation, and these authors highlighted the lack of adequate numbers. They also stated that 'methodologic limitations preclude any evidence-based clinical recommendations'.[57]

CONCLUSIONS

The controversy continues but there has been a shift in emphasis. Albumin is no longer beyond reproach although, despite the excitement of 1998, there is

Key points for clinical practice

- Albumin has several physiological functions including its role as a colloid in plasma (contributing to colloid oncotic pressure), a transport molecule for a large range of different types of molecule, contributing to coagulation and a non-specific role in membrane integrity. It is also an oxygen free radical scavenger.

- Serum albumin may be a useful marker in chronic nutrition and disease states.

- Serum albumin concentrations usually fall following any major insult that involves fluid resuscitation.

- The fall in serum albumin concentration is too large and too rapid to be accounted for by changes in either synthetic or catabolic rate and is almost certainly due to redistribution.

- Albumin solutions function as colloid solutions with 20% albumin having a role as an hyperoncotic solution.

- The theoretical benefits of albumin replacement are not readily demonstrated in clinical studies. The routine measurement of serum albumin is of doubtful merit.

- Systematic review of the use of albumin has fuelled an interesting debate, but has shown little of value beyond recognition that injudicious use of intravenous fluids may be detrimental.

no real reason to discontinue its use. What is more difficult is to assess is when there may be benefits and obviously what is needed is more original work because that is what is lacking. No matter how sophisticated the statistical method, it will still be impossible to make a silk purse out of a sow's ear.

REFERENCES

1. Roberts I. Human albumin administration in critically ill patients: systematic review of randomised controlled trials. BMJ 1998; 317: 235–240.
2. Schierhout G, Roberts I. Fluid resuscitation with colloid or crystalloid solutions in critically ill patients: a systematic review of randomised trials. BMJ 1998; 316: 961–964.
3. Pietrangelo A, Panduro A, Chowdhury JR, Shafritz DA. Albumin gene expression is down-regulated by albumin or macromolecule infusion in the rat. J Clin Invest 1992; 89: 1755–1760.
4. Rothschild MA, Oratz M, Schreiber SS, Mongelli J. The effects of ethanol and hyperosmotic perfusates on albumin synthesis and release. Hepatology 1986; 6: 1382–1385.
5. Hutson SM, Stinson Fisher C, Shiman R, Jefferson LS. Regulation of albumin synthesis by hormones and amino acids in primary cultures of rat hepatocytes. Am J Physiol 1987; 252: E291–E298.
6. Kimball SR, Horetsky RL, Jefferson LS. Hormonal regulation of albumin gene expression in primary cultures of rat hepatocytes. Am J Physiol 1995; 268: E6–E14.
7. Tucker VL, Bravo E, Weber CJ, Wisner DH. Blood-to-tissue albumin transport in rats subjected to acute hemorrhage and resuscitation. Shock 1995; 3: 189–195.
8. Zimmerman RS, Trippodo NC, MacPhee AA, Martinez AJ, Barbee RW. High-dose atrial

natriuretic factor enhances albumin escape from the systemic but not the pulmonary circulation. Circ Res 1990; 67: 461–468.

9. Margarson MP, Soni N. Serum albumin: touchstone or totem? Anaesthesia 1998; 53: 789–803.

10. Bent-Hansen L. Whole body capillary exchange of albumin. Acta Physiol Scand Suppl 1991; 603: 5–10.

11. Parving H, Gyntelberg F. Transcapillary escape rate of albumin and plasma volume in essential hypertension. Circ Res 1973; 32: 643–651.

12. Mulvihill JN, Faradji A, Oberling F, Cazenave JP. Surface passivation by human albumin of plasmapheresis circuits reduces platelet accumulation and thrombus formation. Experimental and clinical studies. J Biomed Mater Res 1990; 24: 155–163.

13. Halliwell B. Albumin – an important extracellular antioxidant. Bichem Pharmacol 1988; 374: 569–571.

14. Li H, Marshall ZM, Whorton AR. Stimulation of cystine uptake by nitric oxide: regulation of endothelial cell glutathione levels. Am J Physiol 1999; 276: C803–C811.

15. Lum H, Siflinger-Birnboim A, Blumenstock F, Malik A. Serum albumin decreases transendothelial permeability to macromolecules. Microvasc Res 1991; 42: 91–102.

16. Ramirez-Vick J, Vargas FF. Albumin modulation of paracellular permeability of pig vena caval endothelium shows specificity for pig albumin. Am J Physiol 1993; 264: H1382–H1387.

17. Suttmann U, Ockenga J, Selberg O, Hoogestraat L, Deicher H, Muller MJ. Incidence and prognostic value of malnutrition and wasting in human immunodeficiency virus-infected outpatients. J Acquir Immune Defic Syndr Hum Retrovirol 1995; 8: 239–246.

18. Cirasino L, Landonio G, Imbriani M. Hypoalbuminemia in human immunodeficiency virus infection: causes and possible prognostic value . J Parenter Enter Nutr 1993; 17: 101–102.

19. Huang CM, Ruddel M, Elin RJ. Nutritional status of patients with acquired immunodeficiency syndrome. Clin Chem 1988; 34: 1957–1959.

20. Morlat P, Bartou C, Ragnaud JM et al. *Pneumocystis carinii* pneumonia in AIDS: retro-spective analysis of 80 documented cases (1985–1993). Rev Med Intern 1996; 17: 25–33.

21. Gottschlich MM, Baumer T, Jenkins M, Khoury J, Warden GD. The prognostic value of nutritional and inflammatory indices in patients with burns. J Burn Care Rehabil 1992; 13: 105–113.

22. Murata GH, Fox L, Tzamaloukas AH. Predicting the course of peritonitis in patients receiving continuous ambulatory peritoneal dialysis. Arch Intern Med 1993; 153: 2317–2321.

23. Volkert D, Kruse W, Oster P, Schlierf G. Malnutrition in geriatric patients: diagnostic and prognostic significance of nutritional parameters. Ann Nutr Metab 1992; 36: 97–112.

24. Daly JM, Dudrick SJ, Copeland EMD. Evaluation of nutritional indices as prognostic indicators in the cancer patient. Cancer 1979; 43: 925–931.

25. Maetani S, Kashiwara S, Kuramoto S, Kanazawa T, Satoh M. Prognostic significance of serum albumin urea ratio in suture line leakage of the alimentary tract. Jpn J Surg 1974; 4: 11–20.

26. Su CH, Tsay SH, Wu CC et al. Factors influencing postoperative morbidity, mortality, and survival after resection for hilar cholangiocarcinoma. Ann Surg 1996; 223: 384–394.

27. Weinstein PD, Doerfler ME. Systemic complications of fluid resuscitation. Crit Care Clin 1992; 8: 439–448.

28. Fleck A, Raines G, Hawker F. Increased vascular permeability; a major cause of hypo albuminaemia in disease and injury. Lancet 1985; i: 781–784.

29. Schott U, Lindbom LO, Sjostrand U. Hemodynamic effects of colloid concentration in experimental hemorrhage: a comparison of Ringer's acetate, 3% dextran-60, and 6% dextran-70. Crit Care Med 1988; 16: 346–352.

30. Hein LG, Albrecht M, Dworschak M, Frey L, Bruckner UB. Long-term observation following traumatic-hemorrhagic shock in the dog: a comparison of crystalloidal vs. colloidal fluids. Circ Shock 1988; 26: 353–364.

31. Karanko MS. Plasma volume substitution. Acta Anaesthesiol Scand Suppl 1988; 89: 54–57.

32. Brock H, Rapf B, Necek S et al. Comparison of postoperative volume therapy in heart surgery patients. Anaesthesist 1995; 44: 486–492.

33. Gallagher JD, Moore RA, Kerns D et al. Effects of colloid or crystalloid administration on

pulmonary extravascular water in the postoperative period after coronary artery bypass grafting. Anesth Analg 1985; 64: 753–758.

34. Boldt J. Volume replacement in critically ill intensive-care patients. No classic review. Anaesthesist 1998; 47: 778–785.

35. Riddez L, Hahn RG, Brismar B, Strandberg A, Svensen C, Hedenstierna G. Central and regional hemodynamics during acute hypovolemia and volume substitution in volunteers. Crit Care Med 1997; 25: 635–640.

36. Stoddart PA, Rich P, Sury MR. A comparison of 4.5% human albumin solution and Haemaccel in neonates undergoing major surgery. Paediatr Anaesth 1996; 6: 103–106.

37. Hankeln K, Siebert Spelmeyer C, Bohmert F, Beez M, Laniewski P. Effect of colloid volume replacement substances and Ringer's lactate on hemodynamics and oxygen consumption of intensive care patients. Infusionstherapie 1988; 15: 33–38.

38. Barclay SA, Bennett D. The direct measurement of plasma colloid osmotic pressure is superior to colloid osmotic pressure derived from albumin or total protein. Intensive Care Med 1987; 13: 114–118.

39. Blunt MC, Nicholson JP, Park GR. Serum albumin and colloid osmotic pressure in survivors and nonsurvivors of prolonged critical illness. Anaesthesia 1998; 53: 755–761.

40. Tone O, Ito U, Tomita H, Masaoka H, Tominaga B. High colloid oncotic therapy for brain edema with cerebral hemorrhage. Acta Neurochir Suppl Wien 1994; 60: 568–570.

41. Zetterstrom H, Hedstrand U. Albumin treatment following major surgery. I. Effects on plasma oncotic pressure, renal function and peripheral oedema. Acta Anaesthesiol Scand 1981; 25: 125–132.

42. Bignall S, Bailey PC, Bass CA, Cramb R, Rivers RP, Wadsworth J. The cardiovascular and oncotic effects of albumin infusion in premature infants. Early Hum Dev 1989; 20: 191–201.

43. Wojtysiak SL, Brown RO, Roberson D, Powers DA, Kudsk KA. Effect of hypoalbuminemia and parenteral nutrition on free water excretion and electrolyte-free water resorption. Crit Care Med 1992; 20: 164–169.

44. Grootendorst AF, van Wilgenburg M, de Laat P, van der Hoven B. Albumin abuse in intensive care medicine. Intensive Care Med 1988; 14: 554–557.

45. Grundmann R, Heistermann S. Postoperative albumin infusion therapy based on colloid osmotic pressure. A prospectively randomized trial. Arch Surg 1985; 120: 911–915.

46. Grundmann R, Von LC. Indications for postoperative human albumin therapy in the intensive care unit – a prospective randomized study. Langenbecks Arch Chir 1986; 367: 235–246.

47. Brown RO, Bradley JE, Bekemeyer WB, Luther RW. Effect of albumin supplementation during parenteral nutrition on hospital morbidity. Crit Care Med 1988; 16: 1177–1182.

48. Foley EF, Borlase BC, Dzik WH, Bistrian BR, Benotti PN. Albumin supplementation in the critically ill. A prospective, randomized trial. Arch Surg 1990; 125: 739–742.

49. Stockwell M, Soni N, Riley B. Colloid solutions in the critically ill. A randomized comparison of albumin and polygeline. 1. Outcome and duration of stay in the intensive care unit. Anaesthesia 1992; 47: 3–6.

50. Golub R, Sorrento Jr JJ, Cantu Jr R, Nierman DM, Moideen A, Stein HD. Efficacy of albumin supplementation in the surgical intensive care unit: a prospective, randomized study. Crit Care Med 1994; 22: 613–619.

51. Salerno F, Badalmenti S, Lorenzano E, Moser P, Incerti P. Randomised comparative study of Hemaccel vs. albumin infusion after total paracentesis in cirrhotic patients with refractory ascites. Hepatology 1991; 13: 707–713.

52. Akcicek F, Yalniz T, Basci A, Ok E, Mees E. Diuretic effect of frusemide in patients with nephrotic syndrome: is it potentiated by intravenous albumin? BMJ 1995; 310: 162–163.

53. Woods MS, Kelley H. Oncotic pressure, albumin and ileus: the effect of albumin replacement on postoperative ileus. Am Surg 1993; 59: 758–763.

54. Greenhalgh DG, Housinger TA, Kagan RJ et al. Maintenance of serum albumin levels in pediatric burn patients: a prospective, randomized trial. J Trauma 1995; 39: 67–73.

55. Sheridan RL, Prelack K, Cunningham JJ. Physiologic hypoalbuminemia is well tolerated by severely burned children. J-Trauma 1997; 43: 448–452.

56. Velanovich V. Crystalloid versus colloid resuscitation: a meta analysis of mortality. Surgery 1989; 105: 65–71.

57. Choi PT, Yip G, Quinonez LG, Cook DJ. Crystalloids vs. colloids in fluid resuscitation: a systematic review. Crit Care Med 1999; 27: 200–210.

Jean-Pierre van Besouw

Risk assessment

Predictions are often wrong, particularly about the future.
Dan Quayle. US Vice President 1989–1993

Risk can be defined as the chance of an adverse outcome[1] and to the man in the street generally implies a degree of danger. To the anaesthetist, risk can be classified in terms of risk of patient death or risk of a peri-operative untoward event. Historically, the medical profession has focused on patient factors as being the major determinants of this risk. Increasingly, however, we must focus on the role of the healthcare providers (including anaesthetists) and the healthcare system and its infrastructure, as also having a major role to play in determining whether a patient undergoing a specific procedure, does so with the best possible outcome. The risk of death from any cause for all procedures and for all categories of patient, within the peri-operative period is around 1 in 1000. Peri-operative deaths, where anaesthetic factors are the major contributor to an adverse outcome, account for 1 in 10,000 procedures. Whilst risk of death from anaesthetic related causes for a patient undergoing day care surgery is around 1 in 22,000 less than those associated with driving a car.[2]

Risk assessment is, therefore, dependent on an analysis of all of the components within the system, both patient and healthcare providers. Risk analysis is the process of evaluation of the risk involved in a given course of action. The two elements of this analysis are identification and quantification of risk. Identification is dependent on information and data collection, whilst quantification is dependent on a combination of clinical judgement and mathematical modelling. The quality and accuracy of the information involved in risk identification can be enhanced by research and audit. Risk analysis is not a static process, assessments need to be revised in the light of new information, treatment strategies and

Dr J-P. van Besouw, Consultant Anaesthetist, Department of Anaesthetics, St George's Hospital, Blackshaw Road, London SW17 0QT, UK

Table 1 How to assess risk in the workplace

Step 1:	Look for the hazards
Step 2:	Decide who might be harmed
Step 3:	Evaluate the risks and decide whether the existing precautions are adequate or whether more should be done
Step 4:	Record your findings
Step 5:	Review your assessment and revise where necessary

techniques. The process of risk analysis is one of assessing probability, whilst the decision to proceed with a given course of action is dependent on how risk-averse a patient or their doctors are.

IDENTIFYING AND QUANTIFYING RISK – GENERAL PRINCIPLES

In the assessment of risk it is important to apply some general principles from without the health service. The Health and Safety Executive (HSE) provides a general guide[3] to employers on reducing risk in the workplace, the precepts outlined in this advice form a ready framework for all situations including healthcare provision, and are a good starting point for the analysis of risk (Table 1).

LOOKING FOR HAZARDS

Adverse events can occur throughout the peri-operative period and as previously mentioned may be patient or operator related (Table 2). Important pre-operative factors are associated with the patients presenting medical condition and pre-existing physical status. Intra-operative risk factors include the type of surgery, choice of anaesthetic and experience of the operators. Postoperative factors can be patient related (e.g. anaemia), medically related (e.g. adequacy of pain relief) or institutional related (e.g. availability of intensive care or high dependency beds). Risk assessment involves a retrospective analysis of any adverse outcomes for a given procedure, patient type, operator or institution.

Table 2 Factors associated with adverse events in the peri-operative period

Pre-operative risk factors
   Medical condition
   Age

Intra-operative risk factors
   Type of anaesthetic
   Type and site of surgery
   Experience of anaesthetist/surgeon/assistants
   Emergency status
   Duration of procedure
   Haemodynamic stability
   Monitoring

Postoperative risk factors
   Pain relief
   Availability of high dependency care facility
   Anaemia
   Oxygen therapy

Patient related risk scores[4-7] have been developed by a process of retrospective analysis followed by prospective application to a similar patient subset for validation of accuracy. Scoring systems are not perfect, they may reflect institutional or practitioner bias and may rapidly become out-dated by advances in technology and therapies. It is, therefore, imperative to be mindful of the innate faults of these systems when implementing them.

The process of identifying risk, within healthcare providers, is a requirement in the implementation of Clinical Governance (see below).[8] Clinical Governance is perceived as a framework within which healthcare organisations can work to improve and assure the quality of healthcare that they provide. Part and parcel of this process involves a self assessment of performance by the individual practitioner, including anaesthetists.[9-11]

DECIDE WHO MIGHT BE HARMED

The anaesthetist in the pre-operative assessment of the patient assesses risk by drawing together information from the history and examination of the patient. This, in conjunction with the results of appropriate pre-operative investigations, allows a patient risk profile to be established. Superimposed upon this will be the nature and complexity of the intended surgery and associated anaesthetic and postoperative management.

EVALUATE THE RISK

This is the process whereby the anaesthetist assimilates the information gleaned from the individual assessment of the patient and compares the given patient against an historical data set, either from published data or from experience and management of similar patients over time. Following this process, the decision to proceed can be taken, or further pre-operative treatments and investigations instituted in order to optimise the patient in an attempt to lower the risks to the patient. If no further pre-operative investigations or treatments are required or delaying surgery will be associated with an increased risk to the patient, then the anaesthetist must decide the most appropriate anaesthetic management. Included in this decision will be a requirement to consider who should be managing the case from both surgical and anaesthetic perspectives, the time of day that the surgery is scheduled and whether the proposed plan, fits in with accepted guidelines for the management of such cases. Evidence from the NCEPOD reports suggests that 'out of hours' operating is associated with a higher mortality.[12]

RECORD YOUR FINDINGS

It is essential that any pre-operative assessment is recorded in the patient record; increasingly, there is a trend for an assessment to be made by one anaesthetist, further investigations requested and the subsequent anaesthesia administered by another anaesthetist. This is particularly a problem where patients are seen overnight and operated on the following day or where patients are seen in a pre-anaesthetic assessment clinic.[13]

Table 3 ASA classification of physical status	
ASA 1	Normal healthy patient – no known organic, biochemical or psychiatric disease
ASA 2	Patient with mild to moderate systemic disease, e.g. mild asthmatic
ASA 3	Patient with severe systemic disease that limits normal activity, e.g. severe rheumatoid arthritis
ASA 4	Patient with severe systemic disease that is a consistent threat to life, e.g. unstable angina
ASA 5	Patient who is moribund and unlikely to survive 24 h

The addition of the letter E, e.g. 2(E), indicates those patients in whom emergency surgery is undertaken.

THE PATIENT AND OUTCOME

The development of patient risk profiles can be traced back to 1941, when the American Society of Anesthesiologists (ASA) first introduced the concept of assessment of physical status of patients presenting for surgery. Subsequent refinements resulted in the publication of the ASA classification of physical status in 1963.[14] The system based upon the pre-operative history, examination and interpretation of available investigations assigned the patient to one of five categories (Table 3).

The ASA classification, however, is simplistic, subjective and fails to take into account the nature of the intended surgery. As a means of accurately predicting an adverse outcome it therefore has limited value. The subjectivity of the ASA classification has led to the development of more objective, risk assessment scoring systems. These newer risk assessment systems focus on single organ dysfunction and, in particular, cardiac[4–7,15–19] and respiratory[20–27] pathophysiology in the patient presenting for surgery. Attempts at developing risk assessment profiles in patients without significant cardio-respiratory disease or in specific patient sub-groups (e.g. the morbidly obese,[28] the elderly or the paediatric patient) or in association with a particular surgical specialty (e.g. obstetrics, urology, etc.) have found limited success,[29] as the majority of untoward peri-operative events are associated with either pre-operative cardiac or respiratory dysfunction. The construction of a systems-based risk assessment index is dependent upon an analysis of patient outcomes, an understanding of statistics and probability, and a flexibility that ensures that changing demographics and practices are reflected in the risk assessment process. Examples of the development of such systems have been the cardiac risk index and the pulmonary risk index.

CARDIAC RISK INDEX

The existence of cardiac disease in a patient presenting for non-cardiac surgery presents a considerable risk of both mortality and morbidity to the patient. The majority of these events, however, take place in the postoperative period.[15] The most widely quoted risk index for patients, with cardiac disease is that first

Table 4 Pre-operative factors relating to the development of postoperative cardiac complications

Factor	Points
Gallop rhythm or elevated jugular venous pressure	11
Myocardial infarction in preceding 6 months	10
Rhythm other than sinus or premature atrial contractions on pre-operative electrocardiogram	7
> 5 premature ventricular contractions per minute	7
Age > 70 years	5
Emergency surgery	4
Intraperitoneal, intrathoracic or aortic operation	3
Poor general physical status	3
Significant aortic stenosis	3
Total possible points	53

After Goldman et al.[16]

described by Goldman in 1977 (Table 4).[16] This was the first real attempt to analyse risk of peri-operative morbid events in a group of 1000 patients with pre-existing cardiac disease.

The number of points, which an individual patient accrues, places them into one of four classes associated with an increasing risk of peri-operative cardiac morbidity (Table 5). This risk index has been widely validated in large populations of patients undergoing various types of non-cardiac surgery.

Concerns over its application, to patients undergoing vascular surgery led to it being modified (Table 6).[17] The American College of Physicians Guidelines incorporates aspects of this revised classification into its algorithm for the peri-operative management of patients with coronary artery disease undergoing non-cardiac, vascular surgery.[7] Evidence supports the notion that patients with a score greater than 16 should undergo further diagnostic testing, especially if major vascular surgery is contemplated.

Major changes in management strategies for the treatment of acute myocardial infarction, including the use of thrombolytic agents, percutaneous transluminal angioplasty and coronary artery stenting, have altered and continue to alter the risk profile of patients presenting for non-cardiac surgery.

Cardiac risk and surgical procedure

As mentioned previously, the nature of the intended surgery can adversely affect outcome. There is little in the literature which helps to define surgery specific related cardiac complications. One study,[6] using data from the Coronary Artery Surgery Study (CASS), has achieved this. In a retrospective analysis of patients with known cardiac disease, randomised to medical treatment or coronary

Table 5 Classification of risk based on points scored in the Goldman risk index cardiac risk index (CRI)

Class 1	0–5 points
Class 2	6–12 points
Class 3	13–25 points
Class 4	> 25 points

Table 6 Detsky modification of the Goldman cardiac risk index

Variables		Points
Angina	Class IV	20
	Class III	10
	Unstable angina < 3 months	10
Suspected critical aortic stenosis		20
Myocardial infarction	< 6 months	10
	> 6 months	5
Pulmonary oedema	< 1 week	10
	Ever	5
Emergency surgery		10
Non sinus rhythm		5
>5 ventricular premature beats		5
Poor general health		5
Age > 70 years		5
Class I	**Low risk**	**0–15**
Class II	**Intermediate risk**	**20–30**
Class III	**High risk**	**> 30**

artery bypass prior to non-cardiac surgery, the incidence of peri-operative cardiac events and their relationship to the type of surgery were noted; the findings are summarised in Table 7.

Cardiac risk indices continue to be modified and updated in the light of changing therapies and advances in the management of cardiac disease coupled with evidence based evaluation of risk strategies.

PULMONARY RISK

Pulmonary complications are frequent causes of peri-operative morbidity and mortality in all types of surgery.[19] Chronic lung disease, frequently caused by

Table 7 Cardiac risk stratification related to non-cardiac procedures

High risk (> 5% chance of death or non fatal MI)
    Emergency operations, especially in the elderly
    Major vascular
    Peripheral vascular
    Procedures associated with massive blood loss or fluid shifts

Intermediate risk (< 5% chance of death or non fatal MI)
    Carotid artery surgery
    Major head and neck surgery
    Elective intra-abdominal or intrathoracic surgery
    Orthopaedic procedures
    Prostatic surgery

Low risk (< 1% chance of death or non fatal MI)
    Endoscopic surgery
    Peripheral surgery
    Ocular surgery
    Breast surgery

Table 8 Pulmonary risk index

Factor
Obesity
Recent history of cigarette smoking
Cough
Diffuse wheeze
Elevated P_aCO_2 > 6 kPa
FEV_1/FVC < 70% predicted

Presence of a factor scores 1 point.

cigarette smoking, is common in the hospital population and, in order to reduce the incidence of peri-operative respiratory complications, it is essential to have a framework for risk assessment. Attempts to produce a unified approach to pulmonary risk have been largely unsuccessful. A number of studies utilising history and clinical examination have identified patients at risk of pulmonary complications; in the same studies, however, pre-operative pulmonary function tests were not identified as being discriminatory independent risk factors.[19–22] This inability to predict accurate peri-operative morbidity for patients with respiratory disease is indicative of the high incidence of co-morbidity in this group of patients. In one study looking at patients undergoing abdominal surgery, 33% of patients had both cardiac and pulmonary complications postoperatively.[23] In such circumstances, it is impossible to attribute the risk due to pulmonary disease independently and overall risk can only be assessed using a multifactorial scoring system. An example of such a multifactorial scoring has been developed for patients undergoing lung resection.[24] The cardiopulmonary risk index (CPRI) is a combination of the Goldman cardiac risk index value – scored from 1 to 4 – plus a pulmonary risk index – scored from 1 to 6 – based on the presence of any number of the factors listed in Table 8. A combined total score of > 4 is highly predictive of postoperative complications; in a subsequent study, pre-operative exercise testing was able to further define patient risk.[25] Critics of this system point out the highly subjective assessment of cough and wheeze and that the nature of intended surgery is not accounted for.[26] A more objective approach to the assessment of postoperative risk of morbidity in patients for thoracic surgery undergoing lung resection has been reported[27] based on the calculation of a predictive respiratory complication quotient (PRQ). PRQ is calculated using a complex mathematical formula from the results of patient spirometry, carbon monoxide diffusion capacity, split lung function testing and an analysis of the effects of exercise on blood gases. A PRQ of less then 2200 was associated with an increased risk of pulmonary complication. Whether or not such a system can be applied to predict respiratory complications in patients undergoing non-thoracic surgery has yet to be evaluated.

THE ANAESTHETIST AND OUTCOME

Much has been written regarding the role of the patient in determining an adverse outcome in respect of surgery. It is only in the last few years that there has been an increased focus on the role of the healthcare professional in the determination of patient adverse outcomes from surgery and anaesthesia.[30,31] The innate conservatism of the medical profession has stifled the development of systems aimed at evaluating individual performance. Anaesthetists as a group are, however, at the forefront of the development of systems aimed at evaluating performance; much information has been obtained from studies carried out with patient simulators.[32,33] These studies indicate that much can be learned about the performance and vigilance of an individual. Training of anaesthetists – both in the UK and abroad – is still largely based on the apprenticeship model. Junior doctors progress through a set path of work experience and examinations to the final end point of a career grade post in anaesthesia. The examination system largely tests factual knowledge; there is, however, no reliable way of testing practical ability and aptitude that ensures a common minimum standard is achieved by all. Of equal concern is the ability of the professional organisations to institute and police a system of continuing professional development and education (CPDE) which tests both learning and practical skills throughout a doctor's career.

One particular development which allows clinical skills to be tested without compromising patient safety has been the anaesthetic simulator. Anaesthetic simulators have been described of varying complexity from 'low' to 'high' fidelity;[34,35] the majority of commercially available systems upon which much of the work in anaesthetic practice is based are so called 'high-fidelity'. Such systems are associated with a higher level of acceptability by the user and are, therefore, more likely to reflect what happens in 'real life'. Many have the advantage of involving the anaesthetic team and are, therefore, capable of assessing the interactions and approach of individuals in a 'true-to-life' scenario. Studies of performance utilising 'intermediate-fidelity' systems – generally where the doctor interfaces with a computer screen – have shown high levels of treatment inadequacy by experienced anaesthetists.[36] Whether this reflects a lack of empathy with the simulator or a true failure to respond to a clinical situation is a point of major conjecture.[37] Attempts have been made to evaluate the assessment of an individual's performance in a simulated setting and to ensure that results are both reliable and valid, with an acceptable level of inter-observer variability.[38,39] In an analysis of performance of 10 test scenarios, 40% of the scenarios had to be eliminated because of a failure of internal consistency. Also of concern and highlighted in another study is the difficulty of measuring an individual's or team's performance which fluctuates within the time frame of the scenario, such that an aggregate score indicates an acceptable level of performance but disguises the fact that potentially dangerous errors have occurred.[40] The results of these studies highlight the difficulty in designing clinical case scenarios, with appropriate levels of sensitivity and specificity, particularly if the results are to contribute to the process of accreditation or re-validation. Undoubtedly simulators will have a part to play in the objective assessment of an anaesthetist's response to a given scenario; it is, however, a major leap forward to assume that lessons learnt from the analysis of performance in a simulator will help to reduce the risk to the patient in the real world.

A number of studies have considered work-place evaluation of the performance of the anaesthetist. The acquisition of some basic anaesthetically related skills (e.g. orotracheal intubation, regional anaesthesia and insertion of arterial lines, in the first year of training) has been studied.[41] Self evaluation of success, as evidenced by the ability to perform a given task without recourse to help from a senior colleague, was recorded. The study results showed that a success rate of 80–90% could be achieved for the tasks under study, after 60–90 cumulative procedures. Whether further years in training and clinical practice leads to an improved success rate or whether a failure rate of 1 in 5 is acceptable are questions that remain unresolved. Attempts to analyse the role of surgeon versus anaesthetist as independent risk factor are fraught with difficulty. An oft quoted study from New Zealand reported that the anaesthetist in contrast to the surgeon was a significant factor in determining outcome for patients undergoing first-time coronary artery bypass grafting.[42] Studies of poor outcome for individual surgeons (see below) often fail to take into account the factors in the genesis of an adverse event other than the surgeon and the pre-operative state of the patient. This highlights the need for continual appraisal of outcomes both at an individual and institutional level.

New technologies and monitoring techniques are often introduced into the operating theatre in the expectation that they will improve outcome by earlier detection of a critical incident; however, they can also result in decreased vigilance on the part of the anaesthetist and paradoxically result in an increased risk to the patient. A good example of this has been the introduction of anaesthetist-operated transoesophageal echocardiography in the cardiac theatres. This technique, on first introduction, has a defined learning curve which even in the hands of an experienced single-handed anaesthetist resulted in decreased vigilance and an increase in near-misses, which was attributed to the distracting influence of the new technology.[43]

Improved data collection of critical incidents and the relationship of these events to an adverse outcome will be necessary if we are to improve risk assessment where the anaesthetist is a factor.[44,45] Information from observational data can be used in the construction of mathematical models of probability risk analysis[46] and, in particular, the application of Bayesian logic. Described in 1763, Bayes' theorem or rule established a mathematical basis for probability inference, a mechanism by which the probability of an event occurring in the future is calculated from the number of times it has not occurred in the past, at the time of analysis. An established data set is used to form a probability matrix of explanatory variables against outcome variables. It is an essential requirement that all the data variables are categorical. The advantage of the Bayesian model is that the data set can be constantly revised over time. This analysis of risk is increasingly favoured to other forms of mathematical analysis, e.g. multiple regression and multiple regression logistic analysis, previously used in quantifying patient risk.

THE SURGEON AND OUTCOME

There is undoubtedly increased interest in the role that the surgeon plays in ensuring a good outcome from an operation. Much of this interest has been generated in the field of paediatric cardiac surgery,[47] where an investigation of the performance of one particular unit has led to a dramatic re-evaluation of the ways in which individual and institutional performance is monitored.

Cardiac surgery as a specialty is an ideal model for the analysis of risk; it comprises a relatively small group of surgeons, undertaking a limited number of procedures in which there is a significant measurable outcome denominator, i.e. death. The Society of Cardiothoracic Surgeons have collected registry data for the past two decades. These data allow an analysis of outcome, notably death within 30 days, and is presented as an annual report; it provides a useful reference against which surgeons can compare their own outcome data. The individual practitioner, however, needs a more refined analysis of self performance in order to identify any decline. One such means of analysis is the cumulative sum method (CUSUM).[48] Sequential outcomes for a given procedure are plotted along the abscissa, an adverse outcome (e.g. death) is plotted as an addition on the ordinate; over a period of time, the slope of the line allows an individual's performance for that procedure to be assessed and to be compared with others. An increasing gradient equates to a worsening performance and is an early indicator of the necessity for further investigation. Such analysis, however, can only take into account a single procedure and makes no reference to potentially important contributory factors (e.g. pre-operative status of the patient, experience of the anaesthetist, quality of ICU care, etc.). A refinement of the CUSUM plot has been proposed which attempts to incorporate patient related risk factors in the analysis of outcome.[49] The variable life adjusted display (VLAD) is a means of displaying cumulative outcomes against that which would be expected from published series. An outcome better than predicted is associated with an upward movement of the plot, whilst an unexpected death is reflected in a downward movement of the plot. The magnitude of the fall or rise is determined by the published prediction of risk for the given procedure. The resulting plot reflects the difference between the expected and actual cumulative survival accounting for established patient risk factors. Although such plots have been used by surgeons to track performance, the same data set can be used to construct similar plots for other members of the team (e.g. anaesthetists, perfusionists and theatre staff).[50] The graphical display allows for the early detection of declining performance by an individual, ensuring that remedial action can be initiated. Such analysis is not without problems; the patient data, upon which predicted outcome is measured, must be contemporary so as be an accurate reflection of risk of an adverse outcome. Although easily applied to cardiac surgery, such a technique may not be readily applicable to other surgical specialties where complications are infrequent. Similarly, the average anaesthetist works in a variety of surgical environments, with different populations of patients and risk profiles, many of which are poorly defined. Detecting a decline in performance for an individual anaesthetist might be a more difficult proposition than for the cardiac surgeon.

HEALTHCARE SYSTEMS AND OUTCOME

To date, the analysis of adverse outcomes has focused on the roles of the patient and their doctors in the final result. Increasingly, attention is being directed towards the part the healthcare system has to play in reducing risks for the patient undergoing surgery and anaesthesia. Medical errors are reported to be the third most frequent cause of death in the UK, resulting in the death of some 40,000 patients. Studies in which the role of the anaesthetist in the genesis of an error has been analysed suggest that human factors were responsible for 61% of adverse outcomes, whilst latent errors accounted for 49% of adverse outcomes. Latent errors or systems-based errors are those errors which exist within the infrastructure of an organisation which can compound the risk to the patient and can be identified as a contributing cause in up to 85% of untoward events in the peri-operative period.[51] Examples of such latent errors include poor equipment design, product labelling or theatre layout, inadequate training and lack of procedures and policies.[52] In an attempt to limit the effects of these latent errors, political initiatives have been instituted. The major tenet of this initiative is promulgated under the banner of 'Clinical Governance',[53] the definition of which is: 'a system through which NHS organisations are accountable for continuously improving the quality of their services and safeguarding high standards of care by creating an environment in which clinical excellence will flourish'. The major components of the Clinical Governance initiative are as follows.

1. Establish clear lines of responsibility and accountability for the overall quality of clinical care.

2. Have in place a comprehensive programme of quality improvement activities which include such issues as audit programmes, national confidential enquiries, evidence-based practice, continuing professional development, quality assurance and effective methods of monitoring clinical care.

3. Establish clear policies for the management of risk which promote self assessment to identify and manage risks and have programmes in place to reduce risk.

4. Have procedures for all professional groups to identify and remedy poor performance including complaints procedures, professional performance procedures and critical incident reporting.

Responsibility for the implementation of the Clinical Governance initiative has been devolved to a number of different organisations. The General Medical Council and the Royal Medical Colleges are seeking to enforce professional self regulation, with the introduction of mandatory continuing professional development programmes for their members. Such programmes aim to weed out the poorly performing doctor. The majority of European countries operate self regulatory programmes, with doctors expected to acquire a set number of CPDE credits from attendance at approved educational activities. In contrast, in the USA, the stimulus to continued learning is the requirement for regular re-certification based on performance in a written exam. Such approaches do not address the issue of clinical competency, which can only be effectively assessed by workplace and practice-based observation of skills and behaviour in action.

Professional associations and colleges have developed good practice recommendations[11] aimed at introducing uniformity of practice across the profession, e.g. in the organisation of anaesthetic departments. An individual anaesthetic department within a given trust will be required to establish a detailed portfolio of the services that it provides and the way in which they should be delivered. The second phase of the process is concerned with setting performance standards, monitoring the process and responding to adverse audit feedback. The development of the process is as follows:

1. Outline the clinical activity of a department.

2. Describe care pathways for the most common procedures undertaken.

3. Support your choice of care pathways by the accumulation of evidence from national guidelines, protocols, etc.

4. Produce guidelines and rules which reflect both local and national practice.

5. Document and disseminate this information to all concerned in the process.

6. Examine activity and identify areas of risk. Prioritise these into a hierarchy of risk.

7. Measure adherence to the policy, positive and negative outcomes, and monitor areas of high risk.

8. Regularly review the whole process and effect change where necessary.

The establishment of this process allows comparison to be drawn between a given department and what will become a national standard. One step removed from this is the analysis of risk for a patient under the care of that department. The introduction of local Clinical Governance will without doubt focus the thoughts and actions of individuals, departments and trusts into assessing the quality of care that they provide. In addition, trusts under the guidance of organisations such as the National Institute for Clinical Excellence (NICE) and the Commission for Health Improvement will be obliged to introduce improved healthcare which is evidence based.

What is less clear is where the resources will come from to effectively implement this process without significant funding from government. The UK already ranks some way behind its fellow European partners in the provision of healthcare services, e.g. for patients with cardiac disease. Needless to say, these initiatives have been met with some scepticism by the medical fraternity,[54] who fear that political rhetoric will not be easily transformed into action, and that these initiatives, when introduced, may have a negative impact on the provision of quality healthcare.

CONCLUSIONS

Risk assessment has come a long way since the attempts of the ASA to identify and categorise patients presenting for anaesthesia and surgery. The progressive development of weighted scoring systems to identify at risk patients presenting for major surgery has rightfully concentrated in those areas where the greatest benefits are to be gained. By definition, high risk patients will be expected to have a worse outcome; increasingly, there is evidence to support the notion that this may be compounded by poorly performing anaesthetists,[52] surgeons,[50] or healthcare systems.[51] A number of initiatives are being developed in an attempt to minimise these risks and to improve patient outcomes. In the future, risk assessment will involve analysis of all of these components before reaching a decision on the appropriate management of the patient.

Key points for clinical practice

- Risk assessment has developed over the years from an analysis of patient related factors in the genesis of untoward or adverse outcomes to an examination of the healthcare system as a whole.

- The aim of any programme of risk assessment should be to improve objectivity and reduce subjectivity of the process. This can often be enhanced by the use of mathematical modelling.

- The presence of pre-existing cardiac or respiratory disease states are associated with the highest risk of adverse outcome. The interplay of co-existing cardiac and respiratory disease states in determining outcome still needs to be further evaluated.

- Audit systems have been developed to examine the relationships between healthcare professionals, patients, institutions and adverse outcomes.

- Increasingly, doctors will be required to show continuing professional development and be the subject of regular programmes of revalidation. The role of new technologies (e.g. anaesthetic simulators and interactive computer programmes) in this process is under continuous development.

- Political initiatives through the guise of clinical governance have been introduced in an attempt to improve healthcare in the public sector.

REFERENCES

1. Risk Management. London: The Association of Anaesthetists of Great Britain and Ireland, 1998.
2. Warner MA, Shields SE, Chute CG. Major morbidity and mortality within 1 month of ambulatory surgery and anesthesia. JAMA 1993; 270: 1437–1441.
3. Health and Safety Executive. An Introduction to Health and Safety. London: HMSO, 1997.
4. Parsonnet V, Dean D, Bernstein AD. A method of uniform stratification of risk for evaluating the results of surgery in acquired adult heart disease Circulation 1989; 79: I-3–I-12.
5. Goldman L, Caldera D, Nussbaum SR et al. Multifactorial index of cardiac risk in non cardiac surgical procedures. N Engl J Med 1977; 297: 845–850.
6. Eagle KA, Rihal CS, Mickel MC et al. Cardiac risk and non-cardiac surgery: influence of coronary disease and type of surgery in 3368 operations. CASS investigators and University of Michigan Heart Care program. Coronary Artery Surgery Study. Circulation 1997; 96: 1882–1887.
7. Palda VA, Detsky AS. Perioperative assessment and management of risk from coronary artery disease. Ann Intern Med 1997; 127: 313–328.
8. Secretary of State for Health, The New NHS. Modern. Dependable. London: HMSO, 1997.
9. General Medical Council. Good Medical Practice. Guidance from the General Medical Council. London: GMC, 1995.
10. General Medical Council. Maintaining Good Medical Practice. London: GMC, 1998.
11. Good Practice: A Guide for Departments of Anaesthesia. London: The Royal College of Anaesthetists and The Association of Anaesthetists of Great Britain and Ireland, 1998.

12. NCEPOD. Who Operates When? London: NCEPOD, 1997.

13. Lee A, Lum ME, Perry M et al, Risk of unanticipated intraoperative events in patients assessed at a preanaesthetic clinic. Can J Anaesth 1997; 44: 946–954.

14. American Society of Anesthesiologists. New classification of physical status. Anesthesiology 1963; 24: Ill.

15. Coriat P. Reducing cardiovascular risk in patients undergoing non-cardiac surgery. Curr Opin Anesthesiol 1998; 11: 311–314.

16. Goldman L, Caldera D, Nussbaum SR et al. Multifactorial index of cardiac risk in non cardiac surgical procedures. N Engl J Med 1977; 297: 845–850.

17. Detsky A, Abrams H, McLaughlin J et al. Predicting cardiac complications in patients undergoing non-cardiac surgery. J Gen Intern Med 1988; 1: 211–219.

18. Rose DK, Cohen MM, DeBoer DP. Cardiovascular events in the postanesthesia care unit: contribution of risk factors. Anesthesiology 1996; 84: 357–370.

19. Pronovost P, Dorman T, Sadovnikoff N et al. The association between perioperative patient characteristics and both clinical and economic outcomes after abdominal aortic surgery. Jour Cardiothorac Vasc Anesth 1999; 13: 549–554.

20. Mitchell CK, Smoger SH, Pfeifer MP et al. Multivariate analysis of factors associated with postoperative pulmonary complications following general elective surgery. Arch Surg 1998; 133: 194–198.

21. Brooks-Brunn JA. Predictors of postoperative pulmonary complications following abdominal surgery. Chest 1997; 111: 564–571.

22. Wong DH, Weber EC, Schell MJ et al. Factors associated with postoperative pulmonary complications in patients with severe chronic obstructive pulmonary disease. Anesth Analg 1995; 80: 276–284.

23. Lawrence VA, Dhanda R, Hilsenbank SG et al. Risk of pulmonary complications after elective abdominal surgery. Chest 1996; 110: 744–750.

24. Epstein SK, Faling LJ, Daly BD et al. Predicting complications after pulmonary resection: preoperative exercise testing vs a multifactorial cardiopulmonary index. Chest 1993; 104: 694–700.

25. Epstein SK, Faling LJ, Daly BD et al. Inability to perform bicycle ergometry predicts increased morbidity and mortality after lung resection. Chest 1995; 107: 311–316.

26. Melendez JA, Carlon VA. Cardiopulmonary risk index does not predict complications after thoracic surgery. Chest 1998; 114: 69–75.

27. Melendez JA, Barra R. Predictive respiratory complication quotient predicts pulmonary complications in thoracic surgical patients. Ann Thorac Surg 1998; 66: 220–224.

28. Buckley FP. Anaesthetic risks related to obesity. Curr Opin Anesthesiol 1997; 10: 240–243.

29. Osswald PM, Swars O, Leufke P. Scores, scoring and outcome: correlation between pre-operative assessment and post-operative morbidity and mortality of non-hospitalized and hospitalized patients. Clin Anaesthesiol 1998; 12: 471–483.

30. Cohen MM, Duncan PG, Poe WD et al. The Canadian four-centre study of anaesthetic outcomes: II Can outcomes be used to assess the quality of anaesthesia care? Can J Anaesth 1992; 39: 430–439.

31. Horan BF, Warden JC. Urgent non-emergency surgery and death attributable to anaesthetic factors. Anaesth Intensive Care 1996; 24: 694–698.

32. Byrne AJ, Hilton PJ, Lunn JN. Basic simulators for anaesthetists: a pilot study of the ACESS system. Anaesthesia 1994; 49: 376–381.

33. Gaba DM, Howard SK, Flanagan B et al. Assessment of clinical performance during simulated cries using both technical and behavioural ratings. Anaesthesiology 1998; 89: 8–18.

34. Norman J, Wilkins D. Simulators for anaesthesia. J Clin Monit 1996; 12: 91–99.

35. van Meurs WL, Good ML, Lampotang S. Functional anatomy of full scale patient simulators. J Clin Monit 1997; 13: 317–324.

36. Byrne AJ, Jones JG. Responses to simulated anaesthetic emergencies by anaesthetists with different durations of clinical experience. Br J Anaesth 1997; 78: 553–556.

37. Gaba DM, Howard SK. Factors influencing vigilence and performance of anaesthetists. Curr Opin Anaesthesiol 1998; 11: 651–657

38. Devit JH, Kurrek MM, Cohen MM et al. Testing the raters: inter-rater reliability of standardised anaesthesia simulator performance. Can J Anaesth 1997; 44: 924–928.

39. Devit JH, Kurrek MM, Cohen MM et al. Testing internal consistency and construct validity during evaluation of performance in a patient simulator. Anesth Analg 1998; 86: 1157–1159.

40. Howard SK, Gaba DM, Fish KJ et al. Anesthesia crisis resource management training: teaching anesthesiologists to handle critical incidents. Aviat Space Environ Med 1992; 63: 763–770.

41. Konrad C, Schupfer G, Wietlisbach M et al. Learning manual skills in anaesthesiology: is there a recommended number of cases for anaesthetic procedures? Anesth Analg 1998; 86: 635–639.

42. Merry AF, Ramage MC, Whitlock RML et al. First-time coronary artery bypass grafting: the anaesthetist as a risk factor. Br J Anaesth 1992; 68: 6–12.

43. Weinger MB, Herndon OW, Gaba DM et al. The effect of electronic record keeping and transesophageal echocardiography on task distribution, workload and vigilance during cardiac anesthesia. Anesthesiology 1997; 87:144–155.

44. Runcieman WB, Sellen A, Webb RK et al. The Australian incident monitoring survey: errors, incidents and accidents in anaesthetic practice. Anaesth Intensive Care 1993; 21: 506–519.

45. Webb RK, Currie M, Morgan CA et al. The Australian incident monitoring survey: an analysis of 2000 incident reports. Anaesth Intensive Care 1993; 21: 520–528.

46. Pate-Cornell ME, Lakats LM, Murphy DM et al. Anesthesia patient risk: a quantitative approach to organizational factors and risk management options. Risk Analysis 1997; 17: 511–523.

47. Treasure T. Lessons from the Bristol case. More openness – on risks and on individual surgeon's performance. BMJ 1998; 316: 1685–1686.

48. de Laval MR, Francois K, Bull C et al. Analysis of a cluster of surgical failures. Application to a series of neonatal arterial switch operations. J Thorac Cardiovasc Surg 1994; 107: 914–924.

49. Lovegrove J, Valencia O, Treasure T et al. Monitoring the results of cardiac surgery by variable life adjusted display. Lancet 1997; 350: 1128–1130.

50. Treasure T, Lovegrove J, Valencia O. The influence of the surgeon on outcome. Clin Anaesthesiol 1999; 13: 295–306.

51. Reason JT. Safety in the operating theatre. Part 2: human error and organisational failure. Curr Anaesth Crit Care 1995; 6: 121–126.

52. Aitkenhead AR. Influence of the anaesthetist on outcome. Clin Anaesthesiol 1999; 13: 279–294.

53. Scally G, Donaldson LM. Clinical governance and the drive for quality improvement in the new NHS in England. BMJ 1998; 317: 61–65.

54. Goodman NW. Sacred cows to the abattoir, clinical governance. BMJ 1998; 317: 1725–1727.

Hugo Van Aken Norbert Rolf

The choice of anaesthesia on outcome

Although there is a general tendency for surgical patients to be older and more ill, very large reductions in peri-operative morbidity and mortality have been achieved during the last decade. Anaesthetists have long since ceased to simply 'put patients to sleep'. However, the relative safety of anaesthesia is one of its most insidious hazards.[1] There is a growing literature indicating that life-threatening complications can be observed not only in the intra-operative period, but also in the postoperative period; therefore, it is still important to evaluate the anaesthetic component in the risk to surgical patients.

There are several reasons why it is very difficult to determine the effect of anaesthetic technique on the outcome after surgery. 'Outcome' is a complex term that may have different meanings, depending on different investigators' points of view.[2] It can be defined in terms of: (i) the side-effects and complications of anaesthetic procedures; (ii) temporary postoperative impairment of mental and physical well-being; (iii) non-specific clinical end-points relative to the surgical procedures (postoperative mortality or clinical morbidity end-points such as myocardial infarction, pneumonia, ileus, pulmonary embolism, or reduced cognitive function); or (iv) improvement in postoperative recovery (quality of life, reduction of hospital stay).

It takes a great deal of effort, energy, and time to assess many of these aspects of outcome in empirical studies. Mortality or clinical end-points such as myocardial infarction are rare events after surgery. Only studies that include large numbers of patients, therefore, will be sufficiently powerful to produce adequate statistical evidence. A variety of aspects affect the variability of non-specific measures of postoperative outcome. Major studies with a complex

Prof. Dr Hugo Van Aken, Director, Klinik und Poliklinik für Anästhesiologie und operative Intensivmedizin, Westfälische Wilhelms Universität, Albert Schweitzer Strasse 33, D-48149 Münster, Germany (for correspondence)

Dr Norbert Rolf, Assistant Medical Director, Klinik und Poliklinik für Anästhesiologie und operative Intensivmedizin, Westfälische Wilhelms Universität, Albert Schweitzer Strasse 33, D-48149 Münster, Germany multifactorial design are, therefore, needed to assess the extent and causes of outcomes that are attributable to anaesthetic techniques.

In spite of all these considerations, there is a certain amount of evidence concerning the effects of anaesthetic technique on different aspects of the outcome. The present review will discuss the following questions:

1. What is the contribution of anaesthesia to postoperative mortality and morbidity?

2. Does the choice of anaesthetic technique reduce transient postoperative impairment of mental and physical well-being?

3. Does the choice of anaesthetic technique affect the overall postoperative morbidity or mortality?

ANAESTHESIA-RELATED COMPLICATIONS

The risk of death due to anaesthesia has declined over the last 50 years. Beecher and Todd reported a death rate of 1 per 2680 anaesthetics. With increasing experience among anaesthetists in the use of new anaesthetic drugs, the mortality rate subsequently declined.[3] At the beginning of the 1980s, the risk of mortality due to anaesthesia was estimated at 1 in 10,000 operations and, in the second half of that decade, figures ranged from 1 in 13,207 to 1 in 185,000.[4-6] This recent significant risk reduction coincided with the introduction of safety standards into modern anaesthesia. Analyses had demonstrated that inadequate pre-anaesthetic assessment and insufficient intra- and postoperative monitoring were major factors in mortality.[6] It has been pointed out that, in most cases, the time between the first symptoms of an anaesthetic problem and the critical incident is sufficient to allow for diagnosis and correction of the problem; however, effective use of this time requires adequate monitoring.[7,8] Subsequently, the incidence of severe anaesthetic accidents decreased, and no deaths attributed to anaesthesia were reported during the study period after the Harvard Medical School introduced safety monitoring standards into its hospitals.[9]

Equipment and training problems are not the only causative factors associated with anaesthesia-related deaths. Studies about the contribution of human error or equipment failure to anaesthetic critical incidents illustrate that, from the mid 1970s to the mid 1990s, the relation of both factors did not change. About 70–80% of complications continue to occur due to human error (Table 1). Not only equipment problems, but preventable human factors have to be considered as risk factors for anaesthetic mortality. According to a study by Cooper and colleagues, seven of the ten most common types of critical anaesthetic accidents

Table 1 Human error or equipment failure

Study	Time interval	Number of critical incidents	Human error %	Equipment error %
Cooper et al[75]	1975–1980	1089	71	17
Cooper et al[76]	1978	359	82	14
Craig et al[77]	1981	81	68	20
Chopra et al[78]	1989–1990	549	75	21
Williamson et al[79]	1993	2000	83	12

were related to respiratory problems.[1] Ross and Tinker, therefore, argue that educational priorities for anaesthesiologists should be restructured toward safety, at least in part through renewed awareness of the basic principles of respiratory and circulatory management.[10] Furthermore, as Sigurdsson stated 'although modern monitoring may detect severe derangement at an early stage, patient safety is only improved when the data are correctly assimilated by the anaesthetist and corrective action is taken ... It appears that the part of the system most likely to fail under stress is the anaesthetist himself'.[11]

The risk of serious complications related to regional anaesthesia has been reported in a recent prospective survey in France.[12] The authors observed 98 severe anaesthesia-related complications in a total of 103,730 regional anaesthetics, corresponding to 40,640 spinal anaesthetics, 30,413 epidural anaes-thetics, 21,278 peripheral nerve blocks, and 11,229 intravenous regional anaesthetics. Cardiac arrest was the most common critical event. It occurred in 32 patients, seven of whom died, and was primarily related to spinal anaesthesia with a relative risk of 6.4 per 10,000. Neurological injury (relative risk 5.9 per 10,000) with radiculopathy (relative risk 4.7 per 10,000) or cauda equina syndrome (relative risk 1.2 per 10,000) was also significantly associated with spinal procedures. Nerve trauma during needle placement, and the use of 0.5% hyperbaric lignocaine, were found to be contributory factors. One patient who underwent epidural anaesthesia suffered paraplegia. He had intra-operative hypovolaemic arterial hypotension, and a computed tomography scan to rule out spinal compression was normal. Spinal ischaemia was, therefore, assumed to be the cause of the incident. Seizure attributed to elevated serum levels of local anaesthetics was observed after peripheral nerve blocks (relative risk 7.5 per 10,000), intravenous regional anaesthesia (relative risk 2.7 per 10,000) and epidural anaesthesia (relative risk 1.3 per 10,000). This study shows that there is a relatively high risk of cardiac arrest and neurological injury after spinal anaesthesia. The authors argue that a disproportionate cardiovascular risk may be strongly associated with confounding factors such as advanced age, ASA physical status, or type of surgery, rather than with regional anaesthesia itself. The higher risk of neurological injury, on the other hand, may be associated with the type of regional anaesthesia used.

Another recent survey in Finland of complications associated with spinal or epidural anaesthesia has been published.[13] By sending questionnaires to every hospital in the country, the authors arrived at an estimated number of spinal anaesthesias during a study period from 1987–1993 of 550,000, with epidural anaesthesias totalling 170,000. Based on patients' insurance claims, the incidence of neurological complications was 1.8 per 10,000 after spinal anaesthesia, and 2.4 per 10,000 after epidural anaesthesia. Differences from the French study may be explained by different strategies in information sampling and different diagnoses being summarized as 'neurological injury'. Epidural haematoma was diagnosed in five patients, all of whom had received spinal anaesthesia. One patient who had an epidural suffered paraplegia after a technically difficult puncture and a spinal tap before the catheter was inserted. Myelography did not show a pathological lesion, and the epidural analgesia together with the patient's arteriosclerotic disease and possible spinal cord ischaemia were, therefore, regarded as the causative factors. Cauda equina syndrome was observed in two patients after spinal and epidural analgesia, respectively. The patient with spinal anaesthesia suffered from spinal stenosis due to spondyloarthrosis, and in the patient with epidural analgesia, no predisposing factor could be identified. He developed cauda equina syndrome on the first postoperative day after the catheter had been removed.

Altogether, these data indicate that, as in general anaesthesia, it is of great importance to implement safety standards in regional procedures, which are regarded by many anaesthetists as being simple and safe.[14] Patients should be carefully observed for a time long enough to identify and treat adverse events.

PAIN, NAUSEA AND VOMITING

A recent investigation concerning the contribution of risk factors to postoperative cardiovascular events has been published by Rose and colleagues.[15] They analyzed the risk of postoperative hypertension, hypotension, bradycardia, or tachycardia in 18,380 patients who had been admitted to a postoperative care unit after general anaesthesia. They pointed out that cardiovascular activation parameters, as surrogates for clinical end-points, are associated with an increased postoperative mortality. A multiple logistic regression model was used to determine significant risk factors for tachycardia and hypertension. The analyses demonstrate that, compared to patient, surgical, and intra-operative aspects, anaesthetic factors only contributed slightly to predicting these events. Interestingly, however, peri-operative anaesthetic aspects such as inadequate ventilation, pain, vomiting, or shivering contribute to hypertension and tachycardia. This finding shows that intermediate factors of postoperative well-being may be of great importance for clinical end-points, and that anaesthetic treatment has to be continued during the early postoperative period.

The most frequent and disturbing postoperative problem is pain. The majority of patients (57%) who have undergone surgery report that postoperative pain was their primary concern before the operation.[16] In the past decade, after the first official guidelines were established in Australia, considerable advances have been made world-wide towards establishing new management techniques and organizing acute pain treatment services.[17] In a recent editorial on acute pain management, Lehmann states that 'the name of the game is individual variability' in the need for analgesics.[18] The most important innovation in overcoming the problem was, therefore, the introduction of 'patient-controlled analgesia' (PCA) techniques and continuous assessment of an adequate level of analgesia. Concomitant monitoring of the therapeutic success of patient-controlled administration of analgesic drugs by specially trained members of an acute pain service tailors the drug dosage directly to the specific needs of an individual patient.[19,20] PCA or regional analgesia, supervised by the members of an acute pain service, is therefore the gold standard for postoperative pain therapy. The most effective regimen is regional analgesia, and the most widespread regional analgesic technique is epidural analgesia.[21] According to a consensus statement from the American Society of Regional Anesthesia, combining epidural opioids and local anaesthetics, and tailoring the site of drug administration to the affected dermatomes, is the optimal technique for obtaining optimal pain control while simultaneously minimizing the side-effects.[22–24]

Recent surveys in the UK and in the US demonstrate that in the meantime some 40% of hospitals have implemented acute pain management programs.[16,25] Nevertheless, 71% of postoperative patients experienced pain even after receiving their first dose of medication, and 93% said they believed it was acceptable to complain about pain after surgery.[16] These data show that, in spite of increased professional and public awareness, there is still need to educate the public, patients, and medical staff in order to reduce the severity of postoperative pain.

One of the organizational problems involved in postoperative pain management seems to be that acute pain therapy specialists are responsible for a highly selected number of surgical patients receiving PCA and regional analgesia techniques. Most patients are still treated using applicable techniques by surgical ward staff members. The problem might effectively be reduced if the low-cost model proposed by Rawal and Berggren is used.[26] Regular recording of each patient's pain intensity and recording the treatment efficacy on a bedside vital-sign chart are the cornerstones of this model. After in-service training, and under the supervision of anaesthesiologists, surgical nursing staff are allowed to administer analgesics by themselves, following an algorithm based on these recordings. Wiebalck and colleagues reported a better quality of pain relief in patients' self-ratings and a positive evaluation by the nursing staff after they introduced a programme based on these principles in the Catholic University Hospital in Louvain, Belgium.[27]

The average incidence of postnarcotic nausea and vomiting varies between 20–30%, depending upon multiple factors, such as: the type of surgery and anaesthesia, sex, and psychological stress and anxiety.[28–35] In patients at high risk, a relative frequency of this complication of up to 85% has been observed.[36] Many patients regard nausea and vomiting as being as debilitating as postoperative pain.[28] A great deal of effort has, therefore, been focused on attempts to reduce the incidence of emesis, and the effects of newer drugs such as the 5-HT-3 receptor antagonists ondansetron and granisetron, or subhypnotic doses of propofol, have been studied. However, definite advantages in comparison with the traditional anti-emetic regimen, e.g. using droperidol or metoclopramide, have not been found. At present, therefore, the progress made in reducing postoperative has still only been gradual.[37–41]

POSTOPERATIVE MORBIDITY OR MORTALITY AS CLINICAL END-POINTS

It has been argued that the so-called 'stress response' is necessary to maintain homeostasis after surgical stimulation, but inadequate and long-lasting stress may contribute to postoperative morbidity.[42] Kehlet hypothesized that undesirable sequelae might be reduced by eliminating the surgical stress response.[43] Epidural analgesia using local anaesthetics is the most effective means of inhibiting the pathophysiological cascade mediating surgical stress. At present, epidural analgesia is a major focus of controversy with regard to surgical outcomes.[44]

CARDIAC MORBIDITY

Cardiac morbidity due to intra-operative or postoperative myocardial infarction, angina pectoris, or heart failure or severe arrhythmia, is the leading cause of postoperative mortality.[45] Sympathetic activation by peri-operative stress increases the myocardial oxygen demand. Simultaneously, paradoxical vasoconstriction in atherosclerotic vessels reduces the oxygen supply in poststenotic regions of the myocardium. The oxygen imbalance, increasing the risk of ischaemia and infarction in critical regions of the myocardium, may impair the long-term cardiac prognosis in patients undergoing surgery.[46–48] Animal studies and clinical investigations have demonstrated a beneficial effect of thoracic epidural anaesthesia on myocardial function and paradoxical vasoconstriction.[49–51] In a controversial study, Yeager and colleagues demonstrated a reduction in morbidity and mortality using a technique combining epidural and general anaesthesia.[52] Despite several methodological problems, their work has been very important, as it initiated further hypotheses and investigations of the effects of epidural analgesia on the cardiac outcome after surgery. Subsequent studies, however, produced inconsistent results, which can be explained by differences in the general study design, selection of patient populations, and the duration and type of postoperative analgesic regimen.[53–56]

COAGULATION

The peri-operative stress response also seems to be a mediator of a postoperative hypercoagulability state, increasing the risk of postoperative morbidity and mortality.[44] Epidural analgesia modifies the postoperative hypercoagulation status through several mechanisms. A reduction of inappropriate fibrin formation or an increase in fibrinolysis have been discussed.[57,58] Clinical markers for thromboses of vascular grafts are reduced when epidural analgesia is used. Tuman and colleagues observed a decrease in the incidence of graft failure after major vascular surgery in patients with intra-operative and postoperative epidural analgesia.[55] Similarly, Christopherson and colleagues observed a reduction in the rate of re-operations due to thromboembolic complications in a prospective randomized study of patients undergoing vascular surgery of the lower extremities.[59] These well-designed studies demonstrate a beneficial effect of epidural analgesia in patients at high risk for vaso-occlusive events. To date, however, it is still unclear whether these data can be transferred to other groups of patients undergoing major surgery. The most important reason for this is that clinical events such as pulmonary embolism due to postoperative hypercoagulability are rare. It is an important task for further investigations to organize the recruitment of a sample size large enough to provide adequate statistical power.

PULMONARY COMPLICATIONS

Postoperative impairment of pulmonary function includes a pain-induced decrease in ventilation and a neural reflex–mediated inhibition of diaphragmatic function.[60,61] Epidural anaesthesia for intra-operative and postoperative pain management reduces pulmonary adverse effects by re-establishing diaphragmatic function, with subsequent optimized ventilation. Warner and colleagues demonstrated increases in the functional residual capacity by caudad motion of the diaphragm and a decrease in intrathoracic blood volume.[62] Diaphragmatic dysfunction can be observed after upper abdominal surgery, and it can be partially reversed by a thoracic epidural block.[63] At present, however, the results of clinical studies are inconsistent.[44] There were no significant differences in clinical pulmonary complications and radiographic chest abnormalities between patients with epidural bupivacaine and morphine compared with parenteral opioids.[64] However, there are many arguments in favour of the view that patients with an increased risk due to pre-existing pulmonary disease may benefit from this procedure.

POSTOPERATIVE BOWEL FUNCTION

Delayed postoperative gastrointestinal recovery mainly depends on neurogenic factors. Noxious stimulation is followed by reflex inhibition of gastrointestinal motility, which is mainly mediated through activation of sympathetic efferents.[44] Another important stimulus affecting this complication occurs after periods of bowel ischaemia. Epidural analgesia with local anaesthetics has been shown to reduce postoperative ileus, improve splanchnic blood flow by sympathetic blockade, and accelerate postischaemic bowel motility.[65,66] In a recent review on epidural anaesthesia and gastrointestinal motility, Steinbrook has pointed out that the site of catheter placement is a major factor affecting the positive effects of the procedure.[67] Thoracic epidural blocks have been shown to improve postoperative recovery of gastrointestinal function, whereas lumbar epidural blocks are not as consistently effective. This result may be due to enhanced sympathetic activity in non-anaesthetized segments of the splanchnic region after lumbar epidural analgesia.[68] Future studies measuring epidural motility and intestinal blood flow should, therefore, include documentation of the level and extent of epidural blockade.

MULTIMODAL POSTOPERATIVE THERAPY

Kehlet points out that, although there has been a great effort to reduce postoperative morbidity and mortality by several unimodal interventions, such as epidural analgesia, the beneficial effects of these approaches are still debatable.[43] This may be because the pain-free status and the reduction in the peri-operative stress response has not been used to control for other important factors contributing to postoperative morbidity. A more rational approach to improve morbidity and accelerate convalescence is, therefore, multimodal intervention using pre-operative information and teaching of patients, attenuation of the stress response, pain relief, exercise, and enteral nutrition. It has been demonstrated that this type of multimodal approach, combining balanced analgesia, early oral feeding, and enforced mobilization, reduces the hospital stay after colonic surgery.[69]

Brodner and colleagues studied the effects of a multimodal approach with intra-operative and postoperative thoracic epidural blocks using balanced analgesia, postoperative adjustment of epidural drug dosage to the individual needs of patients, early extubation, and forced mobilization in patients undergoing abdominothoracic oesophageal resection.[70] They observed better pain relief, less negative nitrogen balances, and earlier discharge from the intensive care unit in comparison to patients receiving a traditional regimen with intra-operative general analgesia and postoperative epidural analgesia, with no use of the further aspects of the adjusted rehabilitation programme.

Further studies should be designed concerning the different aspects of postoperative convalescence. Epidural analgesia will only contribute to postoperative recovery if the following rules are carefully followed (from Brodner and colleagues):[70]

1. Balanced analgesia with different classes of analgesics resulting in effective pain relief by synergistic or additive analgesic action with reduced incidence of side effects.[23,71]

2. Placement of epidural catheters targeting transmission of the nociceptive impulses at the spinal levels that are involved in generating pain. An improved ability to titrate analgesia to the affected dermatomes allows a reduction in drug use.[23]

3. Confirming an adequate level and postoperative maintenance of the epidural blockade to eliminate the surgical stress response.[43]

4. Continuous assessment of adequate analgesia. Monitoring of the therapeutic success of analgesic drugs by specially trained members of an acute pain service tailors the drug dosage directly to the specific needs of an individual patient.[20]

5. Combination of epidural analgesia with other treatments to support recovery (e.g. physiotherapy, forced mobilization).[43]

6. Continuous evaluation of possible adverse effects of epidural local anaesthetics and opioids to confirm a maximum of patient safety.[23,72–74]

Key points for clinical practice

- *Definition of outcome*: the most commonly used outcome parameter is death or severe disability. However, application of 'weaker' outcome parameters are more likely to reveal differences between anaesthetic techniques. These also include 'minor' and transient postoperative complications.

- *Anaesthesia-related complications*: these comprise a spectrum of complications, ranging from minor events, such as nausea and vomiting, to severe and permanent injuries, such as myocardial infarction, cerebral damage or death. It is often impossible to clearly identify the anaesthetic employed as the sole causative agent.

- *Patient controlled analgesia (PCA)*: PCA is the method of choice for postoperative pain treatment, either patient controlled intravenous analgesia (PCIA) or preferably patient controlled epidural analgesia (PCEA). This requires adequate training of personnel and staffing.

- *Thoracic epidural anaesthesia*: adequate segmental intra- and postoperative analgesia can, for most abdominal and thoracic procedures, best be achieved by an epidural catheter inserted at the thoracic level. The catheter should be placed in the central dermatomes involved.

1. Cooper JB, Newbower RS, Kitz RJ. An analysis of major errors and equipment failures in anesthesia management: considerations for prevention and detection. Anesthesiology 1984; 60: 34–42.
2. Rigg JR, Jamrozik K. Outcome after general or locoregional anaesthesia in high-risk patients. In press.
3. Beecher HK, Todd DP. A study of the deaths associated with anesthesia and surgery based on a study of 599,548 anesthesia in ten institutions 1948–1952, inclusive. Ann Surg 1954; 140: 2–35.
4. Lunn JN, Mushin WW. (eds) Mortality Associated with Anaesthesia. London: Nuffield Provincial Hospitals Trust, 1982.
5. Smith G, Norman J. Complications and medicolegal aspects of anesthesia [Editorial]. Br J Anaesth 1987; 59: 834–835.
6. Tiret L, Desmonts JM, Hatton F et al. Complications associated with anesthesia – a prospective survey in France. Can Anaesth Soc J 1987; 33: 336–339.
7. Van Aken H, Rolf N. Does the choice of anesthetic technique influence outcome. Anesth Analg 1996; (Suppl): 128–133.
8. Cote CJ, Rolf N, Liu LM et al. A single-blind study of combined pulse oximetry and capnography in children. Anesthesiology 1991; 74: 980–987.
9. Eichhorn JH. Prevention of intraoperative anesthesia accidents and related severe injury through safety monitoring. Anesthesiology 1989; 70: 572–577.
10. Ross AF, Tinker JH. Anesthesia risk. In: Miller RD. (ed) Anesthesia. New York: Churchill Livingstone, 1990; 715–742
11. Sigurdsson GH, McAteer E. Morbidity and mortality associated with anaesthesia. Acta Anaesthesiol Scand 1996; 40: 1057–1063.
12. Auroy Y, Narchi P, Messiah A et al. Serious complications related to regional anesthesia. Anesthesiology 1997; 87: 479–486.
13. Aromaa U, Lahdensuu M, Cozanits DA. Severe complications associated with epidural and spinal anaesthesias in Finland 1987–1993. A study based on patients' insurance claims. Acta Anaesthesiol Scand 1997; 41: 445–452.
14. Vandermeulen EP, Van Aken H, Vermylen J. Anticoagulants and spinal-epidural anesthesia. Anesth Analg 1994; 79: 1165–1177.
15. Rose DK, Cohen MM, DeBoer DP. Cardiovascular events in the postanesthesia care unit. Anesthesiology 1996; 84: 772–781.
16. Warfield CA, Kahn CH. Acute pain management. Anesthesiology 1995; 83: 1090–1094.
17. National Health and Medical Research Council Management of severe pain. Commonwealth Australia, 1988.
18. Lehmann KA. The name of the game. J Clin Anesth 1996; 8: 1–3.
19. Rauck RL. Cost-effectiveness and cost/ratio of acute pain management. Reg Anesth 1996; 21: 139–143.
20. Rauck RL. Management of postoperative pain. In: Raj PP. (ed) Current Review of Pain. Philadelphia: Current Medicine, 1994; 47–60.
21. Schug SA, Fry RA. Continuous regional analgesia in comparison with intravenous opioid administration for routine postoperative pain control. Anaesthesia 1994; 49: 528–532.
22. Carpenter RL, Abram SE, Bromage PR et al. Consensus statement on acute pain management. Reg Anesth 1996; 21 (Suppl. 6): 152–156.
23. Wiebalck A, Brodner G, Van Aken H. Postoperative patient-controlled epidural analgesia: The effect of adding sufentanil to bupivacaine. Anesth Analg 1997; 85: 124–129.
24. Hansdottir V, Woestenborghs R, Nordberg G. The cerebrospinal fluid and plasma pharmacokinetics of sufentanil after thoracic or lumbar epidural administration. Anesth Analg 1995; 80: 724–729.
25. Windsor AM, Glynn CJ, Mason DG. National provision of acute pain services. Anaesthesia 1996; 51: 228–231.
26. Rawal N, Berggren L. Organization of acute pain services: a low-cost model. Pain 1994; 57: 117–123.

27. Wiebalck A, Vandermeulen E, Van Aken H et al. Konzept zur Verbesserung der postoperativen Schmerzbehandlung. Anaesthesist 1995; 44: 831–842.

28. Watcha MF, White PF. Post-operative nausea and vomiting: do they matter? Eur J Anaesthesiol Suppl 1995; 10: 18–23.

29. Winning TJ, Brock-Utne JG, Downing JW. Nausea and vomiting after anaesthesia and minor surgery. Anesth Analg 1977; 56: 674–677.

30. Van den Berg AA, Lambourne A, Yazji NS et al. Vomiting after ophthalmic surgery. Anaesthesia 1987; 42: 270–276.

31. Watcha MF, Simeon RM, White PF et al. Effect of propofol on the incidence of postoperative vomiting after strabismus surgery in pediatric outpatients. Anesthesiology 1991; 75: 204–209.

32. Palazzo MGA, Strunin L. Anaesthesia and emesis I: Etiology. Can Anaest Soc J 1984; 31: 178–187.

33. Fisher MM, Chin KC. Reduction in postoperative vomiting in high-risk patients. Anaesthesia 1984; 39: 279–281.

34. Parkhouse J. The cure of postoperative vomiting. Br. J Anaesth 1963; 35: 189–193.

35. Faymonville ME, Mambourg PH, Joris J et al. Psychological approaches during conscious sedation. Hypnosis versus stress reducing strategies: a prospective randomized study. Pain 1997; 73: 361–367.

36. Abramowitz MD, Oh TH, Epstein BS et al. The antiemetic effect of droperidol following outpatient strabismus surgery in children. Anaesthesiology 1983; 59: 579–583.

37. Fortney JT, Gan TJ, Graczyk S et al. A comparison of the efficacy, safety, and patient satisfaction of ondansetron versus droperidol as antiemetics for elective outpatient surgical procedures. S3A-409 and S3A-410 Study Groups. Anesth Analg 1998; 86: 731–738.

38. Honkavaara P, Saarnivaara L. Comparison of subhypnotic doses of thiopentone vs propofol on the incidence of postoperative nausea and vomiting following middle ear surgery. Acta Anaesthesiol Scand 1998; 42: 211–215.

39. Monagle J, Barnes R, Goodchild C et al. Ondansetron is not superior to moderate dose metoclopramide in the prevention of post-operative nausea and vomiting after minor gynaecological surgery. Eur J Anaesthesiol 1997; 14: 604–609.

40. Alon E, Buchser E, Herrera E et al. Tropisetron for treating established postoperative nausea and vomiting: a randomized, double-blind, placebo-controlled study. Anesth Analg 1998; 86: 617–623.

41. Fujii Y, Toyooka H, Tanaka H. Prevention of postoperative nausea and vomiting with a combination of granisetron and droperidol. Anesth Analg 1998; 86: 613–616.

42. Minowada G, Welch WJ. Clinical implications of the stress response. J Clin Invest 1995; 95: 3–12.

43. Kehlet H. Multimodal approach to control postoperative pathophysiology and rehabilitation. Br J Anaesth 1997; 78: 606–617.

44. Liu S, Carpenter RL, Neal JM. Epidural anesthesia and analgesia. Their role in postoperative outcome. Anesthesiology 1995; 82: 1474–1506.

45. Mangano DT. Perioperative cardiac morbidity. Anesthesiology 1990; 72: 153–184.

46. Nabel EG, Ganz P, Gordon JB. Dilatation of normal and constriction of arteriosclerotic coronary arteries caused by the cold pressure test. Circulation 1988; 77: 43–52.

47. Meissner A, Rolf N, Van Aken H. Thoracic epidural anesthesia and the patient with heart disease: benefits, risks and controversies. Anesth Analg 1997; 85: 517–528.

48. Mangano DT, Browner WS, Hollenberg M et al. Long-term cardiac prognosis following noncardiac surgery. JAMA 1992; 268: 233–239.

49. Rolf N, Van de Velde M, Wouters PF et al. Thoracic epidural anesthesia improves functional recovery from myocardial stunning in conscious dogs. Anesth Analg 1996; 83: 935–940.

50. Blomberg S, Emanuelsson H, Ricksten SE. Thoracic epidural anesthesia and central hemodynamics in patients with unstable angina pectoris. Anesth Analg 1989; 69: 558–562.

51. Blomberg S, Emanuelsson H, Kvist H et al. Effect of thoracic epidural anesthesia on coronary arteries and arterioles in patients coronary artery disease. Anesthesiology 1990; 73: 840–847.

52. Yeager MP, Glass DD, Neff RK et al. Epidural anesthesia and analgesia in high-risk surgical patients. Anesthesiology 1987; 66: 729–736.

53. Baron J-F, Bertrand M, Barré E et al. Combined epidural and general anesthesia versus general anesthesia for abdominal aortic surgery. Anesthesiology 1991; 75: 611–618.

54. Bode RH, Lewis KP, Zarich SW et al. Cardiac outcome after peripheral vascular surgery. Comparison of general and regional anesthesia. Anesthesiology 1996; 84: 3–13.

55. Tuman KJ, McCarthy RJ, March RJ et al. Effects of epidural anesthesia and analgesia on coagulation and outcome after major vascular surgery. Anesth Analg 1991; 73: 696–704.

56. Christopherson R, Norris EJ. Regional versus general anesthesia. Anesthesiol Clin North Am 1997; 15: 37–47.

57. Bredbacka S, Blomback M, Hagnevik K et al. Pre- and postoperative changes in coagulation and fibrinolytic variables during abdominal hysterectomy under epidural or general anaesthesia. Acta Anaesthesiol Scand 1986; 30: 204–210.

58. Rosenfeld BA, Beattie C, Christopherson R et al. The effects of different anesthetic regimens on fibrinolysis and the development of postoperative arterial thrombosis. Perioperative Ischemia Randomized Anesthesia Trial Study Group. Anesthesiology 1993; 79: 435–443.

59. Christopherson R, Beattie C, Meinert CL et al. Perioperative ischemia randomized anesthesia trial study group: perioperative morbidity in patients randomized to epidural or general anesthesia for lower extremity vascular surgery. Anesthesiology 1993; 79: 422–434.

60. Dureuil B, Viires N, Cantineau JP et al. Diaphragmatic contractility after upper abdominal surgery. J Appl Phys 1986; 61: 1775–1780.

61. Easton PA, Fitting JW, Arnoux R et al. Recovery of diaphragm function after laparotomy and chronic sonomicrometer implantation. J Appl Physiol 1989; 66: 613–621.

62. Warner DO, Warner MA, Ritman EL. Human chest wall function during epidural anesthesia. Anesthesiology 1996; 85: 761–773.

63. Mankikian B, Cantineau JP, Bertrand M et al. Improvement of diaphragmatic function by a thoracic extradural block after upper abdominal surgery. Anesthesiology 1988; 68: 379–386.

64. Jayr C, Thomas H, Rey A et al. Postoperative pulmonary complications. Epidural analgesia using bupivacaine and opioids versus parenteral opioids. Anesthesiology 1993; 78: 666–676.

65. Liu SS, Carpenter RL, Mackey DC et al. Effects of perioperative analgesic technique on rate of recovery after colon surgery. Anesthesiology 1995; 83: 757–765.

66. Hogan Q, Stadnicka A, Stekiel T et al. Region of epidural blockade determines sympathetic and mesenteric capitance effects in rabbits. Anesthesiology 1995; 83: 604–610.

67. Steinbrook RA. Epidural anesthesia and gastrointestinal motility. Anesth Analg 1998; 86: 837–44.

68. Taniguchi M, Kasaba T, Takasaki M. Epidural anesthesia enhances sympathetic nerve activity in the unanesthetized segments in cats. Anesth Analg 1997; 84: 391–397.

69. Moiniche S, Bulow S, Hesselfeldt P et al. Convalescence and hospital stay after colonic surgery with balanced analgesia, early oral feeding, and enforced mobilisation. Eur J Surg 1995; 161: 283–288.

70. Brodner G, Pogatzki E, Van Aken H et al. A multimodal approach to control postoperative pathophysiology and rehabilitation in patients undergoing abdominothoracic esophagectomy. Anesth Analg 1998; 86: 228–234.

71. Akerman A, Arweström E, Post C. Local anesthetics potentiate spinal morphine antinociception. Anesth Analg 1988; 67: 943–948.

72. Liu S, Angel JM, Owens BD et al. Effects of epidural bupivacaine after thoracotomy. Reg Anesth 1995; 20: 303–310.

73. Broekema AA, Gielen MJM, Hennis PJ. Postoperative analgesia with continuous epidural sufentanil and bupivacaine: a prospective study in 614 patients. Anesth Analg 1996; 82: 754–759.

74. Scott DA, Beilby DS, McClymont C. Postoperative analgesia using epidural infusions of fentanyl with bupivacaine. A prospective analysis of 1,014 patients. Anesthesiology 1995; 83: 727–737.

75. Cooper JB, Long CD, Newbower RS et al. Critical incidents associated with intraoperative exchanges of anesthesia personnel. Anesthesiology 1982; 56: 456–461.

76. Cooper JB, Newbower RS, Long CD et al. Preventable anesthesia mishaps: a study of human factors. Anesthesiology 1978; 49: 399–406.

77. Craig J, Wilson ME. A survey of anaesthetic misadventures. Anaesthesia 1981; 36: 933–936.

78. Chopra V, Bovill JG, Spierdijk J et al. Reported significant observations during anaesthesia: a prospective analysis over an 18-month period. Br J Anaesth 1992; 68: 13–17.

79. Williamson JA, Webb RK, Sellen A et al. The Australian Incident Monitoring Study. Human failure: an analysis of 2000 incident reports. Anaesth Intensive Care 1993; 21: 678–683.

Anthony P. Adams Jeremy N. Cashman

Obesity

Persons who are naturally very fat are apt to die earlier than those who are slender.
Aphorisms, II, 44. Hippocrates 460BC–357BC

CONCEPTS AND EPIDEMIOLOGY

Body Mass Index (BMI) or Quetelet's Index, calculated from a subject's height and weight [weight (kg) ÷ height (m^2)], is widely used to indicate obesity.[1] Although the index is acknowledged as an adequate summary of obesity, the thresholds for categorising underweight, normal weight, overweight and obesity have varied. In the past, different thresholds were accepted for men and women, with women broadly requiring a low BMI for inclusion in each category. Underweight was indicated in a man by a BMI of <20.0 and in a woman of <18.6. Obesity was indicated by a BMI of ≥ 30.0 and ≥ 28.6, respectively (Fig. 1). The *Health of the Nation* (relating to Great Britain) now defines obesity as a BMI of > 30.0 for both men and women – thus targets have been altered because of the change in definition.[2] Existing methods of measuring obesity may unfairly penalise women for having plump bottoms and thighs. About one-half the women thought to be dangerously overweight are, in fact, just comfortably shapely. Many classical painters, most notably Rubens, have depicted the ideal woman as being 'pear' shaped. Over the past half-century, doctors believed that people with an 'apple' shape, carrying fat around the stomach, as most overweight men do, are more likely to die young. The 'pear' shape, accumulating weight around the bottom, as most premenstrual women tend to, is generally regarded as safe and not a long-term

Professor Anthony P. Adams, Head of Department, Division of Anaesthetics, Guy's Hospital, London Bridge, London SE1 9RT, UK (for correspondence)

Dr Jeremy N. Cashman, Consultant Anaesthetist, Department of Anaesthetics, St George's Hospital, Blackshaw Road, London SW17 0QT, UK

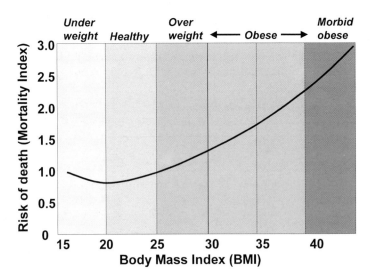

Figure 1 Concept of Body Mass Index (BMI).

risk to health. This is because men's classic 'beer belly' shape stores fat around the internal organs, which is then thought to mobilise into the circulation and raise harmful levels of cholesterol. In contrast, fat around the hips is stored safely between the skin and body wall. Margaret Ashwell, the former scientific director for the British Nutrition Foundation, has devised a simple chart, derived from scientific data,[3–5] that divides waist size by height to illustrate healthy shapes. Obesity and overweight are not synonymous; obesity refers to an excess of fat, whereas overweight may be due to variations in body composition apart from fat.

The prevalence of obesity is increasing at an alarming rate even in non-industrialised countries.[6] In the UK in 1980, 6% of males and 8% of females were deemed to be obese. By 1986/1987 this figure had risen to 8% and 12%, respectively. It may be salutary, now that we have reached the millennium, to determine whether or not the target for obesity of 7% of UK adults by 2000 has been achieved.[7,8] In historical times, when obesity did occur, weight decrease was recognised as difficult. In early Grecian writings, obese people desirous of losing weight were exhorted to eat once a day, perform hard work, take no baths, sleep on a hard bed, and walk naked for as long as possible.[9] These robust, indeed, heroic recommendations, are somewhat matched by some current practices.[10] For example, 14% of a sample of female students, in the US, admitted to self-induced vomiting to lose weight, and in a similar study made in Nigeria on high school and university students, 19% had used laxatives, and 26% had induced vomiting. Vegans (strict vegetarians), compared with meat eaters of the same height, weigh on average about 6 kg less and have a mean BMI of 22 kg/m^2 compared with 24 kg/m^2. Vegetarians, in general, have greater longevity, and a lower mortality rate from ischaemic heart disease. Clearly, only with intense motivation, as prevails in the situation described, is a significantly lower weight practicable. Although some disadvantages of obesity on morbidity and mortality are undoubted, evidence cautions that there are limitations to the benefits that result from weight decrease, especially in the long-term. For example, in an assessment of six major observational studies that reported lowered mortality rates among people who had lost weight, it was concluded that the evidence was equivocal.[11]

Obesity among British children is rising.[12] Most overweight adults gained weight during late adolescence and early adulthood.[13] Measuring BMI at age 5 years is useful to identify the few children who are obese, and who should be encouraged to control their weight.[14] Approximately 50% of obese adolescents with a BMI at or above the 95th percentile become obese adults. Furthermore, the risk factors for adult disease that are associated with obesity in children and adolescents persist into adulthood or increase in prevalence if weight gain occurs.[15] However, there is as yet no agreed measure of obesity in children. The prevalence of obesity increases with age, and the centiles defining adult obesity are unlikely to yield a similar proportion of clinically obese children. Furthermore, targeting obese children is unlikely to identify those most at risk of becoming obese adults; children of different heights show different relations of height to weight.[16] Visceral fat distribution is more likely to prove a better predictor of subsequent mortality than absolute fat mass. Charts for BMI in children have been recommended for clinical use in the UK.[17]

Advances in anaesthesia mean surgery to treat obesity for people previously ruled too high a risk because of their weight. New drugs, improved medical equipment and a better understanding of physiology had reduced the risk associated with surgery. Patients who are obese or morbidly obese have an increased risk from anaesthesia and surgery. It is important to emphasise to surgeons the many problems there are in anaesthetising obese patients so a fully informed discussion can take place. The risks are predominantly anaesthetic: anatomical, physiological and pharmacological (e.g. difficult airway, difficult i.v. access, difficulty maintaining oxygenation and problems of aspiration, etc.) The benefits of surgery from a study in the US are significant but need to be weighed against the risks. The Royal College of Anaesthetists highlighted the problems in a recent report of a nation-wide pilot study of critical incidents in anaesthesia in March 1999. They found that obesity was the most common 'contributing cause' occurring in 42% of incidents.

Carlo Miguel Traico, 32 years, weighing an incredible 401 kg, died of a heart attack in the Argentine province of Cordoba. Apparently Señor Traico, a member of a well-known gypsy family that buys and sells cars and lorries, had spent recent years either sitting down or lying in bed cared for by his parents. Doctors said his weight was the cause of his death.[18] In 1994, a mountainous Brooklyn man, recognised by *The Guinness Book of Records* for losing 50 stone (318 kg) in a diet, had to be lifted from his home by forklift truck and returned to hospital after putting the weight back on. Michael Hebranko, 46 years, now weighs 78 stone (496 kg) after regaining the weight he lost during his last hospital visit three years ago. 'Last Summer he was sitting outside and he looked so good' said his neighbour, Joan Stein. 'Then we started seeing the pizza delivery guys coming to his house and delivering six pizzas at a time'.[19] The sad story of 13-year-old Christina Corrigan made the headlines recently when her body, weighing 309 kg and covered in bed sores, was found in her Californian home. Her mother was convicted of child abuse, despite claims that she had desperately sought help, including 90 visits to a paediatrician who insisted that there was nothing wrong that diet and exercise could not cure.[20]

Many researchers working on the causes of obesity might not have been so sure that dietary recommendations and exercise alone would have helped Corrigan or other chronically obese people. Genetic studies and increasing knowledge of the pathophysiology of obesity paint a complex picture of how normal weight is maintained and what goes wrong in obesity. Claude Bouchard of Laval University, Quebec City, Canada explains the pathways regulating weight form 'a series of redundant regulatory loops, so if one is weakened or attenuated, others can take over. Even when one gene is knocked out, other pathways can compensate'. It is this redundancy that helps the organism regulate calorie storage but the same redundancy makes it hard to get a handle on how to prevent or treat obesity. Put simply, obesity is an ability to balance food intake and energy expenditure. This balancing act involves neural and endocrine signalling, both central and peripheral (Fig. 1). Problems can occur anywhere in this complex system.

The brain controls appetite by means of signals triggered by dietary breakdown products and by autonomic signals produced by distension of the stomach and intestines. The multiple signals generated are processed by complex interactions between neuronal networks and neurotransmitters. Among the neurotransmitters are the cholecystokinins, a family of hormonal and neuronal polypeptides that act on the gut and the brain. Cholecystokinin 8 (CCK-8), the sulphated carboxy-terminal octapeptide of cholecystokinin, is one of the main neurotransmitters involved in appetite control. CCK-8 is released in response to food intake and generates a satiety signal. The gene responsible for leptin, a signal protein for satiety that is produced only in adipose tissue, has been identified in a rodent model.[21] Cholecystokinin (CCK), a factor which limits food intake by inducing satiation, is released at the beginning of a meal, and promotes pancreatic secretion of insulin. The immediate effect of insulin secretion is to lower blood sugar that fosters an increase in appetite. However, circulating insulin crosses the blood–brain barrier and acts on receptors in the hypothalamus to inhibit the secretion of neuropeptide Y. This adds to the fact that the hypothalamus simultaneously juggles many other signals, and the complexity of weight maintenance becomes clear. The goal of research into obesity for the past few years has been to find the genes involved in human obesity. So far, six single-gene mutations have been discovered in obese rodents. Single gene mutations are rare in obese people. However, human obesity has been related to polymorphisms in several genes. An observational study comparing twins reared apart or together has indicated that ~70% of the variance in body mass is due to genetic influences.[22] In addition, the same group has found that the weight of adopted children is related to the BMI of their biological parent rather than their adoptive parent.[23,24] Despite this wide-spread research interest into the inheritability of obesity, environmental influences will probably predominate when it comes to getting fat. On average, 25–30% of human variation in BMI is compatible with a contribution of genetic differences among people. Non-genetic factors account for the rest of the variation. Such estimates indicate a person's genetic susceptibility to their environment; in man, genetic susceptibility is probably related to many genes.

One in three people in Britain carries too much fat and one in 20 is obese; that is 20% or more above maximum desirable body weight. It is estimated that about 100 million people now have a BMI > 30. A receptor in the hypothalamus called the Y5 receptor is the long sought for 'feeding receptor'. Richard Klein, a professor of French at Cornell, author of the best-selling book *Eat Fat*, has noticed that women of authority, even in the university, tend to be large 'their size allows them to impose themselves'.[25]

The world-wide epidemic of obesity is signalled by the rise in the percentage of the population with a BMI of over 30 kg/m², e.g. in Britain from 8% to 15% between 1980 and 1955,[26] and in the US from 12.3% to 20% among men and 16.5% to 24.9% among women between 1976–1980 and 1988–1984.[27] Although BMI is the traditional measure of obesity, the waist to hip circumference was the first index adopted as a measure of the abdominal location of body fat.[28] Waist circumference correlated better with abdominal visceral fat mass. Advocates of using waist circumference to measure obesity argue that it is a straightforward measurement that relates to both body weight and the distribution of fat.[29] Central obesity (waist circumference > 102 cm in males, > 88 cm in females) increases excess mortality and risk of diabetes, heart attacks, and some forms of cancer. Weight gain after age 18 years also predicts increased risk. A gain of more than 10 kg or 1 kg/year signals high risk. Finally, a sedentary lifestyle by itself increases mortality rate from all causes. The life assurance industry has played a key role in making the public aware of the relation between increased weight and earlier death. In 1993, there were 1.25 million American men and women aged 35–74 years with BMIs exceeding 21 kg/m² who died from natural causes.[30] Of these deaths, 325,000 could be attributed to dietary factors, obesity and a sedentary lifestyle, In the US, some 77,315 of 406,973 deaths from coronary heart disease and 34,113 out of 55,110 deaths from diabetes can be attributed to obesity, as can more than 50% of all deaths among the 18 million women and 16.7 million men aged 20–74 years.

However, not all types of obesity are hazardous; it depends in part on where in the body one's fat lies.[31] Individuals with peripheral obesity (i.e. fat distributed subcutaneously around the gluteofemoral region and in the lower part of the abdomen) are at little or no risk of the common medical complications of overweight. Individuals with upper-body (central) obesity (i.e. fat accumulation in the subcutaneous abdominal and visceral depots) are prone to metabolic and cardiovascular complications, especially when there is excess fat in the visceral area. The vascular anatomy and the metabolic activity of visceral fat may be key factors predisposing to complications of obesity.[32]

Supermodels have been criticised for being a bad role model for young women because of unnatural thinness, and have even been linked to the increase in eating disorders, such as anorexia and bulimia.[33,34] Tovée and his colleagues compiled a biometric database (Table 1) on 300 fashion models, 300 glamour models and 300 normal women.[35] Behavioural studies suggest that there is an optimum waist-hip ratio for female attractiveness (Fig. 2); men are supposed to find a waist-hip ratio of 0.7 to be most attractive. This corresponds to a fat distribution which givers optimum fertility.

Fashion models were significantly taller than all the other groups of women – on average 11 cm taller than normal women. Both fashion models and glamour models were significantly underweight on the basis of the BMI, but were consistently heavier than anorexic women. Fashion models and glamour models had a waist-hip ratio close to the optimum of 0.7 and tended to have

Table 1. Biometric characteristics of women[35]

Group	Height (m)	BMI (kg/m²)	Waist-hip ratio	Waist-bust ratio	Bust-hip ratio
Fashion models	1.77 (0.00)	17.57 (0.26)	0.71 (0.02)	0.72 (0.02)	0.99 (0.00)
Glamour models	1.69 (0.00)	18.09 (0.07)	0.68 (0.00)	0.66 (0.00)	1.03 (0.00)
Anorexic women	1.65 (0.01)	14.72 (0.36)	0.76 (0.01)	0.78 (0.01)	0.96 (0.00)
Bulimic women	1.65 (0.01)	23.66 (1.05)	0.77 (0.01)	0.83 (0.01)	0.93 (0.01)
Normal women	1.66 (0.00)	21.86 (0.22)	0.74 (0.00)	0.80 (0.00)	0.92 (0.00)

Reproduced with permission from *The Lancet.*
All values are Mean (±SE)

an hour-glass figure, as shown by the bust-hip ratio. Indeed fashion and glamour models had similar measurements, although glamour models are usually regarded as more curvaceous than fashion models. The key difference may be height: a shorter hour-glass figure may be more curvaceous.

Obesity is associated with a greater likelihood of diabetes, hypertension, hyperlipidaemia, and heart disease as well as increased rates of breast, colon, and uterine cancer.[36] For high-risk patients who fail to respond to diet and exercise, drugs are the preferred method of treatment. In a large cohort of obese persons, the risk of death increased with body weight, but obesity-related excess mortality declined with age at all levels of obesity.[37]

Data obtained from 8960 individuals from the 1970 British Cohort Study suggests that the surge in asthma cases may be linked to rising levels of obesity. The effect is more powerful in women – obese women are twice as likely to suffer from asthma as those of normal weight.[38]

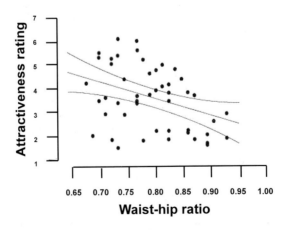

Figure 2 Concept of attractiveness related to waist-hip ratio.[35]Reproduced with permission from *The Lancet.*

The effects of age on excess mortality from all causes associated with obesity are controversial. A prospective cohort study in the US found that the risk of death increased with body weight but obesity-related excess mortality declined with age at all levels of obesity.[39] This study was the largest mortality follow-up of a cohort of obese patients and included a considerable number of grossly obese (BMI 32–40 kg/m^2) and morbidly obese (BMI >40 kg/m^2) subjects. Sixteen years' of follow-up data on 112,822 female nurses aged 30–55 years in the US showed that obesity, cigarette smoking and hypertension were all risk factors for pulmonary embolism. A BMI > 29 kg/m^2 was associated with a 3-fold increase in the prevalence of pulmonary embolism. Obesity predisposes to venous stasis and deep vein thrombosis, which often leads to pulmonary embolism.[40]

Mortality rises exponentially with increasing body weight. The risk of coronary heart disease is doubled if the BMI is >25 kg/m^2 and nearly quadrupled if the index is ≥29 kg/m^2. The risk of developing diabetes increases with increasing weight and people with a BMI >35 kg/m^2 have a 40-fold higher risk of developing the disease. Respiratory disease, particularly sleep apnoea, and osteoarthritis are more common in obese people. They also have higher risks of developing many cancers (e.g. the risks of large bowel and endometrial cancers are increased 2–5-fold). Surgery and anaesthesia are more hazardous, and obesity increases obstetric risk. BMI is an important determinant of lung volumes, respiratory mechanics and oxygenation in anaesthetized patients in the supine position.

CHILDREN

Children with obstructive sleep apnoea (OSA) from adenotonsillar hypertrophy have a diminished ventilatory response to CO_2 stimulation, compared to those without OSA symptoms. Obesity was more prevalent in the children with OSA and with depressed ventilatory responses. Children with OSA undergoing adenotonsillectomy are at risk of respiratory compromise after operation.[41]

A review undertaken to ascertain whether children with the Prader-Willi syndrome present particular problems to the anaesthetist showed that those, in an early stage of the condition, who are below their centile for weight, present no specific problems. Children who are heavier than 97th centile weight have problems associated with their obesity: difficult i.v. access and sleep apnoea.[42]

SURGERY FOR THE TREATMENT OF OBESITY

Surgery is increasingly being used for morbid obesity.[43–48] Banded gastroplasty[49] can lead to serious protein-calorie and vitamin deficiency that may, in turn, lead to serious neurological and other sequelae. Since increasing numbers of people are undergoing surgery – typically, vertical banded gastroplasty – we are likely to see significantly more neurological complications, such as Wernicke's encephalopathy, which occurs as a result of thiamine deficiency and can be prevented by supplementation.[50] Selection of patients, pre-operative pre-paration together with careful anaesthesia and surgery may be expected to reduce the likelihood of postoperative complications. Long-term benefits include regression of the diseases resulting from obesity but electrolytic disturbances occur.[51]

Laparoscopic surgical techniques seem beneficial in obese patients in terms of respiratory morbidity, with a faster return to normal respiratory function. Furthermore, laparoscopic gastric banding (laparoscopic gastroplasty) has a number of advantages from a surgical point of view (viz non-invasive, low morbidity, ease of revision and complete reversibility.[52] There has been little information about intra-operative respiratory mechanics and about patient tolerance to abdominal insufflation in the morbidly obese. A study of morbidly obese patients (mean BMI 45 kg/m^2) undergoing laparoscopic gastroplasty showed alterations in pulmonary mechanics to be less than those observed with comparable degrees of abdominal inflation in non-obese patients, and were well tolerated. From the point of view of intra-operative respiratory mechanics, laparoscopic surgery was judged to be safe in morbidly obese patients.[53,54]

RESPIRATORY FUNCTION

Epidemiological data indicate that the relationship between obesity and OSA is largely explained by variation in neck size. Fat deposits in the neck may predispose to upper airway occlusion during sleep by altering the mechanical properties of the upper airway, particularly at the level of the velopharynx (VP). Obese patients with large necks have a more collapsible VP during wakefulness, which may predispose to upper airway obstruction during sleep.[55]

In addition to the elastic load, obese subjects have to overcome increased respiratory resistance resulting from the reduction in lung volumes related to being overweight.[56] BMI is an important determinant of lung volumes, respiratory mechanics, and oxygenation during anaesthesia with patients in the supine position.[57] Morbidly obese patients, during anaesthesia and paralysis, experience more severe impairment of respiratory mechanics and gas exchange than normal subjects. Sedated-paralyzed morbidly obese patients, compared with normal subjects, are characterised by marked derangements in lung and chest wall mechanics and reduced lung volume after abdominal surgery. These alterations may account for the impaired arterial oxygenation in the postoperative period.[57] With increasing BMI: (i) FRC decreased exponentially; (ii) the compliance of the total respiratory system and of the lung decreased exponentially, whereas the compliance of the chest wall was only minimally affected; (iii) the resistance of the total respiratory system and of the lung increased, whereas the chest wall resistance was unaffected; and (iv) the work of breathing increased, mainly due to the lung component.[57] There is evidence that, in such circumstances, positive end-expiratory pressure (PEEP) improves respiratory function in morbidly obese patients but not in normal patients.[58] However, a study of eight morbidly obese patients (BMI 46 kg/m^2) during general anaesthesia and controlled lung ventilation failed to find any advantage from the use of large tidal volumes from a baseline of 13 ml/kg to 22 ml/kg.[59] Patient and surgical factors are more important determinants of pulmonary gas exchange than were tidal volume or inspiratory gas. Manual hyperinflation is a simple and effective manoeuvre to improve gas exchange.[60]

Changes in respiratory system mechanics over a wide range of postures that may be encountered clinically are relatively small in awake subjects due to adaptability of total chest wall mechanical behaviour.[61] By compressing the abdomen and restricting chest wall movement, the prone position compromises pulmonary compliance. For spine surgery, placing the anaesthetized patient into the prone position increases the risk of improper ventilation. Pulmonary compliance is decreased in the obese by the use of chest rolls or the Wilson frame; however, there was no decrease using the Jackson spinal surgery table.[62] Pelosi's group investigated the effects of the prone position on FRC and of the mechanical properties – compliance and resistance – of the total respiratory system, lung and chest wall and gas exchange in 10 anaesthetized and paralysed obese patients (BMI > 30 kg/m^2) undergoing elective surgery.[63] Measurements were taken in the supine position for 15–30 min, then in the prone position while maintaining the same respiratory pattern and inspired oxygen concentration (V$_T$ 12 ml/kg^1, RR 14 bpm, FIO$_2$ 0.4). The FRC and lung compliance increased from the supine to prone position; however, the prone position reduced chest wall compliance and thus the total respiratory system compliance was unchanged. Turning the patients prone did not modify the resistances of the total respiratory system, lung and chest wall. The increase in FRC and lung compliance was paralleled by a significant improvement of PaO$_2$ from supine to prone although PaCO$_2$ was unchanged. This group had previously demonstrated in normal subjects that the prone position during general anaesthesia does not negatively affect respiratory mechanics and improves lung volumes and oxygenation.[64] The Trendelenburg ('head-down') posture increases the mechanical impedance of the lung to inflation, probably due to decreases in lung volume. This effect may be clinically relevant in obese patients[65] and great care required.

The dietary treatment of morbid obesity is sufficient to induce improvement in lung volumes, but not enough to improve arterial saturation, although ventilatory mechanics is improved sufficiently and the tendency towards small airway closure was decreased; hypoxaemia was significantly relieved by standing up both before and after weight loss.[66]

CIRCULATORY FUNCTION

Morbidly obese patients are at an increased risk for structural and functional abnormalities of the heart.[67] It has been recognized that abnormalities in cardiac structure and function occur more commonly when patients have been obese for 15 years or longer than in those with obesity of shorter duration. Heart weight increases in direct relation to body weight, and extremely obese people have excessive epicardial fat, whereas left ventricular (LV) fat content remains normal. Eccentric LV hypertrophy is the most common abnormality in the heart of morbidly obese patients; it comprises chamber dilation and some wall thickening. When hypertension accompanies severe obesity, a combination of concentric and eccentric hypertrophy is present. The use of non-invasive techniques has provided further insight into the mechanisms of heart disease in the morbidly obese patient. Echocardiographic studies in obese patients have shown LV enlargement in 8–40%, increased LV wall thickness in 6–56%, increased LV mass in 64–87%, left atrial enlargement in 10–40%, and right ventricular enlargement in 32% of patients. It is now established that the BMI strongly correlates with LV mass, wall thickness, and cavity dimension, even after adjusting for age and blood pressure.[68] LV hypertrophy is one of the strongest risk factors for cardiovascular morbidity and mortality, and an increase in relative wall thickness has been shown to increase cardiovascular risk.

Right ventricular function (RVF) has been investigated during gastric bypass in morbidly obese patients. The presence of chronic hypoxaemia and hypercapnia in morbidly obese patients with OSA syndrome while awake did not change during gastric bypass procedures despite decreases in pulmonary artery (PA) pressure, pulmonary capillary wedge pressure (PCWP) and pulmonary vascular resistance (PVR) after opening the abdomen. This decrease in PA pressure and PVR may be caused by decreases in pleural pressure reflected by a concomitant decrease in oesophageal pressure.[69]

The massively obese state is accompanied by marked haemodynamic abnormalities. Extreme obesity causes an increase in blood volume and cardiac output in direct proportion to the amount of weight gained.[70] The blood volume and cardiac output of a person weighing 170 kg are about twice those of a 70 kg subject.[71] The increased cardiac output is due to an increase in stroke volume, stroke work, and cardiac work to serve the metabolic requirements of excessive fat. The increase in the total blood is a result of the increase in size of the vascular bed in the excess adipose tissue. Mean arterial pressure, systemic vascular resistance, pulmonary capillary wedge pressure, pulmonary artery pressure and RV end-diastolic pressure exceed those for healthy subjects.[72] Pulmonary hypertension is a consequence of elevated LV diastolic pressure and, in some cases, the obesity hypoventilation syndrome acts as a second causative factor.

Several epidemiological studies suggest a relation between central obesity and coronary heart disease (CHD). Many of them have demonstrated a relation between central obesity and CHD independent of coexisting CHD. However, there is no consensus about identifying CHD as an independent risk factor. There is strong evidence that severe obesity is associated with arterial hypertension. The presence of hypertension is related not only to excess fat but also to the waist-hip ratio. The adverse effects of obesity and hypertension are additive: the combination significantly increases the development of congestive heart failure.

PROBLEMS IN PREGNANCY

The high incidence of antepartum medical disease and emergency Caesarean section complicate anaesthetic care in morbidly obese parturients.[73] The morbidly obese parturient has a higher incidence of obstetric and perinatal complications. Higher maternal weight before pregnancy increases the risk of late fetal death, although it protects against the delivery of a small-for-gestational-age infant.[74] Anaesthesia in these patients is also associated with an increased frequency and severity of complications. The triennial report on maternal mortality reveals that three of the only four deaths directly attributable to anaesthesia had a common feature, namely obesity.[75] Unfortunately, this aspect is not further discussed in the report.

Epidural anaesthesia is feasible; however, the high initial failure rate necessitates early catheter placement, critical block assessment and catheter replacement when indicated, and provision for alternative airway management.

Case reports provide useful insights into management of the obese. A morbidly obese parturient (150 kg, 150 cm height) with severe pre-eclampsia, generalized oedema and acute respiratory failure was managed by Caesarean section using infiltration lignocaine (0.5–1%) block.[76] A 26-year-old morbidly obese parturient (BMI 62 kg/m²) with pre-eclampsia was successfully managed, with good analgesia and lack of complications, using an epidural anaesthetic – the distance between the skin and the epidural space was 9 cm at the L3-4 interspace via a midline approach. The catheter was inserted 5 cm cephalad in the sitting position and a single dose of 17 ml mepivacaine 1.5% was given in the supine position.[77] Another detailed report, with successful outcome, concerns a woman with acute onset of asthma (39-year-old; 225 kg weight 160 cm tall, BMI 88 kg/m²) who had an abdominal panniculus which extended down to her thighs.[78] The patient was positioned in a sitting position with her feet firmly planted on a high stool and the lumbar pads of fat were strapped firmly out of the way with adhesive tape. A lumbar epidural catheter was inserted using an extra long Tuohy needle (epidural space located at a depth of 13 cm) using lignocaine 2% in a total dosage of 12 ml.

DRUG REGIMENS AND INTERACTIONS

Combination drug therapy can often effectively treat the problem of obesity. The most commonly used combination is a mix of fenfluramine and phentermine. Fenfluramine inhibits the re-uptake of serotonin and acts on the hypothalamic appetite control centre, while phentermine acts as an appetite suppressant. Problems with hypotension during induction, hypoglycaemia, hyperthermia and pulmonary hypertension have been reported. Recently, dexfenfluramine (the dextro-isomer of fenfluramine) has been approved in the US.[79]

ANAESTHETIC MANAGEMENT OF THE OBESE PATIENT

PRE-OPERATIVE MANAGEMENT

1. Avoid respiratory depressants.
2. Give H_2 receptor antagonists to block secretion of gastric acid (ranitidine 150 mg p.o. night before and morning of surgery).
3. Assess difficulty of intubation very carefully: always have a back-up plan ready.

AIRWAY

Although anterior displacement of the mandible during anaesthesia is often helpful to relieve airway obstruction in normal patients, it is less effective in obese patients. Mandibular advancement increases the retroglossal area at a given pharyngeal pressure. However, at a given pharyngeal pressure mandibular advancement increases the retropalatal area in the non-obese but not in the obese.[80]

The management of morbidly obese patients has been described in recent reviews and case reports and depends upon an appreciation of potential problems and a thorough understanding of the pathophysiological changes that accompany obesity.[1,81–88] Although obese patients are often difficult to intubate there does not appear to be a correlation between BMI and the difficulty of laryngoscopy; the obese patient presents a persuasive argument for the insertion of an endotracheal tube before the induction of anaesthesia.[89] The prospect of providing anaesthesia for a morbidly obese patient with intestinal obstruction provides a real challenge. The problems in the management of such an emergency case have been described for a morbidly obese patient (150 kg, 157 cm height, 61 BMI kg/m^2); the SpO$_2$ decreased rapidly down to 30% during induction.[90]

The intravenous induction of anaesthesia is technically difficult because of the lack of suitable veins: there is a particular risk of accidental intra-arterial and extravascular injection. Obese patients are at increased risk of developing hypoxaemia when apnoeic. Patients were pre-oxygenated for 5 min or until expired N$_2$ was < 5%. The time taken for the SpO$_2$ to fall to 90% was 5 min in patients of normal weight, 4 min in a group of obese patients (> 20% but less than 45.5 kg over ideal body weight), and about 2.5 min in a group of obese patients who were more than 45.5 kg over ideal weight.[91]

TRACHEAL INTUBATION

The choice of technique and equipment is a personal one. Choi has designed a flangeless blade that embodies two different curvatures of 20° and 30°.[92] An ingenious blade for difficult intubation is on the Bullard laryngoscope which is a spoon shaped or duck-billed blade using a combined fibre-optic and mirror instrument. It is classified as an indirect instrument because, unlike conventional direct instruments, it uses mirrors and fibre-optic material to look around a corner at the larynx rather than providing a direct view. Adult and paediatric versions have been developed concurrently.[93] Although such devices have been recommended for emergency airway management in the obese,[94] it must be remembered that their use requires sufficient prior practice. An awake tracheal intubation, generally using the fibre-optic approach, should be considered in difficult circumstances. This technique has much to commend it, but the obese patient is not a suitable case for an anaesthetist who is inexperienced to experiment. Capnography is essential to confirm correct placement of the endotracheal tube. Contrary to previous reports, the self-inflating bulb (SIB) device (designed to differentiate oesophageal from tracheal intubation) is associated with a high incidence of false negative results in morbidly obese patients.[95] The mechanism of these false negative results appears to be related to the reduction of calibre of airways secondary to a marked decrease in FRC, and collapse of large airways due to invagination of the posterior tracheal wall when subatmospheric pressure is generated by the SIB.

MAINTENANCE OF ANAESTHESIA

The pharmacokinetic parameters of propofol during operation, and for up to 8 h afterwards, were compared with non-obese subjects. Propofol does not accumulate in morbidly obese patients (body weight 115.5 ± 20.8 kg (range 97–160 kg) using the following dosage scheme in 8 patients receiving a 66:34% mixture of N$_2$O:O2.[96] A stepped infusion of 21 mg/kg/h was given for the first 5 min; then 12 mg/kg/h for 10 min, then 6 mg/kg/h thereafter. Body weight was determined by an empirical formula (corrected weight = ideal weight + 990.4 x excess weight].

Predictions of a reduction in the FRC following the induction of anaesthesia in obese patients have been confirmed, the possible causes being a loss of elastic recoil and premature airway closure: there is a shift of ventilation to the non-dependent lung regions. The elderly obese patient with a reduced FRC may reach a state during anaesthesia where the closing volume (CV) exceeds FRC. Trapped gas behind the closed airways equilibrates with venous blood and contributes to venous admixture in the pulmonary circulation. Inspired oxygen concentrations should be increased to at least 50% in order to maintain arterial oxygen saturation at safe levels; pulse oximetry is essential to check on this.

Sevoflurane is a good agent for bariatric surgery because of its physical and chemical characteristics and its partition coefficient (blood-gas 0.65). Advantages claimed include: quick awakening, a low incidence of nausea and vomiting, a prompt regain of physical and psychological functioning, an early discharge from hospital and a larger turnover of patients with lower costs.[97] Obesity, untreated diabetes mellitus and alcohol abuse increase the hepatic content and activity of cytochrome P450 2E1 and, therefore, enhanced anaesthetic defluorination is to be suspected. Mean serum inorganic fluoride concentrations in obese patients who received sevoflurane increased more rapidly and were significantly higher than in controls. The peak serum fluoride level in the obese patients was 51.7 ± 2.5 $\mu mol/l$ and exceeded 50 $\mu mol/l$ for nearly 2 h.[98] However, another study comparing non-obese with obese (BMI > 35 kg/m^2) patients for a mean of 1.4 alveolar concentration (MAC) hours found peak plasma inorganic fluoride ion concentrations of 30 ± 2 $\mu mol/l$ in obese and 28 ± 2 $\mu mol/l$ in the non-obese, 1 h after discontinuing anaesthesia.[99] Although sevoflurane is deemed to have extremely low hepatotoxic potential compared to isoflurane and thus need not be avoided,[100] studies with sensitive methods in morbidly obese patients do not exist.[101]

Attention to the prevention of hypothermia (by use of a forced air warming system compared to a warmed blanket) in obese patients presenting for major abdominal surgery suggests benefits which include: less blood loss intra-operatively and a higher postanaesthesia Aldrete Score.[102]

ANAESTHESIA AND MONITORING

Meticulous planning of the whole process of surgery and anaesthesia including care both before and after operation is absolutely vital. Nowadays, there are reports of patients with superobesity (e.g. weights of 355 kg and 377 kg) undergoing surgery: the emphasis is on preconceived protocols to treat such patients.[103]

1. Adequate pre-oxygenation is essential.
2. Use cricoid pressure.
3. Consider direct arterial pressure monitoring.
4. Full standard monitoring applied including temperature, peripheral nerve stimulator.
5. Endotracheal tube preferred (awake or asleep).

6. Monitor SpO_2 to determine optimal FIO_2.

7. Intermittent positive pressure ventilation (IPPV) preferred (to prevent atelectasis).

8. Careful positioning (nerve damage).

9. Avoid long acting drugs.

10. Avoid lipid soluble anaesthetics.

11. Prefer drugs that do not require much metabolism (e.g. sevoflurane).

12. Do not extubate until patient fully awake and can control airway with spontaneous ventilation.

13. Consider a period of postoperative IPPV if pain likely to be difficult to control.

USE OF NEUROMUSCULAR BLOCKING DRUGS

An overdosage is likely when neuromuscular blocking drugs (NMBs) are administered on a body weight basis to obese patients. For instance, there have been conflicting reports on the duration of atracurium in the obese due to lack of appreciation of the importance of using lean body mass (LBM) as a basis for dosage (the same applies to other neuromuscular drugs). When LBM is taken into account, there is no difference between obese patients and non-obese in the elimination of atracurium.[104] A study considering anthropometric variables concluded that a dose of atracurium expressed as mg/kg body weight in the obese is prolonged: it is suggested that the dose be reduced to 0.23 mg for each kilogram of total body weight above 70 kg.[105] The dosage of atracurium necessary to maintain a 95% twitch depression (ED_{95}) was 0.34 mg/kg in underweight patients, 0.29 mg/kg in normal weight patients and 0.22 mg/kg in overweight patients.[106] In view of the difficulty in estimating LBM in routine clinical practice, it is emphasized that ED_{95} correlates only slightly less than with normal weight. Moreover, recovery of neuromuscular transmission in the 3 groups was comparable. From a clinical standpoint, a peripheral nerve stimulator must always be used to monitor the effects of the blockade; small doses of muscle relaxants should be used and their effect properly monitored – more drug can be given if required.

The pharmacodynamics and pharmacokinetics of rocuronium in female patients are not altered by obesity.[107] The population pharmacokinetics of doxacurium were investigated: not unexpectedly, obesity is a factor which has to be taken into account.[108] Vecuronium has also been investigated: when the data were calculated on the basis of ideal body weight for obese and control patients, total volume of distribution, plasma clearance and elimination half-life were no different.[109]

The clearance of doxacurium is markedly decreased in patients with renal failure undergoing kidney transplantation. Both obesity and renal dysfunction markedly prolong recovery after doxacurium administration. Obesity decreased both the clearance (CL) of doxacurium, by 1.1% above ideal body weight (IBW) and its neuromuscular junction sensitivity by 0.4% above IBW. Thus dosing of doxacurium should be based on IBW and, although no further adjustment is recommended for renal dysfunction, recovery will take longer in its presence.[110] There are no differences in protein binding of the neuromuscular blocking drugs (atracurium, mivacurium, doxacurium, vecuronium) in obese patients.[111]

OPIOIDS

The characteristics of the new opioid remifentanil suggest it to be the analgesic of choice in obese patients. The pharmacokinetics of the drug are not appreciably different in obese versus lean subjects and the pharmacokinetic parameters are more closely related to LBM than to total body weight (TBW). Hence dosing regimens should be based on IBW (or LBM) and not on TBW.[112] The high lipid solubility of sufentanil probably explains the altered pharmacokinetics of this opioid in obese patients. There is an increased volume of distribution of sufentanil in the obese (9098 ± 2793 ml/kg) when compared to a control group (5073 ± 1673 ml/kg), and a prolonged elimination half life (208 ± 82 min versus 135 ±42 min).[113]

REGIONAL ANAESTHESIA

Spinal and epidural (extradural) anaesthesia have both been recommended in the obese patient either alone[114] or as part of a combined regional analgesia and general anaesthesia technique.[83] Meticulous planning is again vital. The positioning of the patient, palpation of landmarks, and needle location are difficult: an image intensifier is a valuable aid. The combination of general anaesthesia and thoracic peridural block, when it is possible, has been described as an ideal technique for the anaesthetic management of patients presenting for bariatric surgery. It is emphasized that the technique requires specialized personnel working in a specialized environment with the aim of assessing the operative risk and reducing it to an acceptable level taking into account the benefit of the surgical procedure.[115] A technique based on a thoracic epidural block, to avoid general endotracheal anaesthesia, has been used for the surgical treatment of panniculus morbidus, i.e. large pannuliculi where severe problems with hygiene, immobility and chronic infection were caused by the lymphoedematous chronically infected pannus.[116] Previously conduction analgesia has not been recommended for upper abdominal surgery: reductions in cardiac output may occur while levels of regional analgesia conducive to good operating conditions further embarrass respiration and pulmonary gas exchange.

Epidural local analgesic drugs tend not to 'fix' very quickly in the obese patient and there is a tendency for continuing cephalad spread. It has been suggested that the L4-5 rather than the L3-4 interspace be used when extensive spread of the block is to be avoided with bupivacaine.[117] The sitting position limited cephalad spread only in obese parturients and the decrease in spread was in proportion to the obesity. Cephalad spread is positively correlated to the BMI.[118] Intra-operative epidural catheter malfunction is not uncommon. In two cases, the problem was resolved by the anaesthetist placing the palm of both hands under the patients' lumbar area and thoracic area; the epidural catheter with tape and subcutaneous tissue was pulled towards the head – in each case this simple manoeuvre made the catheter function again.[119] Particular care in obese patients is necessary when the glucose-free (hypobaric) preparation of bupivacaine is used for spinal anaesthesia.[120]

Phrenic nerve paralysis is a common complication in interscalene brachial plexus block. The complication is often ignored by most anaesthetists because of lack of clinical symptoms in patients with no underlying lung disease. However, dyspnoea following such a complication has been reported: the decreased respiratory reserve and direct compressing effect of the abdominal organs on the diaphragm in the supine position were thought to be the risk factors.[121]

The main drawback to the use of regional techniques is that of haematoma formation given that it is most desirable for obese patients to be receiving heparin therapy – best given intravenously – to combat the development of deep vein thrombosis and pulmonary embolism; in such cases, it is preferable to introduce an epidural catheter before heparinisation is commenced.

Key points for clinical practice

Conditions caused by or aggravated by obesity

- Diabetes mellitus.
- Hypertension.
- All cardiorespiratory diseases.
- Reflux oesophagitis.
- Malignant disease (uterus and ovary).
- Menstrual irregularities and infertility.
- Sleep apnoea and Pickwickian syndrome.
- Musculoskeletal disorders.
- Benign raised intracranial pressure.
- Poor operative risk.
- Poor postoperative would healing.
- Deep vein thrombosis and thromboembolism.

Special problems relating to anaesthesia

- Obtain help (e.g. another experienced anaesthetist).
- Have all the equipment you may possibly need immediately ready.
- Minimise the risk of acid aspiration (e.g. administer ranitidine before operation).
- Assess the airway and ones ability to correctly place an endotracheal tube.
- Use full monitoring.
- Minimise the risk of damage to peripheral nerves during surgery.
- Take prophylactic measures to reduce the risk of deep vein thrombosis occurring (heparin i.v.), anti-thrombosis leg muscle compression devices.
- Keep the patient warm.

POSTOPERATIVE PROBLEMS

The postoperative period is particularly dangerous for obese patients. Meticulous monitoring is vital and should be continued into the recovery period. Patients with a BMI > 25 kg/m^2 have an increased risk of hypoxaemia in the first hour of recovery.[122] The use of laparoscopy for gastroplasty in morbidly obese patients may significantly improve the immediate postoperative course.[123] Obesity is a significant risk factor for clinically relevant noscomial infections in surgical patients.[124] Particular care is required in the postoperative period after the use of fentanyl or similar drugs because of the risk of respiratory depression developing.[125] Obesity is one of the problems which delays early extubation.[126]

Obese patients seem to have a moderate risk of developing postoperative thrombosis even when an effective prophylaxis has been used. Thrombo-elastography and sonoclot analytical techniques have shown that patients with morbid obesity show accelerated fibrin formation, fibrinogen-platelet interaction, and platelet function compared with lean controls, but no difference in fibrinolysis.[127] High free fatty acids, hypercholesterolaemia and diabetes are not obvious extra risks in obese patients. Thromboprophylaxis should be given to all obesity patients who are to be operated upon regardless of age. Any symptoms suggestive of thromboembolism must be investigated promptly.[128]

REFERENCES

1. Adams AP. Nutritional disorders. In: Vickers MD, Power I. (eds) Medicine for Anaesthetists. Oxford: Blackwell Science, 1999; 266–293.
2. Secretary of State for Health. The Health of the Nation – Specification of National Indicators. London: Department of Health, 1992.
3. Ashwell MA, LeJeune SRE, McPherson K. Ratio of waist circumference to height may be better indicator of need for weight management. BMJ 1996; 312: 37
4. Ashwell MA, Cole TJ, Dixon AK. Ratio of waist circumference to height is strong predictor of abdominal fat. BMJ 1996; 313: 559–560.
5. Cox BD, Whichelow MJ. Ratio of waist circumference to height is better predictor of death than body mass index. BMJ 1966; 313: 1487
6. Bray GA. Obesity: a time bomb to be defused? BMJ 1998; 352: 160–161.
7. Garrow J. Importance of obesity. BMJ 1991; 303: 704–706.
8. Bjorntorp P. Prevalence of obesity 15–20% of middle aged adults in much of Europe. Lancet 1997; 350: 423–426.
9. Atkinson RL. Treatment of obesity. Nutr Rev 1992; 50: 228–239.
10. Walker ARP. Epidemiology and health implications of obesity, with special reference to African populations. Ecol Food Nutr 1998; 37: 21–55.
11. Williamson DF, Pamuk ER. The association between weight loss and increased longevity: a review of the evidence. Ann Intern Med 1993; 199: 731–736.
12. Reilly JJ, Dorosty AR, Emmett PM. Prevalence of overweight and obesity in British children: a cohort study. BMJ 1999; 319: 1039.
13. Power C, Lake JK, Cole TJ. Measurement and short-term health risks of child and adolescent fatness. Int J Obes 1997; 21: 507–526.
14. Cole TJ, Freeman JV, Preece MA. Body mass index reference curves for the UK, 1990. Arch Dis Child 1995; 73: 25–29.
15. Dietz WH. Childhood weight affects adult morbidity and mortality. J Nutr 1998; 128: 411S–414S.
16. Mulligan J, Voss LD. Identifying very fat and very thin children: test of criterion standards for screening test. BMJ 1999; 319: 1103–1104.

17. Prentice AM. Body mass index standards for children. BMJ 1998; 317: 1401–1403.

18. The Times, 29th July 1998.

19. The Times, 9th June 1994.

20. Macready N. The stubborn enigma of obesity. Lancet 1998; 351: 888.

21. Zhang Y, Proenca R, Maffei M, Barone M, Leopold L, Friedman JM. Positional cloning of the mouse obese gene and its human homologue [Erratum Nature 1995; 374; 479]. Nature 1994; 372: 425–432.

22. Stunkard AJ, Harris JR, Pedersen NL, McClearn GE. The body-mass index of twins reared apart. N Engl J Med 1990; 322: 1483–1487.

23. Stunkard AJ, Sorensen TI, Hanis C et al. An adoption study of human obesity. N Engl J Med 1986; 314: 193–198

24. Stunkard AJ, Foch TT, Hrubec Z. A twin study of human obesity. JAMA 1986; 256: 51–54.

25. Klein R. Eat Fat. New York: Vintage Books, 1998.

26. Wilding J. Science, medicine, and the future: obesity treatment. BMJ 1997; 315: 997–1000.

27. Flegal KM, Carroll MD, Kuczmarski RJ, Johnson CL. Obesity and overweight in the United States: prevalence and trends, 1960–1994. Int J Obes 1998; 22: 39–47.

28. Bjorntorp P. Abdominal fat distribution and disease: an overview of epidemiological data. Ann Med 1992; 24: 15–18.

29. Pounder D, Carson D, Orihara Y. Evaluation of indices of obesity in men: descriptive study. BMJ 1998; 316: 1428–1429.

30. McGinnis JM, Foege WH. Actual causes of death in the United States. JAMA 1993; 270: 2207–2212.

31. Byers T. Body weight and mortality [editorial]. N Engl J Med 1995; 333: 723–724.

32. Arner P. Not all fat is alike. BMJ 1998; 351: 1301.

33. Frean A, Bradberry G. Vogue model too thin for Omega. The Times, 31 May 1996; 1.

34. Orbach S. Commentary. The Guardian, 31 May 1996; 1.

35. Tovée MJ, Mason SM, Emery JL, McCluiskey SE, Cohen-Tovée M. Supermodels: stick insects or hourglasses? Lancet 1997; 350: 1474–1484.

36. Calle EE, Thun MJ, Petrelli JM, Rodriguez C, Heath Jr CW. Body-mass index and mortality in a prospective cohort of US adults. N Engl J Med 1999; 341: 1097–1105.

37. Bender R, Jöckel K-H, Trautner C, Spraul M, Berger M. Effect of age in excess mortality in obesity. JAMA 1999; 281: 1498–1504.

38. Shaheen SO, Sterne JAC, Montgomery SM, Azima H. Birth weight, body mass index and asthma in young adults. Thorax 1999; 54: 396–402.

39. Bender R, Jockel KH, Trautner C et al. Effect of age on excess mortality in obesity. JAMA 1999; 281: 1498–1504.

40. Goldhaber SZ, Grodstein F, Stampfer MJ et al. A prospective study of risk factors for pulmonary embolism in women. JAMA 1997; 277: 642–645.

41. Strauss SG, Lynn AM, Bratton SL, Nespeca MK. Ventilatory response to CO_2 in children with obstructive sleep apnoea from adenotonsillar hypertrophy. Anesth Analg 1999; 89: 328–332.

42. Dearlove OR, Dobson A, Super M. Anaesthesia and the Prader-Willi syndrome. Paediatr Anaesth 1998; 8: 267–271.

43. Wilding J. Science, medicine, and the future: obesity treatment. BMJ 1997; 315: 997–1000.

44. Fobi MAL, Lee H, Holness R, Cabinda D. Gastric bypass operation for obesity. World J Surg 1998; 22: 925–935>.

45. Scopinaro N, Adami GF, Marinari GM et al. Biliopancreatic diversion. World J Surg 1998; 22: 936–946.

46. Marceau P, Hould F-S, Simard S et al. Biliopancreatic diversion with duodenal switch. World J Surg 1998; 22: 947–954.

47. Belachew M, Legrand M, Vincent V, Lismonde M, Le Docte N, Deschamps V. Laparoscopic adjustable gastric banding. World J Surg 1998; 22: 955–963.

48. Lönroth H, Dalenbäck J. Other laparoscopic procedures. World J Surg 1998; 22: 964–968.

49. Mason EE, Doherty C, Cullen JJ, Scott D, Rodriguez EM, Maher JW. Vertical banded

gastroplasty: evolution of vertical banded gastroplasty. World J Surg 1998; 22: 919–924.

50. Seehra H, MacDermot N, Lascelles RG, et al. Lesson of the week. Wernicke's encephalopathy after vertical banded gastroplasty for morbid obesity. BMJ 1996; 312: 434.

51. Sedletskii IuI, Lebedev LV, Gostevskoi AA, Mirchuk KK. Vestn Khir Im I I Grek 1999; 158: 61–63.

52. Oria HE. Gastric banding for morbid obesity. Eur J Gastroenterol Hepatol 1999; 11: 105–114.

53. Dumont L, Mattys M, Mardirosoff M, Vervloesem N, Alle JL, Massaut J. Changes in pulmonary mechanics during laparoscopic gastroplasty in morbidly obese patients. Acta Anaesthesiol Scand 1997; 41: 408–413>.

54. Dumont L, Mattys M, Mardirosoff C, Picard V, Alle JL, Massaut J. Hemodynamic changes during laparoscopic gastroplasty in morbidly obese patients. Obes Surg 1997; 7: 326–331.

55. Ryan CF, Love LL. Mechanical properties of the velopharynx in obese patients with obstructive sleep apnea. Am J Respir Crit Care Med 1996; 154: 806–812.

56. Zerah F, Harf A, Perlemuter L, Lorino H, Atlan G. Effects of obesity on respiratory resistance. Chest 1993; 103: 1470–1476.

57. Pelosi P, Croci M, Ravagnan I et al. The effects of body mass index on lung volumes, respiratory mechanics, and gas exchange during general anesthesia. Anesth Analg 1998; 87: 654–650.

58. Pelosi P, Ravagnan I, Giurati G et al. Positive end-expiratory pressure improves respiratory function in obese but not in normal subjects during anesthesia and paralysis. Anesthesiology 1999; 91: 1221–1231.

59. Bardoczky GI, Yernault JC, Houben JJ, d'Hollander AA. Large tidal volume ventilation does not improve oxygenation in morbidly obese patients during anaesthesia. Anesth Analg 1995; 81: 385–388.

60. Tweed WA, Phua WT, Chong KY, Lim E, Lee TL. Tidal volume, lung hyperinflation and arterial oxygenation during general anaesthesia. Anaesth Intensive Care 1993; 21: 806–810.

61. Barnas GM, Green MD, Mackenzie CF et al. Effect of posture on lung and regional chest wall mechanics. Anesthesiology 1993; 78: 251–259.

62. Palmon SC, Kirsch JR, Depper JA, Toung TJK. The effect of the prone position on pulmonary mechanics is frame-dependent. Anesth Analg 1998; 87: 1175–1180.

63. Pelosi P, Croci M, Calappi E et al. Prone positioning improves pulmonary function in obese patients during general anesthesia. Anesth Analg 1996; 83: 578–583.

64. Pelosi P, Croci, Calappi E et al. The prone positioning during general anesthesia minimally affects respiratory mechanics while improving functional residual capacity and increasing oxygen tension. Anesth Analg 1995; 80: 955–960.

65. Fahy BG, Barnas GM, Nagle SE, Flowers JL, Njoku MJ, Agarwal M. Effects of Trendelenburg and reverse Trendelenburg postures on lung and chest wall mechanics. J Clin Anesth 1996; 8: 236–244.

66. Hakala K, Mustajoki P, Aittomaki J, Sovijarvi AR. Effect of weight loss and body position on pulmonary function and gas exchange abnormalities in morbid obesity. Int J Obes Relat Metab Disord 1995; 19: 242–246.

67. Herrera MF, Oseguera J, Gamino R et al. Cardiac abnormalities associated with morbid obesity. World J Surg 1998; 22: 993–997.

68. Lauer MS, Anderson KM, Kannel WB, Levy D. The impact of obesity on left ventricular mass and geometry: the Framingham Heart Study. JAMA 1991; 266: 231–236.

69. Nakatsuka M. Pulmonary vascular resistance and right ventricular function in morbid obesity in relation to gastric bypass surgery. J Clin Anesth 1996; 8: 205–209.

70. Alexander JK. Obesity and cardiac performance. Am J Cardiol 1964; 14: 860–865.

71. Alexander JK, Dennis DW, Smith WG, Amad KH, Ducan WC, Austin RD. Blood volume, cardiac output and distribution of systemic blood flow in extreme obesity. Cardiovasc Res Center Bull 1962; 1: 39–44.

72. De Devitiis O, Fazio S, Petitto, M, Maddalena G, Contaldo F, Mancini M. Obesity and cardiac function. Circulation 1981; 64: 477–482.

73. Hood DD, Dewan DM. Anesthetic and obstetric outcome in morbidly obese

parturients. Anesthesiology 1993; 79: 1210–1218.

74. Cnattingius S, Bergstrom R, Lipworth L, Kramer MS. Prepregnancy weight and the risk of adverse pregnancy outcomes. N Engl J Med 1998; 333: 147–152.

75. Department of Health. Report of confidential enquiries into maternal deaths in the United Kingdom 1988–1990. London: HMSO, 1994.

76. Gautam PL, Kathuria S, Kaul TK. Infiltration block for caesarean section in a morbidly obese parturient. Acta Anaesthesiol Scand 1999; 43: 580–581.

77. Konishi R, Akazawa S, Mitsuhata H et al. Cesarian section in morbidly obese parturient under epidural anesthesia. Masui 1996; 45: 1503–1506.

78. Patel J. Anaesthesia for LSCS in a morbidly obese patient. Anaesth Intensive Care 1999; 27: 216–219.

79. Jeffers LA. Anesthetic considerations for the new antiobesity medications. AANA J 1996; 64: 541–544.

80. Isono S, Tanaka A, Tagaito Y, Sho Y, Nishino T. Pharyngeal patency in response to advancement of the mandible in obese anesthetized persons. Anesthesiology 1997; 87: 1055–1062.

81. Brown BR (ed). Anesthesia and the Obese Patient. Contemporary Anesthesia Practice; vol. 5. Philadelphia: Davis, 1982.

82. Hunter JD, Reid C, Noble D. Anaesthetic management of the morbidly obese patient. Hosp Med 1998; 59: 481–483.

83. Tuteja LV, Vanarase MY, Deval DB. Anaesthetic management of a morbidly obese patient. J Postgrad Med 1996; 42: 127–128.

84. Oberg B, Poulsen TD. Obesity: an anaesthetic challenge. Acta Anaesthesiol Scand 1996; 40: 191–200.

85. Wilson AT, Reilly CS. Anaesthesia and the obese patient. Int J Obes Relat Metab Disord 1993; 17: 427–435.

86. Shenkman Z, Shir Y, Brodsky JB. Perioperative management of the obese patient. Br J Anaesth 1993; 70: 349–359.

87. Trempy GA, Rock P. Anesthetic management of a morbidly obese woman with a massive ovarian cyst. J Clin Anesth 1993; 5: 62–68.

88. Domínguez-Cherit G, Gonzalez R, Borunda D, Pedroza J, Gonzalez-Barranco J, Herrera MF. Anesthesia for morbidly obese patients [Erratum: see World J Surg 1998; 22: 1182.]. World J Surg 1998; 22: 969–973.

89. Bond A. Obesity and difficult intubation. Anaesth Intensive Care 1993; 21: 828–830.

90. Sugano H, Mori M, Miyoshi A. Anesthetic management of a morbidly obese patient with intestinal obstruction. Masui 1999; 48: 280–282.

91. Jense HG, Dubin SA, Silverstein PI, O'Leary-Escolas U. Effect of obesity on safe duration of apnea in anesthetized humans. Anesth Analg 1991; 72: 89–93.

92. Choi JJ-I, A new double-angle blade for direct laryngoscopy. Anesthesiology 1990; 72: 576.

93. Borland M, Casselbrant M. The Bullard laryngoscope. A new indirect oral laryngoscope (pediatric version). Anesth Analg 1990; 70: 105–108.

94. Cohn AI, Hart RT, McGraw SR, Blass NH. The Bullard laryngoscope for emergency airway management in a morbidly obese parturient. Anesth Analg 1995; 81: 872–873.

95. Lang DJ, Wafai Y, Salem MR, Czinn EA, Halim AA, Baraka A. Efficacy of the self-inflating bulb in confirming tracheal intubation in the morbidly obese. Anesthesiology 1996; 85: 246–253.

96. Servin F, Farinotti R, Haberer J-P, Desmonts J-M. Propofol infusion for maintenance of anesthesia in morbidly obese patients receiving nitrous oxide. Anesthesiology 1993; 78: 657–665.

97. Martinotti R, Vassallo C, Ramaioli F, De Amici D, Della Marta ME. Anesthesia with sevoflurane in bariastric surgery. Obes Surg 1999; 9: 180–182.

98. Higuchi H, Satoh T, Arimura S, Kanno M, Endoh R. Serum inorganic fluoride levels in mildly obese patients during and after sevoflurane anesthesia. Anesth Analg 1993; 77: 1018–1021.

99. Frink Jr EJ, Malan Jr TP, Brown EA, Morgan S, Brown Jr BR. Plasma inorganic fluoride levels with sevoflurane anesthesia in morbidly obese and nonobese patients. Anesth Analg 1993; 76: 1333–1337.

100. Schindler E, Hemplemann G. Perfusion and metabolism of liver and splanchnic nerve area under seroflurane anesthetic. Anaesthesist 1998; 47 Suppl. 1: S19–S23.

101. Artru AA. Renal effects of sevoflurane during conditions of possible increased risk. J Clin Anesth 1998; 10: 531–538.

102. Mason DS, Sapala JA, Wood MH, Sapala MA. Influence of a forced air warming system on morbidly obese patients undergoing Roux-en-Y gastric bypass. Obes Surg 1998; 8: 453–460.

103. Sarr MG, Felty CL, Hilmer DM et al. Technical and practical considerations involved in operations on patients weighing more than 270 kg. Arch Surg 1995; 130: 102–105.

104. Varin F, Ducharme J, Theoret Y, Besner JG, Bevan DR, Donati F. Influence of extreme obesity on the body disposition and neuromuscular blocking effect of atracurium. Clin Pharmacol Ther 1990; 48: 18–25.

105. Kirkegaard-Nielsen H, Helbo-Hansen HS, Lindholm P, Severinsen IK, Pedersen HS. Anthropometric variables as predictors for duration of action of astracurium-induced neuromuscular block. Anesth Analg 1996; 83: 1076–1080.

106. Blobner M, Felber AR, Schneck HJ, Jelen-Esselborn S. Dose-response relationship of atracurium in underweight, normal and overweight patients. Anasthesiol Intensivmed Notfallmed Schmerzthner 1994; 29: 338–342.

107. Puhringer FK, Keller C, Kleinsasser A, Giesinger S, Benzer A. Pharmacokinetics of rocuronium bromide in obese female patients. Eur J Anaesthesiol 1999; 16: 507–510.

108. Schmith VD, Fiedler-Kelly J, Abou-Donia M, Huffman CS, Grasela Jr TH. Population pharmacodynamics of doxacurium. Clin Pharmacol Ther 1992; 52: 528–536.

109. Schwartz AE, Matteo RS, Ornstein E, Halevy JD, Diaz J. Pharmacokinetics and pharmacodynamics of vecuronium in the obese surgical patient. Anesth Analg 1992; 74: 515–518.

110. Fisher DM, Reynolds KS, Schmith VD et al. The influence of renal function on the pharmacokinetics and pharmacodynamics and simulated time course of doxacurium. Anesth Analg 1999; 89: 786–795.

111. Cameron M, Donati F, Varin F. In vitro plasma protein binding of neuromuscular blocking agents in different subpopulations of patients. Anesth Analg 1995; 81: 1019–1025.

112. Egan TD, Huizinga B, Gupta SK et al. Remifentanil pharmacokinetics in obese versus lean patients. Anesthesiology 1988; 89: 562–573.

113. Schwartz AE, Matteo RS, Ornstein E, Young WL, Myers KJ. Pharmacokinetics of sufentanil in obese patients. Anesth Analg 1991; 73: 790–793.

114. Friederich JA, Heyneker TJ, Berman JM. Anesthetic management of a massively morbidly obese patient. Reg Anesth 1995; 20: 538–542.

115. Munsch Y, Sagnard P. The anesthetist's point of view in the surgical treatment of morbid obesity. Ann Chir 1997; 51: 183–188.

116. Petty P, Manson PN, Black R, Romano JJ, Sitzman J, Vogel J. Panniculus morbidus. Ann Plast Surg 1992; 28: 442–452.

117. Taivainen T, Tuominen M, Rosenberg PH. Influence of obesity on the spread of spinal analgesia after injection of plain 0.5% bupivacaine at the L3-4 or L4-5 interspace. Br J Anaesth 1990; 64: 542–546.

118. Hodgkinson R, Husain FJ. Obesity, gravity, and the spread of epidural anesthesia. Anesth Analg 1981; 60: 421–424.

119. Leith P, Sanborn R, Brock-Utne JG. Intraoperative epidural catheter malfunction in two obese patients. Acta Anaesthesiol Scand 1997; 41: 651–653.

120. Thage B, Callesen T. Bupivacaine in spinal anaesthesia. The spread of analgesia – dependence on baricity, dosage, technique of injection and patient characteristics. Ugeskr Laeger 1993; 155: 3104–3108.

121. Rau RH, Chan YL, Cheng HI et al. Dyspnea resulting from phrenic nerve paralysis after interscalene brachial plexus block in an obese male – a case report. Acta Anaesthesiol Sin 1997; 35: 113–118.

122. Brown LT, Purcell GJ, Traugott FM. Hypoxaemia during postoperative recovery using continuous pulse oximetry. Anaesth Intensive Care 1990; 18: 509–516.

123. Juvin P, Marmuse JP, Delerme S et al. Post-operative course after conventional or laparo-scopic gastroplasty in morbidly obese patients. Eur J Anaesthesiol 1999; 16: 400–403.

124. Choban PS, Heckler R, Burge JC, Flancbaum L. Increased noscomial infections in obese surgical patients. Am Surg 1995; 61: 1001–1005.

125. Rose DK, Cohen MM, Wigglesworth DF, DeBoer DP. Critical respiratory events in the postanesthesia care unit. Patient, surgical and anesthetic factors. Anesthesiology 1994; 81: 410–418.

126. Stone WM, Larson JS, Young M, Weaver AL, Lunn JJ. Early extubation after abdominal aortic reconstruction. J Cardiothorac Vasc Anesth 1998; 12: 174–176.

127. Pivalizza EG, Pivalizza PJ, Weavind LM. Perioperative thromboelastography and sonoclot analysis in morbidly obese patients. Can J Anaesth 1997; 44: 942–945.

128. Eriksson S, Backman L, Ljungstrom KG. The incidence of clinical postoperative thrombosis after gastric surgery for obesity during 16 years. Obes Surg 1997; 7: 332–335.

János Károvits Helena Scott

Minor sequelae of central neural blocks

Central neural blocks are considered very safe procedures. However, the ghost of 'permanent paralysis' still lingers on and, despite the well-established safety record of such blocks, patients often refuse to accept them fearing neurological consequences.

There is no doubt that the practice of neuraxial blocks has evolved greatly in the last few decades. New drugs and needles have become available and more refined puncture techniques are used. Extensive monitoring has given an extra degree of safety to the application of these blocks. However, expectations have also grown significantly. Anaesthetic mortality figures have improved tremendously and the need to decrease morbidity has now become the issue of today's clinical practice.

Complications associated with these blocks are classified as major and minor. The former consists of meningitis and major nerve or spinal cord injuries. Minor complications are those where only 'transient alteration in physiological function' appears.[1] High spinal blocks, hypotension, postdural puncture headache (PDPH), minor neurological injuries and backache belong into this category.

Neuraxial blocks pose a unique risk for neurological injuries. All the complications associated with central blocks can be divided into two categories: (i) those unrelated to the blocks, but coincident with them temporally; and (ii) those that are direct consequence of the procedure. The cause of this latter type may be direct or indirect trauma, ischaemia, infection and neurotoxicity of local anaesthetic agents.[2] Needles and catheters may cause direct nerve damage. Tumour, haematoma or improper patient positioning, by causing nerve compression, may induce indirect injury. Temporary or permanent alteration of blood supply to the neural structures

Dr János Károvits, Consultant Anaesthetist and Honorary Senior Lecturer, Department of Anaesthetics, Guy's Hospital, St Thomas Street, London SE1 9RT, UK (for correspondence)

Dr Helena Scott, Consultant Anaesthetist, Department of Anaesthetics, Guy's Hospital, St Thomas Street, London SE1 9RT, UK leads to ischaemic injury, and infection of the central nervous system may also have very serious consequences. The importance of toxicity caused by the local anaesthetic agent itself or by the additives has long been recognised.[3–5]

Backache has long been regarded as a complication of epidural analgesia, particularly in obstetrics, on which much of the current research is based. Since back pain is a very common, variable and subjective complaint in the general population, it is essential that the findings are interpreted and compared very carefully.

Several excellent reviews deal with hypotension and postdural puncture headache. In the following, we focus our attention on minor neurological complications and backache since these are still controversial issues and much has been published recently on these problems.

NEUROLOGICAL COMPLICATIONS

ANATOMY AND PHYSIOLOGY OF INJURIES

Spinal nerve roots are the primary sites of these injuries. The ventral root comprises mainly myelinated motor axons, but about one-third of its axons are unmyelinated, nociceptive afferents. The lesion of this root leads to weakness and atrophy in the innervated muscles. The dorsal root is larger in diameter and comprises the axons of neurons in the dorsal root ganglion (DRG). Injury is followed by sensory impairment in a dermatomal distribution. Fusion of the roots forms the segmental spinal nerve. The compression of this nerve thought to cause the radicular pain. The segmental neurological (motor and sensory) deficit and the radicular pain are termed radiculopathy.[6]

Since the lumbar and sacral roots run a long intraspinal course and their exit points are away from their corresponding spinal segment, they are more exposed to injury. This long intraspinal course explains also the difficulty in localising a lesion accurately to a specific level of the spinal column.

Nerve roots contain less endoneurial collagen and have essentially no epineurial compartment. The lack of these protective elements makes them uniquely susceptible to compression injuries. In addition, nerve roots and DRG are covered with only a thin layer of perineurium. This does not provide an effective barrier against toxins or infective agents.

The response of nerve roots to injury is limited. Either segmental demyelination or axonal atrophy, axonal degeneration (Wallerian) will follow any injury. Following demyelination, the recovery is usually rapid and effective over a period of weeks to months. On the other hand, recovery is extremely poor with axonal degeneration.[6]

TECHNICAL CAUSES OF NERVE INJURY

Needles

Nerve damage caused by needles has mostly been investigated in peripheral nerve blocks. Selander suggested the avoidance of eliciting paraesthesiae when performing nerve blocks.[7] Gentily and Wargnier advocated the use of the nerve stimulator instead of eliciting paraesthesiae. They believed that paraesthesia increases the risk of nerve damage.[8] These authors were heavily criticised by Moore in an editorial.[9] He suggested that 'there are no statistically significant clinical data to demonstrate that eliciting paraesthesiae results in neuropathy'. This may well be true for peripheral nerve blocks as far as statistical significance is concerned. Nevertheless, a recent retrospective study of 4767 spinal anaesthetics found that paraesthesia was elicited during needle placement in 298 (6.3%) patients. Six patients had persistent paraesthesiae and four of them reported paraesthesiae during needle placement. The frequency of persistent paraesthesiae was 1.3:1000 (6 patients) with a 95% confidence interval of 0.5–2.7 cases per 1000. Statistical significance was found between paraesthesia during needle placement and the risk of persistent paraesthesiae. It was concluded that elicitation of paraesthesiae during needle placement significantly increased the risk of persistent paraesthesiae.[10] However, none of these six patients suffered permanent neurological damage. The paraesthesiae resolved within a week in four patients and recovery was complete within 12–24 months in the remaining two. Another prospective survey of 103,730 regional anaesthetics gave a very similar warning. Twenty-eight patients had radiculopathy (19 spinal anaesthesia, 5 epidural anaesthesia, 4 peripheral blocks). The radiculopathy had the same distribution as the associated paraesthesiae. In 12/19 cases after spinal, and in all cases of radiculopathy after epidural anaesthesia and peripheral blocks, the needle puncture was associated either with paraesthesia or pain occurred during the injection of the drug. In addition, the topography of paraesthesiae and the extent of radiculopathy that followed were the same in all cases. There were 12 patients who had neurological complications after spinal anaesthetic, but no paraesthesia during needle placement. Intrathecal hyperbaric lignocaine 5% was used in 9 out of these 12 patients.[11]

It is generally accepted that eliciting paraesthesiae during peripheral block procedures is probably harmless provided that no anaesthetic agent is injected intrafascicularly.[12] As far as central neural blocks are concerned, the available evidence clearly indicates that paraesthesia is best avoided when performing the block and no drug should be injected if the needle placement is associated with paraesthesiae. Drug injection should be stopped immediately if pain occurs during the process. However, the lack of paraesthesiae does not give a guarantee of a neurological injury-free course of events.

Catheters

Intra- or extradural catheters can also cause nerve injury. Horlocker reported on Dripps' study of 1950. It was found then that the 'incidence of paraesthesiae was 13% with single dose and 30% with continuous catheter spinal anaesthetic technique'.[2] Laboratory study showed that subarachnoid catheters in rats caused demyelination and inflammation in both the spinal roots and cord of animals.[13]

NEUROTOXICITY OF LOCAL ANAESTHETIC DRUGS

Clinical and laboratory evidence shows that these drugs are potentially neurotoxic. Local anaesthetic agents can cause structural and functional changes in nerves. Even clinically used concentration of local anaesthetics may trigger cytotoxic changes.[14] If the drug is deposited outside the perineurial membrane, dose-related inflammatory changes, myelin and Schwann cell injury may follow. The intrafascicular placement of drugs can possibly cause axonal degeneration. The neuropathy that follows is delayed, but detectable by nerve conduction studies even in the absence of symptoms.[3] The presence of an axonal degeneration, however, is unequivocal.

Ross and colleagues draw attention to the role that intrathecal maldistribution of local anaesthetic agents may play in the development of cauda equina syndrome following continuous spinal anaesthesia.[15–17] It was found that slow injection rates through microcatheters might lead to accumulation of local anaesthetic agent in the dependent areas of the dural sac. The poor mixing of the agent in the CSF results in development of high concentrations of the drug and this may be the cause of the cauda equina syndrome occurring in patients following the use of continuous microcatheter spinal anaesthesia.

Experimental studies proved the neurotoxic effect of different local anaesthetic drugs on nerves and on the spinal cord.[14,18–20] However, these studies used concentrations that greatly exceeded the recommended clinical concentrations or doses.

Lambert used the frog sciatic nerve preparation to study the effects of 5% or 1.5% lignocaine, with or without 7.5% dextrose, and 0.5% tetracaine or 0.75% bupivacaine – without dextrose. He showed that 5% hyperbaric lignocaine and 0.5% tetracaine caused an irreversible total conduction blockade. This inhibition was not due to membrane lysis, since the membrane resting potential remained intact. Neither hyperosmotic–hyperionic solutions nor high dextrose concentration (7.5%) were able to induce the same phenomenon. The 0.75% bupivacaine did not show this irreversible conduction blockade. The observed irreversibility with lignocaine and tetracaine indicates that both amide and ester type of agents may produce this effect.[21]

Subsequently, Bainton established – using frog sciatic nerve – that the non-reversible loss of conduction is dose-dependent.[22] It begins at 40 mmol/l, and 80 mmol/l lignocaine produced complete ablation of activity. A concentration of 40 mmol/l is equivalent to 1% lignocaine. Thus, the use of less than 1% concentration supposedly does not cause irreversible impulse conduction. Meissner produced similar results by using cauda nerves from fresh bovine cadavers. He found that concentrations greater than 2.5% hyperbaric or 0.5% isobaric lignocaine induce an irreversible block after 30 min exposure. Bupivacaine 0.5%, either isobaric or hyperbaric, did not have this effect.[23]

Unfortunately, these studies give no universally accepted explanation of the mechanism of this neurological injury. The most that can be said today is that the mechanisms necessary for depolarisation and propagation of the action potential are somehow permanently disabled. It is obvious that, in clinical practice, the primary target organ of the local anaesthetics is the neural tissue. In view of this, it is remarkable that anaesthetists are generally supplied with data on systemic or cardiovascular toxicity, but hardly any data are given specifically on neurotoxicity. It is also clear that concentrations used for spinal anaesthesia exceed those required for an adequate block.[22,24,25] A standard test model on which the neurotoxic properties of local anaesthetics can be studied needs to be developed. The role of Schwann cells in the neurotoxicity phenomenon also needs to be investigated. Furthermore, well-designed clinical studies on the mechanism of spinal anaesthesia and on dose-response relationship are much in need.

In 1993, Schneider reported on four patients who had transient neurological toxicity following the intrathecal use of 5% hyperbaric lignocaine. He used the term 'transient radicular irritation' to describe the clinical symptoms.[26] Following Schneider's report, a series of papers was published on transient neurological irritation caused by clinical concentrations of commonly used local anaesthetic agents.[24,27-30] Later, Hampl termed it as 'transient neurologic symptoms' (TNS) and defined it as 'pain and/or dysaesthesia in the buttocks, thighs, or lower limbs occurring after recovery from the anaesthetic'.[31] In this prospective, blind, randomised study on 270 patients, the incidence of TNS was found to be 37% ($n = 44$) after lignocaine 5%, and in only one patient after bupivacaine 0.5%. In 34/44 patients (77%), the symptoms persisted less than 3 days and in 98% the symptoms were bilateral. None of the patients had sensory or motor deficits, bladder or bowel dysfunction, or abnormal tendon reflexes. However, all patients receiving lignocaine underwent surgery in the lithotomy position. The following factors were implicated as a possible cause of the TNS: lithotomy position; prolonged duration of surgery; hyperosmolarity-hyperbaricity; glucose; needle type and injection rate.[32,33] The lithotomy position, by stretching the sacral nerve roots and a possible sacral pooling of local anaesthetic agents, may certainly play a role in the development of symptoms.[34] However, 62% of patients receiving bupivacaine were also put into the lithotomy position and yet only one had the same symptoms. Yuen reviewed the clinical features of 12 patients with neurological complications following lumbar epidural anaesthesia or analgesia found that the more severe radiculopathies occurred in patients who had longer duration of anaesthesia.[35] Hyperosmolarity cannot be blamed as a cause of TNS, since similar incidence of symptoms were found with 5% lignocaine in 7.5% glucose (osmolarity 824 mOsm/l) and with 2% lignocaine in 7.5% glucose (osmolarity 614 mOsm/l) when the same dose (1 mg/kg) was administered.[24,31] The role of glucose is still controversial since Jun and Choi showed that dextrose in the usual clinical concentration range (2.5-7.5%) directly depressed peripheral nerve conduction *in vitro*.[36] On the other hand, Lambert and Sakura could not find any additional effect of 7.5% glucose on anaesthetic induced irreversible conduction failure.[21,37] Even anaesthetic-free 10% glucose failed to produce significant histological damage when given intrathecally.[38]

Holman showed that only an injection rate slower than 6 ml/min would minimise the spread of drugs given intrathecally if the needle port was directed caudally.[39] As far as needle characteristics are concerned, probably the size of the orifice is the most important. The 24 gauge Sprotte needle orifice area is 4.3 and 9.1 times greater than the 25 gauge and 27 gauge Whitacre needle areas, respectively. This feature of needles becomes important when a very slow rate of injection is used. In this case, a 24 gauge needle with a large orifice area could minimise the maldistribution of drugs injected.

The epidemiological study of Freedman involving 1863 patients showed that the type, size or direction of the pencil-point needles side-port did not affect the incidence of TNS.[33]

However, diluting the contents of a syringe does not eliminate completely the danger of maldistribution. It was shown that, depending on the order of addition, the final concentration of a tracer varies from 200% more to 50% less than expected.[40] For some time it seemed that TNS only followed the use of lignocaine. However, several studies published recently showed that procaine,[32] prilocaine[41] and mepivacaine[42] could also be implicated. It was suggested that, for short surgical procedures and for out-patient surgery, prilocaine or mepivacaine may be a good alternative agents to lignocaine as the incidence of TNS is lower with these drugs.[41,43]

Summarising the clinical experience with TNS, Dahlgren stated that it follows an uncomplicated spinal that has made a complete regression. The sensory symptoms develop about 6 h after ambulation. The pain is localised to the posterior side of the lower half of the body and it is severe in 30% of patients. No objective signs of any neurological impairment can be detected.[33,42] The question is, 'is this neurotoxicity' really justified? It was suggested that TNS following a single injection for spinal anaesthesia might represent only a milder form of toxicity.[27,44] It is also true that the diagnostic criteria used to attribute this pain to radicular irritation were never disclosed. Indeed, even the group first reported on this phenomenon accepted that the symptoms do not satisfy standard criteria of radicular pain. The term TNS is only used as an 'outcome variable' as they put it.[45] Furthermore, it tends to resolve spontaneously even without treatment and the pain responds well to antispasmodics and analgesics.

Toxicity is partly dose-related.[20–22] Correlation between dose and pain intensity and extent of symptoms could not be established. The only clinical symptom is pain, and motor deficit was never identified. Why would local anaesthetics cause only sensory disturbances? In fact no specific sensory neurotoxin is known. The lithotomy position probably only predisposes, but does not give an explanation as far as cause is concerned. Does it have than a clinical relevance? Probably yes, but not as a form of neurotoxicity. It is possibly rather a form of myopathy caused by the improper handling of patients without protective muscular tone or a consequence of overstretching the lumbosacral nerves and not the neurotoxic effect of a local anaesthetic. Dahlgren put forward a theory and suggested that, when piercing the dura, the spinal needle may cause limited bleeding and can separate the arachnoid from the dura: there is a chance for a small amount of fluid or blood to accumulate subarachnoidally. This blood may haemolyze in about 6 h releasing cytokines, adenosine, prostanoids and potassium, etc. These substances then irritate the sensory nerve root cells when the patient stands up and the fluid is drawn caudally. He draws attention to the fact that 'no case of TRI has been reported in a completely immobilised patient, but is not infrequent in those early ambulated'[42] This is a very attractive theory, but no elements of it have been investigated so far. Furthermore, it does not explain the selective sensory nature and the bilateral occurrence of the complaints, and it is difficult to accept that this 'fluid' moves only into a dorso-caudal direction.

THE INCIDENCE OF MINOR NEUROLOGICAL CONSEQUENCES

Spinal and epidural blocks are widely used to provide surgical anaesthesia, obstetric, postoperative analgesia and chronic pain relief. Usubiaga reported the largest series so far (780,000 surgical procedures) and he gave a neurological complication rate of 1:11,000 cases.[46] Crawford identified a 1:2400 incidence rate for obstetric epidural blocks. The frequency of occurrence of persistently numb patches was 1:27,000 in his series.[47] Horlocker evaluated four other extensive studies reporting over a total of 52,112 spinal anaesthetics and found that the incidence of minor sensory neurological deficits (numbness, persistent paraesthesia) ranged from 0–0.7%. The frequency of motor deficits was 0.005–0.02%.[48–51] In this group, 481 (10.1%) patients had a pre-existing neurological condition. Six patients had persistent paraesthesiae (1.3:1000; CI, 0.5–2.7:1000). Although it is difficult to compare results of different studies because of the differing population and study design, her results are better than, or at least as good as, those previously reported.

Obstetric regional anaesthesia is often blamed for causing different maternal complications.[52] MacDonald puts the risk of epidural analgesia as a cause of neurological complications in parturients to less than 1:11,000, 1:20,000 blocks.[53] However, Donaldson estimated that neurological damage following this type of anaesthetic intervention is 3–4 times less likely to occur than neurological problems associated with parturition.[54]

Scott reported a 1:4000–5000 overall complication rate following obstetric epidural block: the incidence of neuropathy were found to be 1:13,000.[55] The frequency of minor neurological problems after labour and delivery with a duration of less than 72 h was 18.9 in 10,000 deliveries in Ong's study.[56] The prospective study by Holdcroft identified that neurological complications persisting for more than 6 weeks during pregnancy and following delivery occurred with a frequency of 1:2530 deliveries. The majority of these problems were only identified within the community. This means that risk assessments using only hospital outcome data would certainly under-report the frequency of these complications. Neither general nor regional anaesthesia could be singled out as a contributing factor to any particular neurological complication and only 1 patient had a neurological problem attributable to epidural analgesia.[57]

A French prospective, multicentre survey revealed that in 103,730 regional anaesthesia (40,640 spinal, 30,413 epidural anaesthesia, 21,278 peripheral nerve blocks and 11,229 intravenous regional anaesthesia) the incidence of radicular deficit was 2.7:10,000 and neurological injury occurred in 3.3:10,000 cases. The incidence of neurological injury was more than 3 times higher after spinal anaesthesia than after the other techniques combined (6 ± 1:10,000 versus 1.6 ± 0.5: 10,000). Radiculopathy was also more often reported following spinal than epidural anaesthesia.[11] This is in contrast to Dahlgren's work that reported a higher rate of neurological complications after epidural anaesthesia.[58] In the French study, the high risk of spinal anaesthesia is partly attributable to factors independent from the regional anaesthesia procedure, but the higher risk of neurological injury was primarily associated with the blocks. The overall incidence of severe anaesthesia related complication in regional anaesthesia was much less than 0.1%.

The only paper published by a neurologist on neurological deficits following epidural anaesthesia and analgesia surveyed records of all in-patient neurological consultations over a 7-year period.[35] Lumbosacral radiculopathy or polyradiculopathy was diagnosed in 11 patients and one patient suffered a moderately severe thoracic myelopathy (lower extremity weakness, hyperactive reflexes, burning pain in the legs, dysaesthesias to light touch below T_{11} and urinary retention) as a consequence of unintended spinal anaesthesia. The estimated frequency of neurological complications was 1:1100. This is thought to be an underestimate of the true frequency but it is certainly much higher than the 1:11,000 reported earlier.[46] The frequency of severe, persistent neurological deficits was estimated to be around 1:6500 cases. The outcome of the reported 12 cases was very good. Direct injury by needle or catheter was suspected in 3/12 patients. Only one patient with severe polyradiculopathy showed little improvement in 4 years and the patient with myelopathy needed 2 years for a near complete recovery. In all the other patients, the problems resolved within days.

Giebler studied neurological complications related to thoracic epidural analgesia. The prospective-retrospective study of 4185 patient gave a 3.1% (n = 128) overall incidence of complications following thoracic epidural catheterisation.[59] Postoperative radicular pain occurred in 0.2% (n = 9) and peripheral nerve lesion in 0.6% (n = 24). Peroneal nerve palsy that was probably related to positioning, or other problems rather than to the epidural procedure, was found in 14/24 patients. It is of note that the inadvertent dural puncture rate was less in the lower- (3.4%) than in the mid- (0.9%) or upper- (0.4%) thoracic region. The calculated maximum risk at 95% confidence level (the upper band) for permanent neural lesions after thoracic epidural catheterisation was 0.07%.[59] This is better than the 0.3% risk reported earlier.[60] The prospective study of de Leon-Casasola gave also 0.07% as the maximum overall risk rate for neurological injuries in cancer patients undergoing epidural catheterisation for pain relief.[61] In this study, lumbar catheters were used in 2248 (53.2%) and thoracic catheters in 1979 (46,8%) patients and the duration of therapy was 6.3 ± 2.6 days.

Freedman's study collected data from 6092 patients (73% capture rate) undergoing spinal anaesthesia; 2555 (42%) patients were randomly selected for follow-up of which 1,883 (74%) were successfully interviewed. The final number of participants was 1,863; 47% received lignocaine, 40% bupivacaine and 13% tetracaine.[33] The incidence of TNS was significantly higher in the lignocaine group than in the bupivacaine or tetracaine groups, 11.9% versus 1.3% or 1.6%, respectively. This places the relative risk associated with lignocaine at 5.1 (95% CI, 2.5–10.2) compared to those receiving bupivacaine and 3.2 (95% CI, 1.04–9.84) compared to the group receiving tetracaine. The relative risk of TNS with lignocaine spinal anaesthesia in the lithotomy position was 2.6 (95% CI, 1.5-4.5), for outpatient status 3.6 (95% CI, 1.9–6.8) and for obesity 1.6 (95% CI, 1–2.5). It was also calculated that the risk for TNS after spinal anaesthesia with lignocaine has a range from 3.1% (in-patient, supine position) to 24.3% (out-patient, lithotomy position).

Other factors previously thought to increase the risk of TNS – such as gender, age, dose, concentration, vasoconstrictors, needle type and gauge, approach, pre-existing neurological problems – did not affect the risk.

All these data demonstrate that the much-feared neurological complications of these blocks are not a clinically significant threat. The fact that no paper was published on this topic by a neurologist for over 30 years before 1995 also attests to the safety of these procedures. The severe anaesthesia-related complication rate in regional anaesthesia is at worst around 0.1%. Spinal anaesthesia probably carries a higher risk than the other techniques. Fortunately, spontaneous resolution of the symptoms can be expected within a month in most of these complications. The existence of TNS is controversial. However, the occurrence of symptoms that define this syndrome is 7–9 times higher following the use of lignocaine than with tetracaine or bupivacaine. It is, therefore, prudent to avoid the use of lignocaine in central blocks for out-patients, long surgery, obese patients and, above all, if the patient is going to be in the lithotomy position for a prolonged period.

CLINICAL PRESENTATION OF SYMPTOMS

Neurological injuries may be associated not only with central neural blocks but also with surgical conditions (retractor blades, operations on the perineum, hip joint replacement and nerve stretch during positioning, transverse skin incision), long labours, cephalopelvic disproportion (CPD), and forceps delivery.

The risk factors contributing to the development of neurological symptoms are the following: direct trauma, ischaemia, neurotoxicity, sepsis, depressed immune status, corticosteroid treatment, local infection, pre-existing neurological conditions and diabetes mellitus.[10,62] Most textbooks consider pre-existing neurological problems as a relative contra-indication to central blockade. However, the results of Horlocker and of Freedman imply that these are not significant risk factors and the exacerbation of pre-existing or the development of new neurological deficits are unlikely.[10,33] Other observations clearly contradict this. Yuen found that pre-existing lumbar stenosis, injection during general anaesthesia, long surgery and inadvertent intrathecal injection of high volumes or concentrated solutions of local anaesthetics as factors that may increase the severity of neurological complication.[35] Dahlgren also suggest using epidural blocks with extreme care if the patient has generalised vascular degeneration or to use instead spinal anaesthesia in patients with spondylotic backs. Central blocks are not advocated in his view if the intracranial pressure is increased and if the patient has polyneuropathy, spinal cord pathology or spinal stenosis.[58]

Diabetes mellitus is another problem that may facilitate the development of neurological deficits and infection. Neither Kahn nor Horlocker approved it as a strong predictor of these complications.[10,63] Lithotomy position > 4 h, BMI ≤ 20 kg/m^2 and smoking were independent predictors for motor neuropathy but only in peripheral nerve injury. Outpatient status and BMI > 30 kg/m^2 were significant risk factors for TNS after lignocaine.[33]

The symptoms of neurological impairment may range from numbness of a small skin area, mild paraesthesia and muscular weakness to muscular paralysis and paraplegia. The nerves most commonly involved are the lateral cutaneous nerve of the thigh, the ilioinguinal, iliohypogastric, genitofemoral, femoral, pudendal, obturator and sciatic nerves.

DIAGNOSIS AND DIFFERENTIAL DIAGNOSIS

Radiography that demonstrates the role of pathological processes affecting the bones of the spine may help the diagnosis. Myelography is almost totally replaced by non-invasive CT or MRI in the detection of compression injuries. CSF examination is very useful in polyradiculopathy by detecting the high protein level and it is a powerful method applied for the identification of infection or malignant cells. Electromyography in expert hands is the best diagnostic tool for the exploration of nerve injury.[6]

A peripheral nerve lesion is presumed if the functional disturbance appears in areas distal to the lesion with – depending on the nerve's composition – motor, sensory and vegetative deficits. Radiculopathy is suspected if the radiation of pain and diminished sensitivity occurs in the corresponding dermatome. In case of root damage, unlike with peripheral lesions, the hypervalgesic area is greater than the hypo-aesthetic area.[59]

To differentiate radiculopathy caused by epidural block from neuropathies associated with vaginal delivery or positioning problems can be very difficult. Good history taking, careful examination and electrophysiological studies may help. It is suggested that upper lumbar plexopathy as a consequence of labour or delivery is uncommon. The L-2 and L-3 nerve fibres are protected from the descending fetal head because they run posterior to the psoas muscle.[35]

THERAPY

Our therapeutic arsenal for the treatment of minor neurological injuries is very limited. Fortunately, most minor neurological problems disappear in less than 72 h. NSAIDs, oral steroids, antidepressants, anticonvulsants and, in case of severe pain, narcotics have been used with success.[24,30]

BACKACHE

Neuraxial blockade is the most effective method of analgesia for labour. Whilst proponents of 'natural childbirth' may be expected to refuse it for aesthetic reasons, the commonest fear of women who choose otherwise not to have one is that it will cause postpartum backache.[64,65]

BACKACHE IN THE CHILD-BEARING YEARS – EPIDEMIOLOGY

The majority of women report backache during pregnancy. Several studies from Sweden estimate the incidence as much as 75% at some point during pregnancy, of which 60% start during the pregnancy. The prevalence is about 50% from the 24th week onwards and declines to 10% after delivery. However, a year after delivery, 37% of women complain of backache, of which 7% is severe enough to interfere with daily life.

When assessing which women are most prone to postpartum backache, risk factors appear to be backache pre- and during pregnancy, physically heavy work and multiple pregnancy. Younger women also tend to be at greater risk.[66–71]

MECHANISM OF BACKACHE IN PREGNANCY

The physiological mechanisms predisposing backache in pregnancy are well reviewed elsewhere.[72]

Physical and hormonal changes associated with the enlarging uterus accentuate the lumbar lordosis and increase the strain on the lumbar spine. Relaxin, a hormone known to remodel pelvic connective tissue is secreted during pregnancy. Mean serum levels correlate with symphyseal and low back pain in the third trimester. Antenatal pain is 3 times more likely to be located in the posterior pelvic (sacro-iliac) area than in the back.[68,73] Relaxin is undetectable 3 months after delivery, by which time most pregnancy-related backache has disappeared

Relaxin concentration is also higher in women with IVF compared with spontaneous pregnancies, and they also suffer a higher rate of sacral and pelvic pain in late pregnancy.[74]

Whilst ligament laxity and anatomical changes predispose to excessive musculo-skeletal strain, good posture and positioning can reduce the development of backache.[75] Ostgaard reviewed the assessment and treatment of low backache in working pregnant women. Those following guidelines from a physiotherapist could reduce pain in pregnancy and virtually extinguish persistent pain after delivery. In the intervention groups, the expected correlation between backache related to pregnancy and back pain after 6 years were not seen.[69,76]

STUDIES EXAMINING EPIDURAL ANALGESIA AND POSTPARTUM BACKACHE

Table 1 compares the results from 11 studies that examined the relationship between epidural analgesia and the development of postpartum backache.

Two commonly cited British studies firmly associate the provision of epidural analgesia during labour with new long-term backache.[77,78] The results of these studies suggested that epidural analgesia in labour gave a relative risk of new backache of 1.5–1.8. A third study found the incidence to be even higher.[79] In addition, headaches, neck and hand symptoms, and dizziness were also found to be more common.[80]

These results require careful assessment. All the surveys were retrospective; the response rates were low (39% in the Birmingham study) and, despite some meticulous statistical comparisons, it is impossible to rule out response and recall bias to a questionnaire distributed up to 8 years after delivery.

The results also indicated that there was no increase in new backache in women who had had epidural anaesthesia for elective Caesarean section. It was thus hypothesised that new backache was due to the exacerbation of a 'stressed position in labour' by the neuraxial blockade. This is supported by the observation that there is no difference in backache in women who have an elective Caesarean section under regional anaesthesia compared with those who deliver normally without an epidural block despite a similar incidence of backache before and during pregnancy.[81] With no motor block, these women will be better able to detect unnatural positions and protect their backs from undue strain.

These studies specifically assessed patients whose backache was reported as being new. From this point of view, the incidence of pre-existing backache was low when compared with epidemiological studies (9%, 14% and 7%, respectively). Subsequent prospective studies found the incidence of backache in pregnancy similar to epidemiological ones (50%).

In fact, women's recall of backache during pregnancy has been shown to be inaccurate.[82] This must seriously question the true incidence of new backache in these retrospective studies. It is possible that adverse publicity and misinformation causes women to expect backache after their epidural.[83]

Table 1 Studies examining epidural analgesia and postpartum backache

TRIAL Type/duration of study	No. of women/groups examined	Incidence of new backache at conclusion of study	Comments
MacArthur 1990[78] *Retrospective* 1–9 years postpartum	11,701 New backache up to 3 months postpartum	Epidural+ (19%) Epidural– (10.5%) (pre-delivery 9%)	Cause: stressed position in labour secondary to motor blockade
Russell 1993[77] *Retrospective* 18 months postpartum	1015 New backache postpartum	Epidural+ (18%) Epidural– (12%) (pre-delivery 14%)	Backache 'postural and not severe'
MacLeod 1995[79] *Retrospective* 1 year postpartum	1260	Epidural+ (26%) Epidural– (2%) (pre-delivery 7%)	High association with epidural, also linked to obstetric factors: women with problem labours are more likely to have an epidural
Breen 1994[102] *Prospective observational* 2 months postpartum	1042	Epidural+ (44%) Epidural– (45%)	Associated factors: history of back pain, younger age and greater weight. For new-onset pain: greater weight and shorter stature
MacArthur 1995[84] *Prospective cohort* 6 weeks postpartum	329 women with no history of backache	Epidural+ (53%, day 1; 21%, day 7 14%, week 6) Epidural– (43%, day 1; 21%, day 7; 7% week 6	Significant only on the first postpartum day
MacArthur 1997[101] *Follow-up* to 1 year[84]	244 (of original 329)	Epidural+ (10%) Epidural– (14%)	No increased risk of epidural analgesia causing back pain
Patel 1995[103] *Prospective* 6–8 months postpartum	340	Epidural+ (7%) Epidural– (6%) (pre-delivery 64%)	No difference in incidence of backache between regional block & controls
Russell 1996[87] *Prospective randomised controlled trial* 1 year postpartum	450 LA only *versus* LA + opioid *versus* No epidural	7.3% new backache Pre-delivery 26% No differences between groups	Motor block does not affect development of backache
Butler 1998[85] *Prospective observational* 6 weeks postpartum	270	31% > 14 days 8.5% (pre-delivery 11%)	History of back pain increases postpartum risk. Nulliparity decreases risk Epidural – no association
Loughnan 1997[93] *Prospective randomised controlled trial* 6 months postpartum	409 Epidural versus i.m. opioid	Epidural+ (32%) Epidural– (28%) (pre-delivery 28%)	Backache post delivery is common but new backache is not associated with epidural analgesia in primiparae
Breen 1999[94] *Prospective randomised controlled trial* 6 months postpartum	93 (27 at 6 months) Epidural versus i.v. PCA opioid	Epidural+ (27%, day 1; 29% week 8; 31% month 6) Epidural– (33% day 1; 29%, week 8; 27%, month 6) (pre-delivery 75%)	Very high incidence of pre-delivery backache: overall postnatal back ache is not related to epidural analgesia during labour

LA = local anaesthesia; epidural+ = women receiving epidural blockade; epidural– = women not receiving epidural blockade.

PROSPECTIVE STUDIES

In contrast to the previous studies, several prospective surveys have found no direct association between epidural analgesia and new postpartum backache (Table 1), except for the first day after delivery.[84] This is probably the only time that back pain is definitely attributable to the epidural block and is due to local tenderness following insertion of the Tuohy needle.[83] However, these studies do report a much higher incidence of antenatal backache than the retrospective surveys. This symptom is the strongest predictor of the development of pain postpartum.[85]

A possible explanation for the discrepancy in the results of the earlier and later studies lies in the theory of backache being due to stressed positions being adopted in labour because of a profound motor block. Modern techniques of analgesia for labour include the 'low dose' combination of local anaesthetic and opioid instead of local anaesthetic alone. This approach reduces motor block and increases mobility. This means that labouring women can help themselves to move about the bed or delivery room and are not shifted passively into unnatural positions.[86]

Subsequent studies aimed to see if the degree of motor blockade affected the development of backache. No difference was seen in groups with different doses of local anaesthetic.[87] These results agree with a follow-up study by MacArthur and Lewis.[88] They found an excess of new backache in women who had had epidural blockade, and examined the notes further to find any associated anaesthetic characteristics. Against expectations, they found that the only predictor of long-term backache was experiencing backache immediately postpartum. There was no relationship between backache and the duration of the epidural or the extent of the motor or sensory block.

One of the concerns of both women and anaesthetists is the safety of insertion of epidural blocks in women with previous severe back problems. A small series of 66 women with pre-existing backache severe enough to be assessed antenatally were questioned again a year after delivery. The proportion of women whose backache was worse at 1 year was 29.8% in those who had had an epidural block and 26.3% in those who had not.[89]

These prospective studies conclude that epidural analgesia is not associated with postpartum backache, but do find that pain, especially in the first few days, is very common. This may be due to discomfort at the site of insertion of the epidural needle. Two non-obstetric studies have demonstrated a reduction of postepidural 'backache' using tenoxicam or dexamethasone with local anaesthetic for pre-insertion infiltration of the skin of the back.[90,91] They also commented that there was a significant association between backache and number of attempts at needle insertion. This was not found in the obstetric patients reported by Clark.[92]

RANDOMISED TRIALS

Despite the problems incurred with randomising women to receive an epidural block or alternative means of analgesia, two trials have been performed. They used as control groups either intramuscular or intravenous opioid via a patient-controlled pump.[93,94] There were no differences in backache between the groups for the 6-month duration of the studies.

OTHER STUDIES

It is relevant to include studies on patients who have had epidural anaesthesia for operative procedures. Anaesthesia requires full sensory and, consequently, motor blockade, whereas epidural analgesia for labour now minimises motor block, so allowing greater mobility and, theoretically, less likelihood of adopting an unnatural and stressed posture. Three studies examine the development of backache after anaesthesia under epidural.

There was a significantly greater incidence of long-term backache in patients who had an epidural block sited for manual removal of placenta compared with those who had a general anaesthetic (33% and 6%, respectively). Although this study was small, retrospective and non-randomised, it indicated a difference in which the epidural was the main variable in two groups of women who had all undergone the 'stress' of labour without epidural analgesia.[95]

Two studies examined non-obstetric patients. Any new backache would be directly attributable to mechanical factors caused by the neuraxial blockade, rather than changes brought about by pregnancy, labour and delivery. In fact, neither study showed any significant pain other than tenderness at the site of the injection, which lasted about 4 days or that was associated with pre-existing backache (10%).[96,97]

CASE REPORTS

Whilst it appears that backache is not, after all, caused by epidural analgesia, it is appropriate to be reminded that any case of severe or unusual backache, especially if accompanied by neurological symptoms and signs, should always be thoroughly investigated. Abscesses and haematomas, although rare, are neurosurgical emergencies and amenable to appropriate timely referral.[98–100]

CONCLUDING COMMENTS

There appears to be a marked conflict of opinion as to whether or not epidural analgesia causes backache. On closer examination it appears that whilst earlier, retrospective studies[77–79] report a significant association between epidural analgesia and backache, this is not borne out by prospective trials, either observational[84,85,87,88,101–103] or randomised.[93,94] One of the problems with analysing the results of these studies is assessing the methodology. Backache is common before and after delivery. This must be taken into account when considering whether or not it is affected by epidural blockade. Many questions need to be addressed, preferably by means of prospective randomised controlled trials. Only then is it possible to assess whether postpartum backache is new or additional to any suffered before labour. Demographic and obstetric factors (for example, the length of the second stage) must be compared to find out which women are susceptible to backache and to evaluate any associated factors that may explain an apparent link.

A wide spectrum of pathology may be described with the single term 'back-ache'. It is, therefore, important to describe the nature, severity and duration of the backache as well as the incidence. All medical procedures will have side effects and the risk/benefit must be carefully assessed. Pain severe enough to prevent normal daily activities is very different from transitory local bruising.

In conclusion, most women will suffer from some form of backache during their child-bearing years. Health workers should stress the importance of good posture and back care both ante- and postnatally. They may confidently re-assure women that having an epidural will not cause backache.

Key points for clinical practice

- Observe for pain and paraesthesiae during needle insertion and injection; stop immediately if any of these complaints occur.

- Always use the lowest effective concentration of a local anaesthetic drug, avoid inadvertent intrathecal injection of high volumes or concentrations.

- Consider the dose, the use of a vasoconstrictor, the length of surgery, the presence of spinal stenosis and the positioning of the patient.

- Use prilocaine or mepivacaine as alternatives to lignocaine for spinal anaesthesia in short surgical procedures or in out-patient surgery (these drugs are not approved for spinal administration in Britain).

- An injection speed of > 6 ml/min (0.1 ml/s) is desirable for intrathecal blocks.

- Monitor the patient for complications. Early diagnosis and intervention are the most important determinants of a good clinical outcome.

- Nerve damage is a major source of anaesthetic liability, good documentation is essential.

- Backache occurs in at least 50% of women during pregnancy, which is underestimated in retrospective surveys.

- Backache before and during pregnancy is the most accurate predictor of subsequent backache.

- Pregnant women are rendered vulnerable to backache by the on-going physiological and hormonal changes. Education and postural adjustments can minimise the risk both before and after delivery.

- Backache after delivery is also very common, but normally resolves rapidly. Much is related to posture and is not particularly severe.

- Epidural analgesia is not demonstrably associated with the development of new long-term backache.

- Epidural analgesia is safe and effective in women with pre-existing severe backache.

REFERENCES

1. Covino B G, Lambert D H. Epidural and spinal anesthesia. In: Barash P G, Cullen B F, Stoelting R K. (eds) Clinical Anesthesia. Philadelphia: J.B. Lippincott, 1989; 755–786.

2. Horlocker T T. Neurologic complications of spinal anesthesia. Techniques Reg Anesth Pain Manage 1998; 2: 211–218.

3. Löfström B, Wennberg A, Widen L. Late disturbances in nerve function after block with local anaesthetic agents. Acta Anaesthesiol Scand 1966; 10: 111–122.

4. Pollock J E. Toxicity of spinal agents. Techniques Reg Anesth Pain Manage 1998; 2: 194–201.

5. Hodgson P S, Neal J M, Pollock J E, Liu S S. The neurotoxicity of drugs given intrathecally (spinal). Anesth Analg 1999; 88: 797–809.

6. Parry GJ. Diseases of spinal roots. In: Dyck P J. (ed) Peripheral Neuropathy. Philadelphia: Saunders, 1993; 899–910.

7. Selander D, Edshage S, Wolff T. Paresthesiae or no paresthesiae?: nerve lesion after axillary block. Acta Anaesthesiol Scand 1978; 23: 25–33.

8. Gentili M E, Wargnier J P. Peripheral nerve damage and regional anaesthesia. Br J Anaesth 1993; 70: 594.

9. Moore D C, Mulroy M F, Thompson G E. Peripheral nerve damage and regional anaesthesia. Br J Anaesth 1994; 73: 435–435.

10. Horlocker T T, McGregor D G, Matsushige D K, Schroeder D R, Besse J A, and the Perioperative Outcomes Group. A retrospective review of 4767 consecutive spinal anesthetics: central nervous system complications. Anesth Analg 1997; 84: 578–584.

11. Auroy Y, Narchi P, Messiah A, Litt L, Rouvier B, Samii K. Serious complications related to regional anesthesia. Anesthesiology 1997; 87: 479–486.

12. Hogan Q. Local anesthetic toxicity: an update. Reg Anesth 1996; 21: 43–50.

13. Myers R R, Sommer C. Methodology for spinal neurotoxicity studies. Reg Anesth 1993; 17: 439–447.

14. Myers R R, Kalichman M W, Reisner L S. Neurotoxicity of local anesthetics: altered perineural permeability, edema and nerve fiber injury. Anesthesiology 1986; 64: 29–35.

15. Ross B K, Coda B, Heath C H. Local anesthetic distribution in a spinal model: a possible mechanism of neurologic injury after continuous spinal anesthesia. Reg Anesth 1992; 17: 69–77.

16. Rigler M, Drasner K, Krejcie T et al. Cauda equina syndrome after continuous spinal anesthesia. Anesth Analg 1991; 72: 275–281.

17. Lambert D H, Hurley R J. Cauda equina syndrome and continuous spinal anesthesia. Anesth Analg 1991; 72: 817–819.

18. Adams H J, Mastri A R, Eicholzer A W. Morphologic effects of intrathecal etidocaine and tetracaine on the rabbit spinal cord. Anesth Analg 1974; 53: 904–908.

19. Li D R, Bahar M, Cole G. Neurological toxicity of the subarachnoid infusion of bupivacaine, lignocaine or 2-chloroprocaine in the rat. Br J Anaesth 1985; 57: 424–429.

20. Ready L B, Plumer M, Haschke R. Neurotoxicity of intrathecal local anesthetics in rabbits. Anesthesiology 1985; 63: 364–370.

21. Lambert L A, Lambert D H, Strichartz G R. Irreversible conduction block in isolated nerve by high concentrations of local anesthetics. Anesthesiology 1994; 80: 1082–1093.

22. Bainton C, Strichartz G R. Concentration dependence of lidocaine-induced irreversible conduction loss in frog nerve. Anesthesiology 1994; 81: 657–667.

23. Meissner K, Holst D, Mädler S, Stricharzt G R. Potential neurotoxicity of lidocaine and bupivacaine for continuous spinal anaesthesia. Int Monit Reg Anaesth 1997; 9: 8.

24. Hampl K F, Schneider M C, Pargger H, Gut J, Drewe J, Drasner K. A similar incidence of transient neurologic symptoms after spinal anesthesia with 2% and 5% lidocaine. Anesth Analg 1996; 83: 1051–1054.

25. Selander D. Neurotoxicity of local anesthetics: animal data. Reg Anesth 1993; 18: 461–468.

26. Schneider M C, Ettlin T, Kaufmann M et al. Transient neurologic toxicity after hyperbaric subarachnoid anesthesia with 5% lidocaine. Anesth Analg 1993; 76: 1154–1157.

27. Fenerty J, Sonner J, Sakura S, Drasner K. Transient radicular pain following spinal anesthesia: review of the literature and report of a case involving 2% lidocaine. Int J

Obstet Anaesth 1996; 5: 32–35.

28. Hampl K F, Schneider M C, Bont A, Pargger H. Transient radicular irritation after single subarachnoid injection of isobaric 2% lignocaine for spinal anaesthesia. Anaesthesia 1996; 51: 178–181.

29. Liguori G A, Zayas V M. Repeated episodes of transient radiating back and leg pain following spinal anesthesia with 1.5% mepivacaine and 2% lidocaine. Reg Anesth Pain Med 1998; 23: 511–555.

30. Martinez-Burio R, Arzuaga M, Quintana J et al. Incidence of transient neurologic symptoms after hyperbaric subarachnoid anesthesia with 5% lidocaine and 5% prilocaine. Anesthesiology 1998; 88: 624–628.

31. Hampl K F, Schneider M C, Ummenhofer W, Drewe J. Transient neurologic symptoms after spinal anesthesia. Anesth Analg 1995; 81: 1148–1153.

32. Carpenter R L. Hyperbaric lidocaine spinal anesthesia: do we need an alternative? Anesth Analg 1995; 81: 1125–1128.

33. Freedman J M, Li D, Drasner K, Jaskela M C, Larsen B, Wi S. Transient neurological symptoms after spinal anesthesia. An epidemiologic study. Anesthesiology 1998; 89: 633–641.

34. Wong C, Slavenas P. The incidence of transient radicular irritation after spinal anesthesia in obstetric patients. Reg Anesth Pain Med 1999; 24: 55–58.

35. Yuen E C, Layzer R B, Weitz S R, Olney R K. Neurologic complications of lumbar epidural anesthesia and analgesia. Neurology 1995; 45: 1795–1801.

36. Jun H J, Choi Y. Dextrose perfused on isolated rat sciatic nerve decreased A-fiber compound action potential. Anesth Analg 1999; 88: S213.

37. Sakura S, Chan V W S, Ciriales R, Drasner K. The addition of 7.5% glucose does not alter the neurotoxicity of 5% lidocaine administered intrathecally in the rat. Anesthesiology 1995; 82: 236–240.

38. Hashimoto K, Sakura S, Ciriales R, Bollen A W, Drasner K. The functional and histologic effects of glucose administered intrathecally in the rat. Anesthesiology 1995; 83: A829.

39. Holman S J, Robinson R A, Beardsley D, Stewart S F C, Klein L, Stevens R A. Hyperbaric dye solution distribution characteristics after pencil-point needle injection in a spinal cord model. Anesthesiology 1997; 86: 966–973.

40. Dull R O, Peterfreund R A. Variations in the composition of spinal anesthetic solutions: the effects of drug addition order and preparation methods. Anesth Analg 1998; 87: 1326–1330.

41. Hampl K F, Heinzmann-Wiedmer S, Luginbuehl I et al. Transient neurologic symptoms after spinal anesthesia: a lower incidence with prilocaine and bupivacaine than with lidocaine. Anesthesiology 1998; 88: 629–633.

42. Dahlgren N. Lidocaine toxicity: a technical knock-out below the waist? Acta Anaesthesiol Scand 1998; 42: 389–390.

43. Liguori G A, Zayas V M, Chisholm M F. Transient neurologic symptoms after spinal anesthesia with mepivacaine and lidocaine. Anesthesiology 1998; 88: 619–623.

44. Youngs E J. Rate of injection and neurotoxicity of spinal lidocaine. Anesthesiology 1999; 90: 323.

45. Hartrick C T, Hampl K F, Schneider M C, Drasner K. Transient radicular irritation: a misnomer? Anesth Analg 1997; 84: 1392–1393.

46. Usubiaga J E. Neurological complications following epidural anesthesia. Int Anesthesiol Clin 1975; 13 : 1–153.

47. Crawford J S. Some maternal complications of epidural analgesia for labour. Anaesthesia 1985; 40: 1219–1225.

48. Phillips O C, Ebner H, Nelson A T, Black M H. Neurologic complications following spinal anesthesia with lidocaine: a prospective review of 10440 cases. Anesthesiology 1969; 30: 284–289.

49. Dripps R D, Vandam L D. Long-term follow-up of patients who received 10098 spinal anesthetics. Failure to discover major neurological sequelae. JAMA 1954; 156: 1486–1491.

50. Sadove M S, Levin M J, Rant-Sejdinaj I. Neurological complications of spinal anaesthesia. Can J Anaesth 1961; 8: 405–416.

51. Moore D C, Bridenbaugh L D. Spinal (subarachnoid) block. JAMA 1966; 195: 123–128.

52. Reynolds F. Maternal sequelae of childbirth. Br J Anaesth 1995; 75: 515.

53. MacDonald R. Problems with regional anaesthesia: hazards or negligence? Br J Anaesth 1994; 73: 64–68.

54. Donaldson J O. Neurology of Pregnancy. London: Saunders, 1989.

55. Scott D B, Hibbard B M. Serious non-fatal complications associated with extradural block in obstetric practice. Br J Anaesth 1990; 64: 537–541.

56. Ong B Y, Cohen M M, Esmail A, Cumming M, Kozody R, Palahniuk R J. Paresthesias and motor dysfunction after labor and delivery. Anesth Analg 1987; 66: 18–22.

57. Holdcroft A, Gibberd F B, Hargrove R L, Hawkins D F, Dellaportas C I. Neurological complications associated with pregnancy. Br J Anaesth 1995; 75: 522–526.

58. Dahlgren N, Törnebrandt K. Neurological complications after anaesthesia. A follow-up of 18000 spinal and epidural anaesthetics performed over three years. Acta Anaesthesiol Scand 1995; 39: 872–880.

59. Giebler R M, Scherer R U, Peters J. Incidence of neurological complications related to thoracic epidural catheterization (clinical investigation). Anesthesiology 1997; 86: 55–63.

60. Scherer R U, Schmutzler M, Giebler R M, Erhard J, Stocker L, Kox W J. Complications related to thoracic epidural analgesia. Acta Anaesthesiol Scand 1993; 37: 370–374.

61. de Leon-Casasola O A, Parker B, Lema M J, Harrison P, Massey J. Postoperative epidural bupivacaine-morphine therapy. Experience with 4227 surgical cancer patients. Anesthesiology 1994; 81: 368–375.

62. Wedel D J, Horlocker T T. Risks of regional anesthesia – infectious, septic. Reg Anesth 1996; 21: 57–61.

63. Kahn L. Neuropathies masquerading as an epidural complication. Can J Anaesth 1997; 44: 313–316.

64. Gajraj N M, Sharma S K, Souter A J, Pole Y, Sidawi J E. A survey of obstetric patients who refuse regional anaesthesia. Anaesthesia 1995; 50: 740–741.

65. Millett S V, Lucas D N, Yentis S M, Rubin A P, Robinson P N. An investigation into maternal attitudes to epidurals for pain relief in labour. Int J Obstet Anaesth 1997; 6: 209–210.

66. Turgut F, Turgut M, Cetinsahin M. A prospective study of persistent back pain after pregnancy. Eur J Obstet Gynecol Reprod 1998; 80: 45–48.

67. Brynhildsen J, Hansson A, Persson A, Hammar M. Follow-up of patients with low back pain during pregnancy. Obstet Gynecol 1998; 91: 182–186.

68. Kristiansson P, Svardsudd K, Von S B. Back pain during pregnancy: a prospective study. Spine 1996; 21: 702–709.

69. Orvieto R, Achiron A, Ben-Rafael Z, Gelernter I, Achiron R. Low-back pain of pregnancy. Acta Obstet Gynecol Scand 1994; 73: 209–214.

70. Ostgaard H C, Andersson G B. Postpartum low-back pain. Spine 1992; 17: 53–55.

71. Ostgaard H C, Andersson G B, Karlsson K. Prevalence of back pain in pregnancy. Spine 1991; 16: 549–552.

72. MacEvilly M, Buggy D. Back pain and pregnancy: a review. Pain 1996; 64: 405–414.

73. Kristiansson P, Svardsudd K, Von S B. Serum relaxin, symphyseal pain, and back pain during pregnancy. Am J Obstet Gynecol 1996; 175: 1342–1347.

74. Kristiansson P, Nilsson-Wikmar L, Von S B, Svardsudd K, Wramsby H. Back pain in in-vitro fertilized and spontaneous pregnancies. Hum Reprod 1998; 13: 3233–3238.

75. Ostgaard H C, Roos-Hansson E, Zetherstrom G. Regression of back and posterior pelvic pain after pregnancy. Spine 1996; 21: 2777–2780.

76. Ostgaard H C, Zetherstrom G, Roos-Hansson E. Back pain in relation to pregnancy: a 6-year follow-up. Spine 1997; 22: 2945–2950.

77. Russell R, Groves P, Taub N, O'Dowd J, Reynolds F. Assessing long-term backache after childbirth. BMJ 1993; 306: 1299–1303.

78. MacArthur C, Lewis M, Knox E G, Crawford J S. Epidural analgesia and long term backache after childbirth. BMJ 1990; 301: 9–12.

79. MacLeod J, Macintyre C, McClure J H, Whitfield A. Backache and epidural analgesia. Int J Obstet Anaesth 1995; 4: 21–25.

80. MacArthur C, Lewis M, Knox E G. Investigation of long term problems after obstetric

epidural anaesthesia. BMJ 1992; 304: 1279–1282.

81. Wang C H, Cheng K W, Neoh C A, Tang S, Jawan B, Lee J H. Comparison of the incidence of postpartum low back pain in natural childbirth and caesarean section with spinal anesthesia. Acta Anaesthesiol Sin 1994; 32: 243–246.

82. MacArthur C, MacArthur A, Weeks S. Accuracy of recall of back pain after delivery. BMJ 1996; 313: 467.

83. Russell R, Reynolds F. Back pain, pregnancy, and childbirth. BMJ 1997; 314: 1062–1063.

84. MacArthur A, MacArthur C, Weeks S. Epidural anaesthesia and low back pain after delivery: a prospective cohort study. BMJ 1995; 311: 1336–1339.

85. Butler R, Fuller J. Back pain following epidural anaesthesia in labour. Can J Anaesth 1998; 45: 724–728.

86. Collis R E, Baxendall M L, Srikantharajah I D, Edge G, Kadim M Y, Morgan B M. Combined spinal epidural (CSE) analgesia: technique, management and outcome of three hundred mothers. Int J Obstet Anaesth 1994; 3: 71–81.

87. Russell R, Dundas R, Reynolds F. Long term backache after childbirth: prospective search for causative factors. BMJ 1996; 312: 1384–1388.

88. MacArthur C, Lewis M. Anaesthetic characteristics and long-term backache after obstetric epidural anaesthesia. Int J Obstet Anaesth 1996; 5: 8–13.

89. Lucas D N, Nel M R, Dob D, Yentis S M. Obstetric regional analgesia in women with pre-existing backache. Br J Anaesth 1999; 82: A519.

90. Wang Y L, Hsieh J R, Chung H S et al. The local addition of tenoxicam reduces the incidence of low back pain after lumbar epidural anesthesia. Anesthesiology 1998; 89: 1414–1417.

91. Wang Y L, Tan P P, Yang C H, Tsai S C, Chung H S. Epidural dexamethasone reduces the incidence of backache after lumbar epidural anesthesia. Anesth Analg 1997; 84: 376–378.

92. Clark V A, McQueen M A. Factors influencing backache following epidural analgesia in labour. Int J Obstet Anaesth 1993; 2: 193–196.

93. Loughnan B A, Carli F, Romney M, Dore C, Gordon H. The influence of epidural analgesia on the development of new backache in primiparous women: report of a randomized controlled trial. Int J Obstet Anaesth 1997; 6: 203–204.

94. Breen T W, Campbell M D, Halpern S H, Muir H A, Blanchard W. Epidural analgesia and back pain following delivery: a prospective randomized study. Anesthesiology 1999; 90: A7.

95. Vickers R J, May A E. Long-term backache after extradural or general anaesthesia for manual removal of placenta: preliminary report. Br J Anaesth 1993; 70: 214–215.

96. Chan S T. Incidence of back pain after lumbar epidural anaesthesia for non-obstetric surgery – a preliminary report. Med J Malay 1995; 50: 241–245.

97. Kock S, Hopf H B. Incidence and predisposing factors of persistent backache after lumbar catheter epidural anesthesia in a non-obstetrical setting. Anasth Intens Notfall Schmerz 1998; 33: 648–652.

98. Tham E J, Stoodley M A, Macintyre P E, Jones N R. Back pain following postoperative epidural analgesia: an indicator of possible spinal infection. Anaesth Int Care 1997; 25: 297–301.

99. Nay P G, Milaszkiewicz R, Jothilingam S. Extradural air as a cause of paraplegia following lumbar analgesia. Anaesthesia 1993; 48: 402–404.

100. Raj V, Foy J. Paraspinal abscess associated with epidural in labour. Anaesth Int Care 1998; 26: 424–426.

101. MacArthur A J, MacArthur C, Weeks SK. Is epidural anesthesia in labor associated with chronic low back pain? A prospective cohort study [see comments]. Anesth Analg 1997; 85: 1066–1070.

102. Breen T W, Ransil B J, Groves P A, Oriol N E. Factors associated with back pain after childbirth. Anesthesiology 1994; 81: 29–34.

103. Patel M, Fernando R, Gill P, Urquhart J, Morgan B. A prospective study of long-term backache after childbirth in primigravidae – the effect of ambulatory epidural analgesia during labour. Int J Obstet Anaesth 1995; 4: 187.

Index